Praise for *The Triumph of*

"In the NFL, team doctors answer to the organization; players joke that it's like Dracula running the blood bank. It's a microcosm of what David Michaels brilliantly illuminates in *The Triumph of Doubt*: When corporations manipulate science and launch marketing campaigns to sow doubt, they ensure human suffering. Michaels's work is vital reading for everyone to understand these industry tactics."—**CHRIS BORLAND, former NFL player**

"David Michaels is that rare combination: the fearless expert. He not only knows where the bodies are buried, he knows who buried them. *The Triumph of Doubt* and its predecessor, *Doubt Is Their Product*, are timely, readable, and essential guides for anyone seeking to understand how the corruption of science is damaging the health of everyone from football players and factory workers to soda drinkers and truck drivers—in short, anyone with a pulse."—**DAN FAGIN, author of the Pulitzer Prize–winning** *Toms River*

"A page-turner—one you'll wish was fiction. From hired guns to dark money, *The Triumph of Doubt* unravels corporations' playbook for deceiving the public through misinformation."—**MONA HANNA-ATTISHA, author of** *What the Eyes Don't See*

"Scientist, public servant, and passionate advocate for health and safety, Michaels has written an absorbing sequel to his path-breaking work on manufactured doubt. He documents how powerful corporations have turned 'product defense' into a new political strategy, using dark money to pummel good science and keep dangerous products on the market. A must-read in the fight to restore public trust in regulatory science."—**SHEILA JASANOFF, Harvard Kennedy School**

"No one has done more to expose the deep corruption in American safety regulation that harms us all—and especially our kids. After spending seven years as America's chief safety regulator, David Michaels offers a beautifully crafted argument for how much more we need to do. Required—if frightening—reading for anyone who cares about a clean and safe environment for America and the world."—**LAWRENCE LESSIG, author of** *Fidelity and Constraint*

"Whether it's the tobacco industry, the pharmaceutical industry, or the fossil fuel industry, vested interests have repeatedly sought to attack and discredit scientific findings that have revealed the public endangerment by their products. David Michaels should know—he's been fighting the good fight for more than a decade to expose the bad actors and bring them to justice. Read this book to learn what we're up against and how to fight back." —**MICHAEL E. MANN, author of** *The Madhouse Effect*

"Poisoning the well of public debate is the ultimate act of cynicism. As David Michaels makes breathtakingly clear, one industry after another has lied and manipulated in order to make more money, and the rest of us have borne the terrible costs."—**BILL MCKIBBEN, author of** *Falter*

"David Michaels lays bare the dark money and the corporate science racket that kept the lethalities of tobacco, asbestos, lead, silica, pesticides, and scores of other life- and health-destroying products on the market and in the workplace, escaping the reach of the law. He names names of people and companies fronted by their so-called 'product defense' business and its corporate attorney enablers; delays, obfuscation, falsehood, and retaliation against ethical whistleblowers are the coins of their insidious realms. This book is written to get you angry enough to want to learn how to defend yourselves, your communities, and our vulnerable planet. Let it grip you toward detection and defiance."—**RALPH NADER**

"*The Triumph of Doubt* is an industry-by-industry account of how corporations manipulate science and scientists to promote profits, not public health. Nothing less than democracy is at stake here, and we all should be responding right away to David Michaels' call for action."—**MARION NESTLE, author of** *Unsavory Truth*

"While the truth can be inconvenient, corporations and government leaders cannot continue to manufacture alternative narratives that place their interests and profits above our humanity; this culture, if left unchallenged, will result in our doom. *The Triumph of Doubt* reminds us that there can only be one truth."—**BENNET OMALU, author of** *Truth Doesn't Have a Side*

"Few people have done more to document disinformation about science than David Michaels. His new book is an important addition to the growing literature on doubt, disinformation, and deception."—**NAOMI ORESKES, author of** *Merchants of Doubt*

"It takes real courage to speak out against entrenched corporate interests and big industry. I saw that courage firsthand when I worked alongside Dr. Michaels in the Obama administration to protect workers at construction sites from cancer-causing silica dust. *The Triumph of Doubt* doesn't just tell the story of how we overcame the falsehoods of industry-funded studies, it shines a disinfecting light on the ways corporations obscure the truth and downplay risk to pump up their bottom line. This is a must-read."—**TOM PEREZ, former U.S. Labor Secretary**

"As a society, it's vital we properly debate issues using data and research. *The Triumph of Doubt*, David Michaels's wonderfully deep dive into the well-funded war on scientific consensus and certainty, makes the stakes clear: our planet. Read this."—**ADAM SAVAGE,** *Mythbusters*

"A compelling and necessary work for anyone interested in the truth and those who seek to bury it. Michaels details the methods used by those in power to hide the truth—and the moral bankruptcy at work when they do so."—**DEMAURICE SMITH, National Football League Players Association Executive Director**

"As a third-generation coal miner from a family who has suffered the deadly consequences of Black Lung, I know firsthand that worker safety should never be politicized. David Michaels's book is a must-read for business, labor and the scientific community."—**RICHARD TRUMKA, AFL-CIO President**

"David Michaels provides well-written evidence in his book about how corporations that produce dangerous products—tobacco, big oil, chemicals, pharmaceuticals—use 'product defense' science to sow doubt about the hazards hidden in their products to consumers. His evidence highlights the important role unbiased government scientists play in protecting the public health of Americans and our environment from exposure to toxic materials and from corporate deceit."—**SENATOR TOM UDALL**

"From the pharmaceutical industry's role in the opioid crisis to the Koch brothers' climate denial apparatus, Michaels examines big industry's jarring history of manufacturing false scientific doubt in the name of profit. This is an important book that will serve as a tool in exposing corporate deceit."—**SENATOR SHELDON WHITEHOUSE**

THE TRIUMPH
OF DOUBT

THE TRIUMPH OF DOUBT

Dark Money and the Science of Deception

DAVID MICHAELS

OXFORD
UNIVERSITY PRESS

OXFORD
UNIVERSITY PRESS

Oxford University Press is a department of the University of Oxford.
It furthers the University's objective of excellence in research, scholarship,
and education by publishing worldwide. Oxford is a registered trade mark of
Oxford University Press in the UK and certain other countries.

Published in the United States of America by Oxford University Press
198 Madison Avenue, New York, NY 10016, United States of America.

First issued as an Oxford University Press paperback, 2022

Library of Congress Cataloging-in-Publication Data

Names: Michaels, David, 1954- author.
Title: The triumph of doubt : dark money and the science of deception /
David Michaels.
Description: Oxford ; New York : Oxford University Press, [2020] |
Includes bibliographical references and index.
Identifiers: LCCN 2019019548 | ISBN 9780190922665 (hardback : alk. paper) |
ISBN 9780197675311 (Paperback)
Subjects: | MESH: Public Health | Research Support as Topic |
Industry—ethics | Public-Private Sector Partnerships—ethics |
Deception | Public Policy | United States
Classification: LCC RA427.8 | NLM WA 20.5 | DDC 362.1—dc23
LC record available at https://lccn.loc.gov/2019019548

1 3 5 7 9 8 6 4 2

Paperback printed by Lakeside Book Company, United States of America

For the countless people harmed or endangered by
the work of mercenary scientists and the industry that
manufactures doubt and disinformation

It is difficult to get a man to understand something when his salary depends upon his not understanding it.

—Upton Sinclair

Whoever has the gold makes the rules.

—Brant Parker and Johnny Hart

No matter how cynical you become, it's never enough to keep up.

—Lily Tomlin

CONTENTS

1. Introduction   1

2. The Science of Deception   15

3. The Forever Chemicals   27

4. The NFL's Head Doctors   41

5. A Spirited Denial   57

6. The Deal with Diesel   77

7. On Opioids   103

8. Deadly Dust   117

9. Working the Refs   141

10. Volkswagen's Other Bug   161

11. The Climate Denial Machine   181

12. Sickeningly Sweet   199

13. The Party Line   217

14. Science for Sale   233

15. Future in Doubt   251

Disclosures and Acknowledgments   273
Notes   277
Index   317

I

Introduction

AT HALFTIME OF the National Football League's 2015 AFC champion-ship game, the New England Patriots led the Indianapolis Colts 17–7. The game's stakes were high: the winner would advance to the Super Bowl. When the players returned to the field for the second half, the Patriots proceeded to score touchdowns on their first four possessions, blow the game open, and coast to a 45–7 victory.

Within days, however, a strange rumor explaining the Patriots' second-half explosion spread among fans, trollers, and news media. As the rumor went, someone in the Patriots locker room tampered with the footballs during halftime, then sneaked them into the game—perhaps at the direction of the team's famed quarterback Tom Brady, who re-portedly prefers underinflated footballs. Was this how he was able to work his second-half magic against the unwitting Colts? The national intrigue that followed was immediately and predictably labeled "Deflategate." Media scrutiny centered on the sport's most famous player, and required a vigorous response in order for the league to show it was committed to ensuring fair play.

The competitive context in this story was more complicated than an investigation of alleged cheating. Led by Brady, perhaps the best active quarterback (and, at age 38 at the time, also the oldest), the New England Patriots had dominated pro football over the previous 13 years, winning three Super Bowls and losing two others. In an era of parity in the league, this success was unprecedented, affording the Patriots a large and devoted fan base—as well as utter contempt from fans of other teams. The Deflategate allegations fit a pattern of competitive misbehavior that, fairly or not, had followed the Patriots for years; in

2007, the team was publicly judged guilty of cheating after an episode in which they videotaped opposing teams' play-calling signals. This prompted many owners of other teams, as well as some of the league's fans, to believe that at least some of their rival's remarkable sustained success was unearned. Now it seemed the Patriots were doctoring footballs, too.

According to most reports, there was no love lost between Patriots owner Robert Kraft and the other 31 team owners, who together pressured league commissioner Roger Goodell to use the deflated footballs as justification to punish the storied franchise. But Goodell couldn't do this without sufficient proof that Brady and, presumably, a confederate in the locker room, had deflated the balls. Toward that end, Goodell did what many corporate leaders have done for decades when they desperately need "science" to be on their side: he turned to the professionals who produce reports that predictably reach conclusions favorable to their clients.

This book is not about Deflategate. None of the episodes and issues I'll discuss here are as trivial as the allegation that a celebrated quarterback may have cheated in a big football game. The subjects here are deadly serious (including a different NFL story: brain injuries). The knee-jerk behavior demonstrated by the NFL in Deflategate is pertinent only because it's a notorious episode that vividly demonstrates the *reach* of an instinctive, systemic corporate behavior, one that flies mostly under the media's and the public's radar.

Rare is the CEO today who, in the face of public concern about a potentially dangerous product, says, "Let's hire the best scientists to figure out if the problem is real and then, if it is, stop making this stuff." In fact, evidence from decades of corporate crisis behavior suggests exactly the opposite. The instinct is to take the low road: deny the allegations, defend the product at all costs, and attack attack attack the science underpinning the concerns. Of course, corporate leaders and anti-regulation ideologues will never *say* they value profits before the health of their employees or the safety of the public. They'll never *say* they care less about our water and air than environmentalists do. But their actions belie their rhetoric. Decision-makers atop today's corporate structures are responsible for delivering short- and long-term financial returns, and in the pursuit of these goals a certain dissonance creeps in: profits and growth above all else. Avoidance of financial loss, to many corporate executives, is an alibi for just about any ugly decision.

Of course, decisions at the highest level are also not black-and-white or remotely simple. They're dictated by factors such as the cost of possible government regulation, perhaps combined with loss of market share to less hazardous products. And, of course, the companies are afraid of being sued by people sickened by their products, which costs money and can result in serious damage to the brand. All of this is part of the corporate calculus.

Most people, especially Americans, have come to expect corporations to demonstrate mercenary behaviors. It's in the corporations' DNA. We don't expect mercenary scientists. Science is supposed to be constant, apolitical, and above the fray. This book is about those science-for-sale specialists and the "product defense industry" that sustains them—a cabal of apparent experts, PR flaks, and political lobbyists who use bad science to produce whatever results their sponsors want. It's a version of the old garment center joke: "Turn on the blue light, the man wants a blue suit!"

There are a handful of go-to firms in this booming field. In the example of the NFL and Deflategate, Commissioner Goodell hired Exponent, one of the nation's best-known and most successful product defense firms. These operations have on their payrolls (or can bring in on a moment's notice) toxicologists, epidemiologists, biostatisticians, risk assessors, and any other professionally trained, media-savvy experts deemed necessary (economists too, especially for inflating the costs and deflating the benefits of proposed regulation, as well as for antitrust issues). Much of their work involves production of scientific materials that purport to show that a product a corporation makes or uses or even discharges as air or water pollution is just not very dangerous. These useful "experts" produce impressive-looking reports and publish the results of their studies in peer-reviewed scientific journals (reviewed, of course, by peers of the hired guns writing the articles). Simply put, the product defense machine cooks the books, and if the first recipe doesn't pan out with the desired results, they commission a new effort and try again.

I describe this corporate strategy as "manufacturing doubt," or "manufacturing uncertainty." My objective is to identify, characterize, and illuminate this strategy so readers can see exactly what these mercenary scientists and the firms that hire them are doing. In just about every corner of the corporate world, conclusions that might support regulation are always disputed. Studies in animals will be deemed irrelevant, human data are dismissed as not representative, and exposure data are discredited as unreliable. Always, there's too much doubt about the evidence, not enough proof of harm, not enough proof of *enough* harm.

It is public relations disguised as science. The companies' PR experts provide these scientists with contrarian sound bites that play well with reporters, who are mired in the trap of believing there must be two sides to every story equally worthy of fair-minded consideration. The scientists are deployed to influence regulatory agencies that might be trying to protect the public, or to defend against lawsuits by people who believe they were injured by the product in question. The corporations and their hired guns market their studies and reports as "sound science," but actually they just *sound like* science. Such bought-and-paid-for corporate research is sanctified, while any academic research that might threaten corporate interests is vilified. There's a word for that: Orwellian.

Individual companies and entire industries have been playing and fine-tuning this strategy for decades, disingenuously demanding *proof over precaution* in matters of public good. For industry, there is no better way to stymie government efforts to regulate a product that harms the public or the environment; debating the science is much easier and more effective than debating the policy. In earlier decades, we have seen this play out with tobacco, secondhand smoke, asbestos, industrial pollution, and a host of chemicals and products. These industries' strategy of denial is alive and well today. Nor is this practice of hiring experts and hiding data about harms limited to health concerns and the environment. Beyond toxic chemicals, we see it with toxic *information* as well. (Consider the corporate misbehaviors of Facebook, which serve as a pertinent sidebar to my story.)

I am not asserting that the conclusions of every study or report produced by product defense experts are necessarily wrong; it certainly is legitimate for scientists to work to prove one hypothesis in the cause of disproving another. One means by which science moves toward the real truth is by challenging and disproving supposed truth and received wisdom. Maybe there are two sides to every story—but maybe not two *valid* sides, and definitely not when one has been purchased at a high price, and produced by firms whose financial success rests on delivering the studies and reports that support whatever conclusion their corporate clients need.

The strategy of manufacturing doubt has worked wonders as a public relations tool in the current debate over the use of scientific evidence in public policy. In the long run, product defense campaigns rarely hold up; some don't pass the laugh test to begin with. But the main motivation all along has been only to sow confusion and buy time, sometimes lots of time, thereby allowing entire industries to thrive or individual companies to maintain market share while developing a new product. Doubt can delay or obstruct public health or environmental protections, or just convince some jurors that the science isn't strong enough to label a product as responsible for terrible illnesses.

Eventually, as the serious scientific studies get stronger and more definitive, and as the corporate studies are revealed as unconvincing or simply wrong (then generally forgotten, with the authors paying no penalty for their prevarications), the manufacturers give up and acknowledge the harm done by their products. Then they submit to stronger regulation, sometimes even costing themselves more money than they would have paid in the first place. But they can do the math: they have also been *making* a lot of money for all those years. Their wealth compounds. And as for the people who have been sickened or worse in the interim? Or the despoiled environment? Well, those are unfortunate. Sorry.

And what happens to the product defense firms? There's always another opportunity to manipulate the vulnerabilities at the intersection of science and money. In Deflategate, Exponent's official report enabled the NFL's attorneys to assert, four months after the game in question was played, that experts found "no set of credible environmental or physical factors" that could completely account for the change in pressure of the Patriots' footballs. Combined with other circumstantial evidence, "it was more probable than not" that the balls were intentionally deflated. To be fair, the NFL also relied on texts and other evidence suggesting that the game balls may, in fact, have been deflated.[1] But Exponent had done its job, providing the conclusion that was useful to the NFL to build the case for the quarterback's guilt. Goodell suspended Brady for four games in the ensuing 2015 season, fined the Patriots $1 million, and stripped the team of its next first-round draft pick. One can imagine the legal wrangling that followed the suspension: the case ended up in federal court, and the legalities spilled into the new season starting that fall. Brady's suspension was therefore held in abeyance, he played the entire 16-game season and playoffs, and the Patriots were defeated in the AFC Championship game. He served the four-game suspension in 2016. His team won three of the four games in his absence and eventually, with Brady back at the helm, the Super Bowl yet again. (They returned to the Super Bowl in 2019 and won, for a total of six wins and three losses—nine total appearances—in 17 years, which is beyond ridiculous.)

Exponent's report to the owners ended up being an embarrassment to the NFL. John Leonard, a roboticist and mechanical engineering professor at the Massachusetts Institute of Technology, was one of the early skeptics about Exponent's work and conducted a series of analyses that demonstrated that the original calculations were incorrect and that "no nefarious deflation actually occurred."[2] Leonard's very compelling lecture on YouTube has been viewed more than 300,000 times.[3] Since he lives and works in Massachusetts, Leonard could be suspected of bias, but he turns out to be a turncoat in this regard: he roots for the Philadelphia Eagles. Nor is he alone in his criticisms of the Exponent report. Faculty at Carnegie Mellon, the University of Chicago, Rockefeller University, and other academic centers have all pointed out errors in the report.[4] So this was not the product defense industry's finest hour—just an indicative one, and one that received more national attention than most.

Early in my career, I practiced and taught epidemiology, which is the study of the health of populations. I specifically studied the links between disease and workplace exposures, including substances like asbestos, lead, and other chemicals. In 2001, I decided to shift the focus of my research to public policy and the application of the findings of epidemiology to disease prevention. Since then I have written extensively about public health harms and environmental degradations perpetrated by various industries and defended with boilerplate "uncertainty" campaigns. This career-within-the-career was launched—maybe I should say inspired—by the years I served under President Bill Clinton as assistant secretary for environment, safety, and health, at the U.S. Department of Energy (DOE). The agency's name suggests engagement with issues involving oil and electricity generation (reportedly the initial understanding of President Donald Trump's DOE secretary, former Texas governor and presidential candidate Rick Perry), but those are actually minor considerations for this agency. Its primary activities are the production of nuclear weapons and cleaning up the messes resulting from their production. I was, in effect, the chief safety officer for this weapons program. The job there was a particularly challenging one: to protect the workers, community residents, and environment in and around the nation's nuclear weapons complex. These facilities had harbored—and in some cases still do harbor—huge amounts of the toxic chemicals required to make the plutonium and highly enriched uranium at the core of nuclear weapons. Manufacturing and testing these weapons almost necessarily exposed thousands of workers to chemicals and radiation and created some of the most dangerously polluted locations in the country.

This was a very exciting period to be at the Department of Energy. The United States and its allies had won the Cold War, and it was time to reassess the nation's need for a large nuclear weapons arsenal. It was also time to revisit the DOE's unstated policy to pretend that these exposures never made workers sick—"Deny and Defend" was the sardonic label used around headquarters, if not in the paperwork. Workers at sites all around the country believed that their exposures had made them sick, and their government did nothing to help them. I visited with many of these workers and saw that, in many cases, they were right. Clearly, those with chronic beryllium disease had developed this disabling condition in machining the beryllium (a toxic metal) used to help maximize the power of an atomic explosion. For other workers, it was less clear that workplace exposures were responsible for their conditions, but none of them trusted DOE to honestly adjudicate their claims. And they had good reason. Apparently, the agency's institutional leaders had feared that simply acknowledging that workers were being overexposed to radiation or toxic chemicals would have damaged the nation's ability to make the weapons needed to first win World War II, then the Cold War.

Secretary of Energy Bill Richardson asked me to find a solution to this unfair catch-22; our new initiative resulted in President Clinton's apology to these workers. More important, legislation passed by Congress and signed by the president set up a workers' compensation program that to date has awarded more than $16 billion to workers and the families of workers who became sick following exposure in these weapons facilities. (The saga is a lengthy chapter, "Making Peace with the Past," in my previous book, *Doubt Is Their Product*.)

Of course, the weapons program did not end with the Cold War, and controlling worker exposures and limiting pollution going forward would not be easy. Many of the facilities were old and technologically outmoded. Under my leadership, we issued a series of new safety and health regulations. Several of them improved nuclear safety in the weapons industry; the most important was a strengthened beryllium standard, which DOE staff, with the help of academic experts, had been working on for several years. Then it was full steam ahead, and as we developed and then finalized the workplace beryllium exposure regulation, I witnessed firsthand exactly how corporations that make dangerous products can manufacture uncertainty to slow down the regulatory process.

Even though the strengthened DOE rule governing beryllium would apply only to government facilities, the beryllium industry opposed any change at all. Why? Because a new DOE standard, especially one developed with great care and caution, would increase the likelihood that the Occupational Safety and Health Administration (OSHA) would follow with new rules that reduced exposures at the private-sector facilities under that agency's jurisdiction. (There are many such facilities, because beryllium is a remarkable metal—lighter than aluminum yet stronger than steel—and its alloys and compounds exhibit all kinds of unusual characteristics, making it valuable in all kinds of industrial applications.)

The beryllium industry engaged a product defense firm (Exponent, again) to convince the DOE that there was too much uncertainty to move forward.[5] It was clear to me that they were applying the model perfected by the tobacco industry: manufacture uncertainty about the science to avoid having to reduce exposure or compensate victims. That was a long, hard-fought battle—truly scientific and legal trench warfare—but in the end we substantially won.

With the election of President George W. Bush, I left the federal government and returned to academia. Now knowing all too well what tactics to look for, I saw that the beryllium industry's efforts were not unique; tobacco's model was alive and well. In fact, many of the same scientists who had worked for the cigarette makers were now plying their product defense trade on behalf of asbestos, benzene, chromium, and a host of other toxic chemicals. And the new Bush administration was using the arguments provided by these mercenary scientists to slow down implementation of public health and environmental protections.

As I uncovered more and more about these efforts, I published several articles and commentaries in *Science* and other academic journals, identifying the problem and suggesting policy solutions. I titled my piece in *Scientific American* "Doubt Is Their Product," a phrase from the memo of the tobacco industry executive who candidly described that industry's efforts to refute the studies that demonstrated the deadly effects of cigarette smoking. "Doubt is our product," he wrote, "since it is the best means of competing with the 'body of fact' that exists in the minds of the general public. It is also the means of establishing a controversy."[6] The piece in *Scientific American* led me to write the book of the same title, with the subtitle "How Industry's Assault on Science Threatens Your Health." That evolved into a massive research effort. There was no end to the evidence left behind by beleaguered industries: 85 pages of footnotes; 1,100 references.

The book was well received in the scientific community, but it clearly hit some nerves in the corporate world. I was asked by the Defense Research Institute, the attorneys who defend corporations and their uncertainty campaigns, to debate Dennis Paustenbach, one of the product defense scientists whose work I pilloried in the book. I accepted the challenge. If I was willing to say something on paper, I should be willing to say it in public, including in front of an audience of a few hundred attorneys who represent some of the nation's leading polluters (a roster that includes some of the country's largest and most powerful corporations). The debate would have been the opportune moment for Paustenbach to identify the many mistakes I had made in *Doubt Is Their Product*. It must have been frustrating for him—and the audience—that he could not identify a single one.[7] To this day, no one has. I say that not to be self-aggrandizing, but to convey that there is a factual bottom to every issue, and that's what *Doubt Is Their Product* conveyed—and what this book conveys, too. In both, some of the stories of industry's malfeasance are so flagrant some readers may think "Oh, come on, this can't possibly be true." Alas, every story is true.

After I left the Department of Energy, I was happy in the private sector, teaching and writing at George Washington University. I had not planned to go back into government service until President Barack Obama asked me to take the reins at OSHA. I could not refuse. This position—technically, assistant secretary of labor for the Occupational Safety and Health Administration—is the single most important position in the area of worker safety and health in the nation, and the one from which I could make the greatest contribution to public health.

The average tenure for an OSHA administrator is about two years; before me, no chief had served for even four. (Too often, political appointees to federal regulatory agencies hold the office for two or three years, time enough to add the position to their résumé, gain name recognition for speaking and consulting gigs later on, then head for the revolving door—and a far bigger salary—in the private sector. This is especially true of attorneys, who use both their knowledge of an agency's internal procedures and the contacts they have made to switch sides and now cynically fight the agency's attempts to protect the public's health and safety.) I stayed at OSHA for more than seven years—until Donald Trump was inaugurated. I'm often asked how I made it so long in such a difficult job. Well, my situation was different. First, I loved the job, and, also, I had tenure at George Washington University's Milken Institute School of Public Health. Most academics are granted a two-year leave of absence by their universities to take a government post, after which they must return to teaching or give up tenure. GW administrators were very generous to me, extending my initial two-year leave of absence year after year after year. The eventual seven-plus years is virtually unheard of in academia.

Running OSHA was a dream job for me, one that my entire career helped me prepare for. Working for President Obama was a great honor.

I was part of a remarkable, dedicated team of colleagues across the government, committed to working closely together to improve the lives and well-being of the nation. As senior administration leadership, we held ourselves to the highest standards for integrity and commitment to the mission of our agencies, and there were very few cases where our expectations were not met. OSHA was filled with highly competent professionals who shared that dedication to protecting the safety and health of the nation's workers.

When I returned to GW to teach epidemiology and environmental health policy, I planned to focus my research on the relationship of workplace safety and health management and operational excellence. In manufacturing, no production system is *designed* to injure workers. If they are being injured nevertheless, something is awry with the design and/or management. I had seen plenty of examples of firms whose executives told me that their safety programs made them better, more successful companies. Because they managed for safety, their operations ran more smoothly, there was less wastage of labor or materials, and their employees had higher morale and lower turnover, meaning less money was spent on recruiting and training new employees. Safety management made them more productive and therefore more profitable.[8] Take Hasbro, one of the largest toy and board game manufacturers in the world. When I was at OSHA, Hasbro had only one manufacturing plant remaining in the United States. All other production had been shifted to countries in Asia with lower labor costs. That one remaining plant was a unionized operation in Massachusetts, a high-cost state. But a Hasbro executive explained to me that the OSHA voluntary safety program in which that facility was enrolled made the plant so productive, and therefore so profitable, there was no reason to move it overseas. In fact, Hasbro has recently returned Play-Doh production from Turkey and China to Massachusetts.[9]

But the inroads of progress in protecting the science underpinning our public health and environmental protections have not been sustained. Once again, tobacco's uncertainty campaign dating from the 1950s is serving as the template for corporate behavior in 2020. Dark money rules. Corporations or rich individuals pour money into organizations set up as "educational" nonprofits, whose objective is to sow confusion and uncertainty on climate change, toxic chemicals, or the health effects of soda or alcoholic beverages. There is no way to easily find out the hidden funders of some of these groups. Secrets abound, and much of what we've learned comes from either lawsuits or, occasionally, careless mistakes in which donors are identified by accident.

Manufactured doubt is everywhere, defending dangerous products in the food we eat, the beverages we drink, and the air we breathe. The direct impact is thousands of people needlessly sickened. There is no question that if these "uncertainty" campaigns had not been waged, we'd have a far healthier population and a cleaner environment. Following the U.S. election of Donald Trump, the fundamentals of evidence-based policymaking came under unprecedented attack. Just as unwelcome news automatically became fake news, unwelcome science became fake science. Incredibly, the federal government elevated studies conjured by product defense specialists over the studies done by independent, academic scientists. Worse, perhaps, the scientists whose careers have been defined by their science-for-sale studies exonerating toxic chemicals were brought inside, running or advising the very agencies that regulate those chemicals.

All this backsliding inspired me to write this book. It is not a memoir of my tenure at OSHA, but the perspective I acquired in that office did impact my thinking about science and its role in policymaking and regulation. The scientific enterprise is at a crossroads, I believe. We as a society are at a crossroads. We need to understand what is still going on—now more than ever, really—and what the consequences have already been for public health. This is an opportune moment—the necessary moment—to again look hard at how science can be used to protect our health and planetary well-being—but also *misused* to damage them. I'll focus in detail on several of the leading public health concerns that have been targeted by product defense campaigns. Two of my topics—the opioid epidemic and revelations about the long-term impact of head trauma on professional football players (an NFL story a lot more important than Deflategate)—have jolted the national psyche. Others—sugar, alcohol, toxic chemicals, air and water pollution, and of course climate change—directly impact the health of millions of people in the United States and billions around the globe. Climate change, a particular target of President Donald Trump and his administration, will likely end up trumping all of the others in global importance. And

I have no choice but to write bluntly about the impact of the Trump administration on the interface between public policy and lobbying and science, with evidence-based policymaking on the run, alternative facts all the rage. To support the assertions I make in this book, every primary source I reference is on the web, with many of the previously unavailable documents now posted on the "Triumph of Doubt" Special Collection at the Toxic Docs website (toxicdocs.org) operated by Columbia University and the City University of New York.

Other topics could have been discussed in this book. There are analyses to be done, for example, of the corporate efforts to manufacture uncertainty around the causes of earthquakes in Oklahoma ("dewatering"— pumping into the ground water left over from oil drilling); or the dangers of mass-feeding antibiotics to bulk up the animals confined in concentrated feeding operations (and therefore developing antibiotic resistant superbugs); or pesticides, flame retardants, artificial flavors, sterilants, or dozens of other substances that cause untold havoc on the human body. For now, I hope that shining a light on these few instances of harmful, misleading industry behavior will increase awareness, both of what manufactured doubt looks like and where it is leveraged against the public good.

2

The Science of Deception

THE FOOTHOLD OF tobacco in American life and culture began a century ago, when the doughboys of World War I were allotted free cigarettes in their rations. Soldiers kept up the habit when they returned home from the war, passing it along to families, friends, and neighbors. In these early days before tobacco research and tobacco regulation, the only real concern about smoking came from the smokers themselves: that nasty cough that came with the habit.

From the beginning, the tobacco industry used misdirection—in particular, the co-opting of science and medicine—to assuage consumer health concerns. One early cigarette advertisement read "More doctors smoke Camels than any other cigarette!" Another claimed "no adverse effects on the nose, throat, and sinuses of the group smoking Chesterfield." (The Chesterfield claim is a bait-and-switch maneuver; cigarette smoke is a *lung* irritant.)

It took decades—at least two or three, sometimes four or five—for the cancers to appear. Just like with the habit itself, lung cancer existed before World War I, but it was rare. In 1919, Alton Ochsner, founder of the New Orleans medical center that still bears his name, famously wrote of his experience in medical school being summoned to witness the autopsy of a man who had died from lung cancer. Ochsner's professor believed it would be the opportunity of a lifetime, with the students unlikely to see another case. Ochsner later became a surgeon and didn't see his next lung cancer case for seventeen years. He then saw eight more over the next six months. Each man had started smoking while serving in the war. Ochsner was one of the first observers to put two and two together.[1]

As the lung cancer rate among men continued to increase through the 1940s (the rate for women didn't take off until decades later, as more women became addicted), other physicians pointed to pollution and smoking as possible explanations. Once World War II ended, British and American physicians pioneered the new field of epidemiology, which focuses on the distribution and determinants of disease. Lung cancer was a clear and urgent subject for the field's early studies. A famous one, published in 1950 and conducted by British physician Richard Doll and statistician Austin Bradford Hill, compared the smoking rates of lung cancer patients to those of patients hospitalized with other illnesses. The cancer patients smoked more cigarettes each day, and for longer periods of time. Once the statistical analysis was completed, the study found that heavy smokers were fifty times as likely as nonsmokers to contract lung cancer. Three other similar studies appeared that same year. The evidence continued to pile up: In 1952, researchers demonstrated that cigarette smoke "tar" painted on the backs of mice produced tumors, and by the following year, another dozen studies produced results similar to those reported by Doll and Bradford Hill.[2]

The cigarette industry was in trouble. Even though its product and business model produced the highest profit margins of any legal industry, and even though its addicted customers would spend whatever it took to maintain the habit, there was no guarantee that smokers and prospective smokers would be completely dismissive of their health forever. The industry had to do something to stem the tide of attention.

That something came in the form of John W. Hill, founder of the advertising firm Hill & Knowlton (now Hill+Knowlton Strategies), who is widely recognized as saving the tobacco industry from having to take responsibility for killing thousands of smokers each year (a number that has today grown to millions). In December 1953, fresh from helping the chemical industry respond to a congressional investigation into carcinogens in the nation's food supply, Hill warned tobacco industry officials of the problem they were about to face. While industry executives were confident that they had "comprehensive and authoritative scientific material which completely refutes the health charges," Hill had his doubts—and wisely so. The tobacco industry needed more science, he warned. They needed better, or at least different, science, plus

an all-out pro-cigarette PR campaign assuring the public that, for cigarette manufacturers, "public health is paramount to all else." On Hill's
watch, the Tobacco Industry Research Committee (TIRC) started operations, later rebranding as the Council for Tobacco Research. In 1966,
Hill & Knowlton set up its division of scientific, technical, and environmental affairs, and would brag in solicitation brochures that the
founding was "years before the first 'Earth Day' or the establishment of
the Environmental Protection Agency."[3]

And so cigarette manufacturers—by then bound under the unoffi-
cial handle Big Tobacco, a nod to their shared interests—situated themselves as guardians of the public interest by producing their own studies
and reports about the effects of tobacco. Doubt truly was their product.
The manufacturers never failed to remind everyone that some people
who get lung cancer never smoked, and most smokers never develop
lung cancer. There are other causes of lung cancer, like asbestos and
radon. Blame them.

As the evidence linking cigarette smoking with lung cancer (and
heart attacks, and then a host of other diseases) became incontrovert-
ible to all parties except Big Tobacco, the larger playbook for manufacturing doubt was unveiled. And with it, an industry of product defense
firms was born.

For much of the twentieth century, Big Tobacco's defense of its product was steeped in a call for personal responsibility: Even if it were true
that smoking caused lung cancer, no one is forcing anyone to smoke.
It's a free country. You do you. This personal-responsibility dodge,
which would later become useful for industries like sugar and alcohol,
conveniently ignores the engineering of cigarettes to make them more
addictive. It also ignores—because no one understood at the time—
that smoking increases the risk of lung cancer for *nonsmokers*. The tobacco industry recognized the threat of secondhand smoke as early as
the 1970s, and a confidential industry report by the Roper polling organization in 1978 warned that a campaign by antismoking forces targeting secondhand smoke would be "the most dangerous development
to the viability of the tobacco industry that has yet occurred."[4] In 1981,
Takeshi Hirayama, then the chief epidemiologist of the National
Cancer Center Research Institute in Tokyo, published the first important epidemiologic study showing that nonsmoking women whose

spouses smoked had a higher rate of lung cancer than those married to nonsmokers.[5] Public attention and regulation followed.

By 1984, 37 states and the District of Columbia had restricted smoking in some public facilities such as auditoriums and government buildings. These laws had an immediate, marked impact: cigarette manufacturers sold fewer cigarettes in jurisdictions that had imposed restrictions, and internal industry documents attributed as much as 21 percent of the geographic variation to restrictions on smoking in public places. And these restrictions were likely to become even more numerous and more onerous in the future.[6] As the EPA moved to categorize secondhand smoke as a carcinogen, and as OSHA considered restricting smoking in public spaces and workplaces, the tobacco industry declared a red alert. What followed was a new chapter in "doubt science." The new studies that had found the dangers of secondhand smoke had to be declared hopelessly flawed.

The initial focus of tobacco's campaign was Hirayama's study; discrediting him and his team was essential to avoid losing additional market ground. One action was to generate a competing Japanese spousal study, this one concluding—*quelle* surprise—that the studies of nonsmoking spouses have "little scientific basis."[7] An important element of the tactic was to hide the fact that this competing study was conceived and supported by the cigarette makers; the manufacturers worked through a prominent Washington, DC, law firm, Covington and Burling, and claiming it was a "privileged and confidential work product" to conceal the manufacturers' intimate involvement in every aspect of the job.[8] (This kind of "disclosure" subterfuge is endemic in the product defense field, as we will see.)

The second tactic applied to Hirayama's study—and a play that has been copied by product defense professionals countless times since— was to attack its calculations as flawed. Through the Center for Indoor Air Research (CIAR), a new Big Tobacco front group, the industry obtained Hirayama's raw data and hired a product defense firm, ENVIRON, to reanalyze the numbers and declare them all wrong. (Following an apparent product defense turf battle, the job was taken from ENVIRON and bestowed on another firm, Failure Analysis, which was then renamed Exponent, which years later would handle the Deflategate study for the NFL.[9])

It's important to acknowledge here that any single epidemiological study can be flawed, and that any study of great importance can and likely will be subjected to independent confirmation examining the same question using different populations and dissimilar methods. But there are honest reanalyses, and there are disingenuous ones. The second variety is an essential trick of the trade for product defenders and will be discussed in depth shortly.

In the end, Hirayama's results were validated by several other independent studies. Later, in 1985, with support of the National Cancer Institute, a group of researchers under the leadership of Elizabeth Fontham of Louisiana State University launched a large study designed to minimize problems that had been present in the earlier studies around secondhand smoke. One result of this research was explosive enough: nonsmoking wives of male smokers had an increased risk of lung cancer of *30 percent*. The second result was potentially catastrophic (for the tobacco industry): secondhand smoke in workplaces and other locations outside the home increased lung cancer risk by *40 to 60 percent*.[10] Living in a society with smokers had effectively been proven hazardous for people who didn't smoke.

Forget Hirayama. The industry now had to go all out to discredit Fontham's ominous conclusions, which posed an even greater existential threat. Trouble was, Fontham had watched what had happened with Hirayama, and she had no desire to watch the industry hirelings twist her results and make her findings disappear. She refused the entreaties of the tobacco companies to give up her data for their mercenary reanalysis. She would not cooperate, and they could not make her.[11]

The industry's product defense efforts were now in uncharted territory. They would have to proceed without the raw data to reinterpret, which would mean finding a structural flaw in the methods of the study or making do with the small amounts of data published in the study. For that they hired William Butler, a veteran staffer at Failure Analysis. At the subsequent hearing the National Toxicology Program, Butler predictably testified that Fontham's study was flawed and should not be used to designate secondhand smoke as a carcinogen.[12] (As it happened, Fontham's unwillingness to give up her raw data led directly to Congress's passage of the Data Access Act, also known as the Shelby Amendment, which requires all federally supported researchers to give up their raw data. Who on Capitol Hill realized that this legislation was a Trojan horse for corporate interests? Who realized that Big Tobacco was the driving force behind its passage? The legislators who sponsored it and the staffers who wrote it, that's for sure. I discuss this effort, and how it turned out, in Chapter 13).

By the 1990s, the methods of product defense had been operationalized and were available, at a price, from a variety of firms and consultants in the United States. In 1994, when OSHA initiated the laborious process of adopting a new indoor air quality standard for workplaces across the country, the tobacco industry's challenge was led by two product defense specialists: H. Daniel Roth, an epidemiologist who had previously worked for the beryllium industry in its successful opposition to an effort to strengthen the beryllium standard; and Myron Weinberg, president of the consulting firm the Weinberg Group. It was Weinberg who coordinated the unprecedented effort to overwhelm OSHA's regulation writers. In notes from a conference call involving Weinberg and the tobacco company's attorneys, Weinberg's team is described as having "experts in 'deductive meta-analysis' that reveals confounders and identifies the real risk involved, if any." Knowing that OSHA, when preparing a final rule, is required by law to respond to *all* public comments submitted during the review period, Weinberg and his staff planned a "line by line analysis raising scientific questions that OSHA would have to respond to.... [This] attack could take [the agency] two to three years to respond to" and "put the bureaucratic machinery on overload."[13] It was the ultimate implementation of the tactic of creating uncertainty, and its effects were enhanced by Philip Morris's introduction of more than 120 witnesses to testify at OSHA's hearings.

And it all worked. In the end, the science behind the secondhand smoke regulations was irrelevant. OSHA capitulated, and with that lesson of the power of the tobacco industry withdrew the proposal.

To some extent, Big Tobacco's success in the United States eventually tapered. To settle lawsuits demanding reimbursement from the industry for smokers' medical expenses borne by the state Medicaid program, the manufacturers have written checks for more than $150 billion, which is actually only a small fraction of the true costs of smoking-related disease. Presumably more checks are still to come. As lawsuits from the victims

THE SCIENCE OF DECEPTION 21

of tobacco keep mounting, and new scientific questions arise, what's clear is that the industry's legacy isn't its product, but rather its defense. Today's product defense firms, apparently unconcerned about the ugly history and the millions of deaths of the field's innovators, line up at the trough to provide their expertise to help industries new and old—but most all of them dangerous—skate free of responsibility and delay regulation. The playbook remains mostly the same.

In 1999 I was working at the Department of Energy to strengthen the regulation on workplace exposure to beryllium, a metal that causes both lung cancer and chronic beryllium disease, even at very low exposure levels. I came across a 1989 proposal from Hill & Knowlton—the same firm that made its pitch to the tobacco industry in 1953—offering its assistance to Brush Wellman (now called Materion), the primary manufacturer of beryllium products in the United States. In his sales pitch, Howard Marder, the PR firm's senior vice president, wrote:

> Beryllium undoubtedly continues to have a public relations problem. We still see it cited in the media, as well as in our conversations with people who should know better, as a gravely toxic metal that is problematic for workers.... We would like to work with Brush Wellman to help change these common erroneous attitudes. We envision a public relations program designed to educate various audiences... to dispel myths and misinformation about the metal.

The document went on for 37 pages. In it the defense experts offered to prepare "an authoritative white paper... [that] would serve as the most definitive document available on beryllium." They also suggested projects to engage outside scientists in "independent" review of Brush Wellman materials "to nurture relations with the Environmental Protection Agency" and "to challenge all unfair or erroneous treatment in the media to set the record straight." Juicy material, and the promise crystal clear: we'll provide what you need. Appended to this letter was a document in which Hill & Knowlton boasted of its success assisting other corporations that faced regulatory difficulties stemming from their production of an impressive collection of toxic materials, including asbestos, vinyl chloride, fluorocarbons, and dioxin. Oddly, no mention was made of the firm's herculean work on behalf of the cigarette manufacturers.[14]

PR firms like Hill & Knowlton have earned their place in the ecosystem of product defense, but their work is secondary to the more valuable work of product defense scientists. Today's corporations and trade associations may utilize their own PR people for the messaging, but to secure the dissenting data, they need outside help. And in this space, specialists in the production of "sound science" have flourished.

The term "product defense" isn't a disparaging term I invented to write books; the field came up with it on its own. The Weinberg Group has even used it as a Twitter hashtag.[15] And product defense firms are *everywhere*. They cross industries and clients, and the same names keep popping up. The Weinberg Group from the tobacco wars (the one that oversaw the takedown of OSHA) would later help DuPont address the problems with the chemical used to produce Teflon. Roth, the tobacco veteran, would later prepare studies for the alcoholic beverage industry, purporting to show that booze intake has no relationship to breast cancer[16] (it does, I'm afraid), as well as for the coal industry, claiming that the evidence on the health effects from mercury released by burning coal was inconclusive[17] (it's not). Defending assorted toxic products—it would not be much of a reach to say *any* toxic product—has become a lucrative, niche expertise.

Perversely, every scientific advance in understanding the health effects of toxic exposures assures more work for the product defense firms. The field of epidemiology was founded in the nineteenth century but it wasn't until the last few decades that scientists honed the techniques that allow us to recognize and measure the illness and premature death toll associated with, say, specific components of air pollution. And as a general rule, the more we as scientists know, the more clear it becomes that regulation is required. Some industry and free-market ideologues despise this fact, of course, and work strenuously to keep regulations at the less protective levels associated with older, more limited scientific knowledge. This is tantamount to ignoring the health impact of consumer products and toxins altogether. And in cases where the damage is too great to ignore, industry will seek to buy time by drumming up public debate about the evidence of health effects.

When a chemical manufacturer (or trade group representing manu-facturers) is defending itself in a lawsuit from workers or community residents who claim they've been made sick by one of the companies' products, the corporation doesn't go to companies like Cardno ChemRisk or Gradient for an *independent* assessment. They need an exonerating assessment, and they will get one. "Litigation support"—also the in-dustry's own term, one that exactly describes the purpose of this work—is a booming specialty. Global firms that provide environmental consulting services to corporations, especially ones that assist with "environmental management issues" (that is, pollution), now see litiga-tion support as one of their core services. Cardno, originally Australian but now "a global infrastructure, environmental, and social develop-ment company" acquired ChemRisk in 2012; two years later, ENVIRON (which had become Environ, Inc.) was purchased by Ramboll, a global engineering firm headquartered in Denmark. The company's majority owner is the Ramboll Foundation, an organization whose self-branded "Ramboll Philosophy" includes assertions antithetical to the work of product defense: "We act honestly, decently and responsibly.... We avoid conflict of interest and do not collude in corruption; nor do we undertake projects with an aggressive, destructive, or suppressive pur-pose towards nature or people.... [O]bservance of our values must always come before growth in size and short-term financial gain."[18]

The heart of the product defense charade is its claim to produce and publish scientific *research*. Research is the benchmark for true scientific expertise, and publication in a peer-reviewed journal is what makes re-search different from mere argument. The industry understands this very well. To help its clients who manufacture hazardous products or engage in dangerous activities, the industry has taken this model and subjected it to contortions that yield what appears to be real science. But the "studies" done by these specialists have little or nothing to do with advancing science. Their purpose is to manufacture material that will convince juries to spare corporations from paying people who allege their illnesses are caused by the corporation's products or activi-ties. We could as well call it "litigation science": deceptive studies (or re-analyses of other, real studies) that are laundered through academia's flawed publication structures to create the appearance of reasonable doubt.

So is the problem here the academic journals? In part, yes. Academic journals are a big business, both for professional societies that sponsor them and for publishers that produce them. They also serve a deeply entrenched function within the academic establishment, where careers are built on publishing studies in prestigious journals. And in this symbiotic relationship, peer review is the mechanism that is meant to ensure quality and integrity.

But the system of review by other scientists—presumably "peers"—before publication in a scientific journal is one that is widely misunderstood by the public and by some individuals in the regulatory and legal systems. Even rigorous peer review by honest scientists does not guarantee a study's accuracy or quality. Peer review is just one component of a larger quality control process through which scientific knowledge is developed and tested—a process that never really ends. Nevertheless, it has been granted an important role in both the regulatory and legal systems. Some agencies, including the International Agency for Research on Cancer (IARC or "eye-ark," part of the World Health Organization), will not consider using in its deliberations any paper that has not undergone peer review.

It does not—or should not—follow that any article that has been peer-reviewed is of high quality. In the case of product defense publications in journals, the peer review is often conducted by other scientists who are themselves committed to exonerating toxic chemicals from regulation. Any such review is of little value. Part of the proliferation of academic journals in recent decades has been the rise in what are in essence vanity journals—publications whose editorial boards are controlled by scientists who are united in their financial relationships with industries. These journals are just a different kind of front group. And they are the product defense industry's vehicle for speaking their wishes into scientific existence.

Take, for example, the journal *Regulatory Toxicology and Pharmacology*. For many years, the editor-in-chief was Gio Batta Gori, who went from heading the National Cancer Institute's Smoking and Health Program to being a well-paid defender of secondhand smoke for Big Tobacco. The journal's editorial board would meet at the offices of Keller and Heckman, the law firm that represented the trade association for the plastics industry (Society for the Plastics Industry) and other industry groups.[19] The board is filled with prominent product defense consultants. Not everyone on the editorial board is in the consulting business—a few are government and academic scientists—and not *all* the papers published are product defense efforts. The result is that, to the uninitiated judge or jury member, articles in *Regulatory Toxicology and Pharmacology* look credible.

A rival journal that shares *Regulatory Toxicology and Pharmacology*'s approach is *Critical Reviews in Toxicology*. Although these journals publish legitimate science alongside the work of the product defense industry, an analysis by the Center for Public Integrity found that since 1992, half of all review articles authored by the product defense firm Gradient's top scientists were published in one of these two journals.[20] One notable characteristic of many of their papers—it's hard to call them studies—is their length. Many of the papers are so long that it's doubtful more than a few attorneys with litigation interests actually read them. These weighty offerings may not fool regulators and certainly not scientists, but they do look very impressive to their real audiences: judges and juries.

Is product defense actually science? Do the studies prepared by Exponent and Gradient and TERA and Cardno ChemRisk and Ramboll and the other product defense specialists and published in scientific journals or presented at scientific conferences actually contribute to advancing scientific knowledge? I would say relatively few. How can I be so confident? First, their origin as work-for-hire, bought and paid for by the companies with a financial stake in their result, means that their conclusions cannot be considered without skepticism. Second, on issue after issue, tobacco, lead, asbestos, benzene, silica, and many more, they've been proven wrong by subsequent studies done by better scientists without financial conflicts of interest. In terms of actual science, the weight of the scientific evidence eventually sinks them. But in the meantime, they have earned a great deal of money and often set back efforts to protect the public from harm.

The guiding principle in these doubt studies: there is never enough proof; more study is always needed. When an agency like OSHA wants to reduce worker exposures to a chemical, that agency has to prove significant risk. It must demonstrate that the science shows the chemical is harmful and that it is, in fact, hurting people. In trying to prove a positive association between toxin and illness, agencies can't engage in gamesmanship—by law, their efforts and products must be open to public scrutiny. That's not the case for the product defense folks. Their work is always, no matter what venue, regulatory or legal, to argue that the evidence isn't strong enough. Theirs is not a burden of reasonable doubt, yet they demand guilt beyond a shadow of doubt—especially when the challenge is to identify low actual risks. It is difficult, for example, to determine if a widely used product causes cancer in one person out of every 10,000 exposed, and too easy to poke holes in any positive study. (Does the one-out-of-10,000 disease sound almost inconsequential, almost acceptable? The 25,000 adults in the United States with the disease might disagree.)

Unlike humans accused of crimes, chemicals should not be innocent until proven guilty. If anything, the record of new chemicals in the marketplace justifies a reversed presumption: that chemicals and toxins do more to harm health than we initially estimate, and it takes time to determine the nature and extent of those harms. Under U.S. law, manufacturers are supposed to test new chemicals before they are brought on the market. But many older chemicals, even ones we now know are extremely toxic, were grandfathered in under an extremely weak Toxic Substances Control Act, and it is only with recent legislation updating that law that there is a limited effort to actually test the toxicity of products to which we are already being exposed. What's more, laboratory tests really aren't enough, and one can only do epidemiology long after exposure has started. As it plays out in the real world, therefore, the system does tilt toward chemicals being innocent until proven guilty, instead of ensuring that people are protected from harm.

3

The Forever Chemicals

THE NAME DUPONT is synonymous with American industrialism and wealth. What began in 1802 as a gunpowder manufacturer is, since its 2017 merger with Dow Chemical, now the world's largest chemical manufacturer and developer. Many of the oddly named substances that are a part of today's American life—brand names like freon, nylon, and Lycra—were born in DuPont laboratories.

That list of substances includes Teflon, the nonstick material used as a coating on cookware, food wrappers, electrical cables, and waterproof clothing. Today, everyone knows the product by its trademarked name; as the ads say, *not even geckos can stick to Teflon*. It was discovered in 1938 by a chemist working for DuPont who in researching refrigerant gases accidentally synthesized a waxy material with an interesting property: almost nothing would stick to it. This laboratory creation was perhaps the first example of a class of chemicals known as per- and polyfluoro-alkyl substances, or PFAS. They are not found in the natural world, but chemists have created literally thousands of variants in the lab. It was soon apparent to those at DuPont that their new chemical could be used to manufacture a coating in an assortment of products, and mass production of Teflon began almost immediately at the company's Washington Works plant in Parkersburg, West Virginia. Sales followed. By 1948, the company was producing 2 million pounds of the substance per year.[1]

During the same period that DuPont was ramping up Teflon, scientists working to develop an atomic bomb for the Manhattan Project during World War II were desperate for an efficient way to isolate the required U-235 isotope from the raw uranium found in nature; isolating

U-235 was the first step in weaponizing it. A researcher named Joseph H. Simons had a "Eureka" moment in this quest when he passed raw fluorine—a greenish-yellow natural gas known as the "wildest hell-cat" of elements—through a carbon arc and providentially produced a carbon-fluorine compound that worked beautifully for making bombs. After World War II, Minnesota Mining and Manufacturing (later named 3M, another iconic American research and manufacturing company) bought Simons' patent and brought in some of the Manhattan Project's scientists for the company's "Fluorochemical Project." The most famous product of this scientific incubator was created by accident in 1953, when a mixture of chemicals splashed on a lab assistant's canvas shoes. Just as the DuPont chemists found with Teflon, the 3M team learned that the chemical splashed on the assistant's shoes repelled water and grease. Later patented under the name Scotchgard, this was a new PFAS, one that would be heralded by the company as one of its greatest inventions.[2]

A note on PFAS nomenclature, which can be confusing: two of the most prominent types of PFAS are often referred to by their own acronyms, PFOS (used in Scotchgard) and PFOA (used to manufacture Teflon—and also known as C8). All four abbreviations will feature in this story. The overriding point is that it's all one big family of organic compounds with amazing (and valuable) characteristics. Because PFAS repel oil and water, are stable at high and low temperatures, and reduce friction, the list of commercial uses is now virtually countless, including all manner of textiles, paper goods, and automotive and aerospace components. PFAS are almost perfect for leak-proof food wrapping and packaging. The compounds are also terrific in fighting fires where the flames are fueled by a combustible liquid, like gasoline, which water is ineffective at extinguishing. Accordingly, PFAS compounds have been used widely in fire protection at military bases and commercial airports.

The chemical bonds in PFAS are almost impossible to break down Their "half-life"—basically a measure of how long a molecule lives—in the environment is very, *very* long, so long the scientists have not been able to even estimate the length.[3] For that reason, and because the PFAS-intensive, fire-suppressing foams tested or applied at hundreds of airports and military bases have inevitably, inexorably seeped into the wells and water systems in hundreds of nearby communities in the United States, it is all around us, especially in the water we drink. This problem of what is now widely labeled the "forever chemical" is not exclusive to the United States: contaminated drinking water systems have caused outrage from Australia to Italy to Japan, with many more certain to be discovered in years to come. PFAS also enters our food, and therefore our bodies, through migration from packaging (like fast food containers, microwave popcorn bags, and pizza boxes) and from eating fish and other animals that have bioaccumulated PFAS from the environment. There is also exposure, particularly to infants and toddlers, through hand-to-mouth contact with furniture, carpets, and other surfaces treated with PFAS to prevent staining.

Of course, the ubiquity of PFAS in the environment would not be a major health concern if PFAS were not also, by now, ubiquitous in human bodies. Even if these chemicals were not in our drinking water (and data suggest that, for almost all of us, they are), all of us have also been exposed through food and environmental contact.

In 1998, 3M's own scientists undertook a series of studies to determine exactly how widespread the chemicals had become, testing blood samples from numerous studies in the United States and abroad, both recently and in the past. This included samples remote in time (1957, Sweden) and place (1994, rural China)—intersections of time and place where Scotchgard, Teflon, fire extinguishers, and other accouterments of industrial society would hypothetically have been relatively distant. The researchers' findings were sobering: PFAS had migrated everywhere. Only one of the 11 population samples showed *no* presence of PFAS in the subjects. That outlier was a group of 10 U.S. military recruits whose blood had been drawn and tested between 1948 and 1951.[4] Today, detectable levels of PFAS can be found in the blood of virtually all residents of the United States.[5]

The next and most important question: do these chemicals have effects on humans and other animals? In short, yes. And whereas most studies of human exposures to chemicals present ethical and funding challenges to conduct, we now know quite a lot about the health effects of PFAS—more than for almost any of the thousands of products that have provided consumers with "Better Things for Better Living through Chemistry," DuPont's advertising slogan for many years.

As recognition of the toxic effects of PFAS exposure has grown, it has prompted greater national interest in addressing the issue, including efforts to rid food and packaging of them and to produce cleaner water supply infrastructure for communities whose systems are contaminated. Some federal and state agencies are mobilizing. People who are sick and believe their illnesses are related to exposure are suing for compensation. As the industries have dug in to protect their interests, their tactics in doing so have checked all the boxes of a classic misinformation and "uncertainty" campaign: money, toxic exposures, hidden documents, mercenary scientists, lawsuits, government agencies trying to protect the public, and political interference in those efforts.

DuPont is among the foremost offenders in the PFAS saga, responsible for one of the most extensive and harmful drinking-water supply contaminations in American history. At the company's Washington Works plant in West Virginia, some 2.5 million pounds of the substance were lost in processing or discharge, with most of that occurring in the 1980s and 1990s. Much of it was released into the atmosphere as steamy air emissions, while some was dumped carelessly along the banks of the Ohio River or buried in nearby landfills. Such landfills were not suitable depositories of dangerous waste, and enough PFAS waste entered the ground to infiltrate the water supplies of surrounding communities. Over time, residents near the Washington Works had elevated blood levels of PFAS.

Early indications of the adverse health effects of this exposure were seen in farm animals. One farmer in Parkersburg, Wilbur Tennant, had previously sold a portion of his grazing land to DuPont, which in turn used it to dispose of waste from the Washington Works. When Tennant saw his cows (who continued to graze nearby on the farmer's remaining land) becoming deranged and then dying from a strange, inexplicable condition, he suspected chemicals from DuPont's nearby plant were the cause. He contacted an attorney, Rob Bilott, who brought suit against DuPont in 1998.

In 2000, while reviewing the thousands of DuPont documents obtained in discovery, Bilott found reference to a chemical, PFOA (or C8), with a name similar to PFOS—the Scotchgard chemical that 3M had just pulled from the market. He requested that DuPont further provide him with all their internal documents on this chemical. Teflon's manufacturer obliged, sending 110,000 documents—perhaps in an attempt to overwhelm the attorney. The effort was not successful. After months of digging through the documents, some of them more than 50 years old, Bilott pieced together a powerful indictment of a company that was aware of how toxic PFOA actually was, how widespread the exposure, and then took strides to cover it up.

The internal documents from DuPont illustrate both the company's acknowledgment of and attempts to contain the problem with PFOA. When the company tested its factory workers in the 1970s, the workers were found to have high concentrations of PFOA in their blood. In 1981, DuPont was informed by 3M (from which DuPont actually purchased much of its PFOA) that the chemical had been shown to cause birth defects in rats; DuPont then looked at data from its Washington Works Teflon division employees and found that, of the employees' seven most recent births, two babies had eye defects. Ten years later, DuPont's own scientists set an internal safety limit for PFOA concentration in drinking water at one part per billion; later that same year, DuPont measured the concentration in one local water district at three times that level. These are only a few examples of what DuPont learned—and what it kept secret from its workers, nearby residents, and public health agencies—until forced to reveal it by attorney Bilott's suit.[6]

Bilott's work was just starting. Seeing proof that that C8 had contaminated far beyond Tennant's farm, the attorney filed another lawsuit, this a class action on behalf of 80,000 residents in six water districts of Ohio and West Virginia. The suit alleged that humans—not just cows—were being sickened by PFAS and demanded medical monitoring as a part of any financial restitution. Recognizing the larger public health implications of these documents, in March 2001 Bilott sent letters to the EPA and the Justice Department informing them of what he learned. DuPont's response? The firm went to federal court, requesting a gag order to block Bilott from speaking to the EPA. After a federal judge denied the request, Bilott shipped his entire file to the regulatory agency, and in 2004, the EPA also filed suit against DuPont for violating the Toxic Substances Control Act. Federal regulations require that firms disclose information about the toxic effects of their products to the EPA upon discovery; DuPont had clearly failed to do that.

Facing this onslaught of legal action, DuPont did not face the music. Instead, the company set out to convince both the public and government agencies charged with protecting the public that exposure to PFOA was simply not that dangerous for humans. Predictably, DuPont hired a product defense scientist to lead this campaign—a company called ChemRisk, led by Dennis Paustenbach. After performing an initial retrospective assessment of the available research on PFOA, Paustenbach wrote, "The predicted historical lifetime and average daily estimates of PFOA intake by persons who lived within five miles of the plant over the past 50 years were about 10,000-fold less than the intake of the chemical not considered as a health risk by an independent panel of scientists who recently studied PFOA."[7]

The phrasing is rather opaque, but Paustenbach meant to argue that the West Virginia and Ohio residents' cumulative exposure to PFOA would have been well below the level that was identified as dangerous by an independent panel of experts. Readers may have already flagged the telltale word in that statement: "independent." It is rare to see manufacturers hire truly independent panels of scientists. Typically that's the last thing they want. In this case, the allegedly independent panel had been set up for the state of West Virginia by *another* product defense firm, Toxicology Excellence for Risk Assessment (TERA), which was recommended to the state government *by DuPont* because TERA could "assemble a package and then sell this to EPA, or whomever we desired." (That admission is thanks to an internal company email.) TERA's "independent" panel included scientists working for DuPont, ostensibly charged with working in the interests of the state. And the panel gave DuPont what it needed. In 2002, West Virginia set a safe level in drinking water at 150 parts per billion (ppb)—some 150 times the safe level that had been determined earlier by DuPont's scientists for the company's internal use.[8] The faulty state standard of 150 ppb served to lessen DuPont's legal obligation to provide clean drinking water to West Virginians, who continued to be exposed at levels soon found to be dangerous. (Also noteworthy: Michael Dourson, at the time the head of TERA, was later nominated by President Trump to head the chemical safety office of EPA. As I recount in Chapter 15, that nomination failed.)

Another product defense firm, the Weinberg Group, provided DuPont with further assistance in navigating the federal and civil claims related to PFAS. In a 2003 letter signed by Weinberg's vice president of product defense, P. Terrence Gaffney, and uncovered by journalist Paul Thacker, the consultant group outlines its comprehensive strategy for defending DuPont—and in doing so more or less opens the product defense playbook for public edification. All emphases are original:

> The constant theme which permeates our recommendations on the issues faced by DuPont is that DUPONT MUST SHAPE THE DEBATE AT ALL LEVELS. We must implement a strategy at the outset which discourages governmental agencies, the plaintiff's bar, and misguided environmental groups from pursuing this matter any further than the current risk assessment contemplated by the Environmental Protection Agency (EPA) and the matter pending in West Virginia. We strive to end this now.

Weinberg's experts would also seed the scientific literature "with papers and articles dispelling the alleged nexus" between PFOA and health problems that were claimed by community residents. The Weinberg Group would further undertake to "develop 'blue ribbon panels' of thought leaders on issues related to PFOA…to create awareness of safety regarding PFOA in areas of likely litigation, and in particular where medical monitoring claims may be brought…; begin to identify and retain leading scientists to consult on the range of issues involving PFOA so as to develop a premium expert panel and concurrently conflict out experts from consulting with plaintiffs…; reshape the debate by identifying the likely known health benefits of PFOA exposure…; coordinate the publishing of white papers on PFOA, junk science and the limits of medical monitoring…; [and] provide the strategy to illustrate how epidemiological association has little or nothing to do with individual causation."[9]

DuPont denies hiring the Weinberg Group to work on PFOA, although this claim appears to be contradicted by documents, including invoices that surfaced in the litigation.

The advice and work of the product defense firms turned out to be of limited value to DuPont.[10] The EPA's action against the company was easy to address because it arrived at a very advantageous moment in history: 2005, a period of notoriously weak EPA enforcement under the George W. Bush administration. Without admitting liability (as is common in such deals—the EPA accepts such terms in order to get the outcome without a risky court fight), DuPont settled with the federal agency. The company paid a $16.5 million fine, which was the largest civil penalty the EPA had ever obtained to that date. It amounted to pennies for the company, especially given the profits it made from Teflon and related products.[6]

In the civil claims, DuPont evidently lacked confidence that the analyses from ChemRisk and TERA would be enough to overcome the multitudes of victims who were claiming injury. (Civil justice proceedings can be much more diligent enforcers than actions by regulatory agencies, especially in the matter of penalties incurred.) The company agreed to pay $107 million to these plaintiffs, a sum that included measures to improve water treatment facilities and to fund research to determine if there was a "probable link" between C8/PFOA exposure and human disease.

This last stipulation was fraught with danger for DuPont, because the discovery of any such direct link would require it to fund an expensive medical monitoring program and to financially compensate for exposure victims. Three renowned and truly independent epidemiologists, chosen jointly by the attorneys representing the claimants and the company, were given *carte blanche* to study the health effects of PFOA in this population. These "C8 Studies," as they are called, are why we know a great deal about the health effects of exposure to this class of chemicals. They also represent a massive scientific undertaking involving 69,000 subjects, most of whom provided one or more blood samples and filled out extensive questionnaires to help catalog health and exposure histories.[11] The project has resulted in dozens of scientific publications.

The C8 Studies found that PFOA exposure increases human risk of testicular cancer, kidney cancer (among workers at the manufacturing plant), ulcerative colitis, thyroid disease, pregnancy-induced hypertension, and elevated cholesterol levels. This last morbidity is of great concern because it is a risk factor for cardiovascular disease, the nation's leading killer. At the same time, the panel also rejected links with many other diseases.[12] In the end, DuPont and a company it spun off, Chemours, later paid out an additional $670 million to 3,550 residents of West Virginia and Ohio exposed to PFOA.[13]

In 2012, Harvard epidemiologist Philippe Grandjean published a study in the *Journal of the American Medical Association* (*JAMA*) reporting that PFAS exposure appeared to interfere with children's antibody responses to routine childhood immunizations. (This would be bad. The body's antibody response is what provides humans with immunity to the diseases for which we're vaccinated.) His research found that children with higher PFAS levels in their blood had lower concentrations of antibodies, which suggested that PFAS exposure was limiting the function of the immune system.[14] In response, 3M scientists wrote a letter to *JAMA* critical of the Grandjean paper, citing several other published studies and asserting that these findings offered by the company should be "reassuring to those concerned with the immune system, childhood infectious diseases, and [perflourinated compounds]."[15]

Years later, Grandjean, preparing to testify as an expert witness in a lawsuit against 3M, uncovered evidence of a longstanding disinformation campaign: studies conducted by 3M and other manufacturers as far back as 1978, all showing the impact of PFAS exposure on immune system function. *None* of these results was revealed to regulatory agencies or the scientific community for decades; in coverage of the revelation in 2018, Grandjean told an interviewer, "Had I found out in 1978 that this industrial chemical was toxic to the immune system, I could see all sorts of examinations of exposed kids that could be done, but I was not told, so it had to wait, [in] this case 30 years, before I turned my attention to this."[16] Ensuing reporting by the *Intercept*'s Sharon Lerner corroborated and expanded on the discoveries in the lawsuits.[17] By 2016, the U.S. National Toxicology Program had reviewed the extensive human and animal evidence that had been published in the scientific literature (including Grandjean's 2012 study) and concluded that the PFOA used in Teflon and PFOS in Scotchgard are presumed to be immune hazards to humans.[18]

DuPont and 3M were not alone in seeing the wheels fall off their campaigns to evade financial responsibility for cleaning contaminated water systems and toxic dumps (as mandated under the "polluter pays" model of Superfund program administered by the EPA). Nor were they alone in their efforts to defeat a host of civil lawsuits alleging broad PFAS-related liability. PFAS manufacturers of every size and scale have paid hundreds of millions of dollars toward settlements, with many more likely to come. These firms also face threats to their future business. To stem this tide, the industry has returned time and again to the tobacco industry's playbook: manufacture uncertainty about the science, then attack the public health agencies trying to protect the public.

Big Tobacco demonstrated for all hazardous industries that scientists are needed to produce the source material for misinformation campaigns. For manufacturers producing PFAS and countless other chemicals, this means employing firms that will churn out papers, present them at scientific conferences, and publish them in journals edited and peer-reviewed by other product defense scientists. These papers are rarely primary research—studies in which scientists collect new data in the field or the laboratory and analyze the results. Instead, they are reviews and re-analyses of the existing literature, relying on manipulation of the numbers to reach the preordained conclusions. In the case of PFAS, the product defense studies almost uniformly minimize effects of toxic exposures: *The chemical in question is not nearly as dangerous as those biased public health agencies are saying; these exposure levels won't make anyone sick; there's no corporate liability; there's no need to clean up dumps, landfills, and water supplies.*

Alongside the alternative "science" sowed to defend PFAS compounds, an organization called the American Council for Science and Health has carried water for the industry in public debates. Based on the group's history, this is not a surprise. ACSH is an industry-funded organization with a typically rosy-sounding name that specializes in inserting itself at the middle of many public health controversies, with particular expertise in downplaying the risk of exposure to toxic substances. On its website it has published articles opposing regulation of mercury emissions from coal-burning power plants[19] as well as diesel exhaust emissions,[20] while promoting climate change deniers[21] and attacking the science that finds harm from consumption of sugar[22] and alcoholic beverages.[23] For PFAS, one ACSH report concluded that "the current data indicate that we can expect no risk to human health associated with the levels of PFOA exposure found in the general population."[24] This was issued before the C8 studies were published, but ACSH has defended their report even after the independent scientists found significant health effects in exposed humans.[25] Such is the fundamental problem for these product defense specialists and their industry patrons: their arguments age terribly, becoming more suspect and harder to defend in the face of the accumulating counterevidence.

The findings of the early PFAS studies that were suppressed for decades by the companies producing the substances have motivated scientists across the world—epidemiologists, toxicologists, exposure assessment experts—to conduct more research. Hundreds of new studies on PFAS appear in the scientific literature annually, and today it is clear that the health effects of these ubiquitous, dangerous chemicals are profound and diverse. So are many of the routes through which human exposure to these substances can occur. In 2014, for example, scientists working with the data gathered in the C8 study showed that breastfeeding is a major source of PFAS exposure.[26] This discovery lends particular importance to the work of Grandjean, who has demonstrated that PFAS exposure during infancy is associated with subsequent immune deficiency.[27]

DuPont, 3M, and other companies, and their product defense collaborators, can back and fill as hard and as fast as possible, but the weight of this evidence is overwhelmingly against the manufacturers. There is a limit to how much uncertainty mercenary scientists can manufacture, and the PFAS industry may have reached it. It becomes clearer by the day that the level of safe exposure to PFAS (if there is one) is far lower than industry's scientists claim.

Recall the misbegotten episode in which the product defense firm TERA, working for DuPont, helped West Virginia set a safe level of PFAS in drinking water of 150 parts per billion. That was in 2002. Since then, independent science has driven that number down repeatedly. The European Food Safety Agency has expressed concern that PFAS exposure is pushing up cholesterol levels and therefore increasing heart attacks, so in 2018 the organization started a process to decrease PFAS intake through food.[28] Recognizing that drinking water levels must be lowered substantially to avoid PFAS transmission through breast milk, in 2016 the EPA published an advisory that stipulated a maximum of 70 parts per trillion (ppt—the *t* is *trillion*, not billion) for PFOA and

PFOS in water.[29] The amount is almost unimaginably small: the equivalent of 70 drops of water in an Olympic-sized swimming pool. This is also more than 2,000 times lower than TERA's proclaimed "safe" level.

In other words, there appears to be virtually no safe level of exposure to these chemicals, and new studies keep finding new health effects. Researchers in Veneto, a region in Italy with contaminated water, found that young men exposed to PFAS had lower sperm counts, lower sperm mobility, and shorter penises (!) than unexposed men.[30]

These extremely cautionary, restrictive numbers put both the manufacturers and the military (especially the Air Force, which has to clean up the contamination around its bases all over the world) in a difficult position. The Trump White House and its EPA actually tried to block release of a lowered exposure standard from the Centers for Disease Control and Prevention, with one staffer calling it "a public relations nightmare."[31] The ensuing public outcry was enormous and prompted serious pushback from both Democratic and Republican legislators representing districts with military bases and otherwise PFAS-contaminated water supplies. The administration had no choice but to release the report, increasing the pressure on the EPA to tighten regulations—and on the military to focus more resources on either cleaning up the toxic material or providing bottled water on and around the bases.[32]

———

3M stopped manufacturing PFAS in 2002.[33] Of course, this cessation didn't resolve the company's legal problems. Because PFAS persists in the environment, the lawsuits persist in the courtrooms. The state of Minnesota sued 3M, accusing the local company of dumping large amounts of these chemicals while knowing that they were extremely hazardous and covering up the dangers of exposure.[34] 3M's attorneys countered this action by hiring Barbara Beck (of yet another product defense firm, Gradient) to provide a report for the court in which she claimed that the state overestimated any risk and that current exposures are far below a level that could make people sick.[35] Gradient also teamed with Exponent to challenge the National Toxicology Program's decision to categorize PFAS as an immune hazard. Exponent's scientists published their evaluation in *Critical Reviews in Toxicology*, one of the favored product defense journals, asserting, not surprisingly, that "available evidence is insufficient to conclude that a causal relationship has been established between PFOA or PFOS exposure and any immune condition in humans."[36]

In 2018, 3M settled the Minnesota law suit for $850 million without admitting any liability. It was the third-largest payment for an environmental damage claim, after the Deepwater Horizon and the Exxon Valdez spill. After the settlement, the Minnesota attorney general released many of the documents that she would have used in trial, providing fascinating insight into 3M efforts to defend PFOA—including payments of millions of dollars to academic scientists to produce papers that were intended, at least in part, as "defensive barriers to litigation."[37]

DuPont, unable to purchase PFOA from 3M after 2002, built its own factory to manufacture GenX, a PFOA replacement, and other PFAS in Fayetteville, North Carolina. Chemours, the DuPont spin-off that inherited the facility, continues to produce the products that are central to Teflon manufacture. DuPont may be out of the business of producing PFAS, but with Chemours, the drinking water saga continues. Chemours was sued by the state of North Carolina for dumping GenX and contaminating the water supply of 250,000 residents of the area who get their drinking water from the Cape Fear River.[38] In 2018, the firm settled with the state, agreeing to pay $12 million, improve the pollution controls at the plant, commit to regular environmental monitoring, and conduct testing on five PFAS chemicals whose toxicity has not been adequately characterized.[39] That was not even a slap on the wrist, but I have already reported on the earlier DuPont settlements in West Virginia for real money—hundreds of millions of dollars total.

Some manufacturers that once used PFOA and PFOS in their products have now substituted new, presumably safer compounds—although the safety of all PFAS compounds is very much in question.[40] In 2020, we even have a *new* product defense organization defending the manufacturers of the old PFAS products. It's the Responsible Science Policy Coalition, funded by 3M and other producers, and two of its professed goals are very much on-brand for a corporate front group: "Provide scientific resources to public policy decisions at federal and state level"; and "Coordinate investments in research with other stakeholders to maximize value and to accelerate results."[41]

The beat goes on.

4

The NFL's Head Doctors

BASED ON THEIR total number of workplace fatalities, the most dangerous "regular" jobs in America are logging and commercial fishing. But football players (and before them, boxers) are arguably the best-known victims of work-related disease of any kind. No other profession—not one—outranks professional football in causing life-altering injuries.

For professional football players, one severe work-related condition is chronic traumatic encephalopathy, or CTE. The following members of the NFL Hall of Fame have been diagnosed with the disease posthumously: Frank Gifford, Kenny Stabler, Mike Webster. Recent CTE victims from the pro ranks whose cases have garnered significant attention include Junior Seau, Dave Duerson, Terry Long, and Aaron Hernandez. Battered by thousands of jarring hits, these players' brains no longer function normally; they undergo a type of progressive degeneration that actually kills brain cells. These men are damaged beyond repair: no cast, no surgery, no medicine, no rehab can change their fates.

The mental anguish and suffering from CTE is enormous and sometimes unbearable, leading inexorably to a host of side effects and consequences, including depression, memory loss, impulsivity, violent outbursts (a particular problem given the size and strength of some football players), drug abuse, homelessness, and premature death, sometimes by suicide.

In the case of Aaron Hernandez, the star tight end for the New England Patriots between 2010 and 2012, his death in 2017 came after a long line of violent off-the-field incidents. Released by the Patriots in June 2013 after his arrest on suspicion of murder, Hernandez was convicted of first-degree murder in one case, then accused but acquitted in two others. Five days after the acquittal, in April 2017, Hernandez hanged himself in his jail cell outside Boston. Examining his brain, researchers subsequently found CTE of a severity never before seen in anyone younger than their mid-forties. Hernandez was 27 at the time of his death.

Hernandez's brain was one of 111 former NFL players' brains studied by the CTE Center at Boston University, under the direction of neuropathologist and neurologist Anne McKee. Standard imaging of the living brain cannot conclusively identify CTE; it can be diagnosed only by an autopsy, during which the pathologist slices the brain into thin sections and examines the tissue at the cellular level. Here, the damage is startling. Some areas may have deteriorated and atrophied, losing mass. There is often a buildup of a protein called tau, which in the normal brain works to stabilize brain cells' cellular structure. With CTE, that same protein accumulates in excess and can alter the functioning of brain cells—or kill them altogether. Junior Seau and Dave Duerson, all-pro defensive standouts who committed suicide, were convinced that a damaged brain was the cause of their behavior and despair. Desperate to preserve their evidence for researchers, both players chose to shoot themselves in the chest.

The results of the Boston University brain study were overwhelming and distressing: 110 of the 111 NFL players' brains were found to have CTE. Granted, this was a sample of convenience, and not at all representative of all players. Neither was there any comparison population, but given how exceedingly rare CTE is as a disease, none was needed. So while the true risk of CTE if you've played in the NFL may not be the 99 percent found here—and I certainly hope it's not—the study suggests rather convincingly that at least hundreds, and perhaps thousands, of former NFL players have this brain disease.[1] In some cases it is mild, in others severe, and in some totally debilitating. (Nor does the disease disable only the pros. That same study found CTE among some men who had played only in high school, not college or the NFL.[2])

Faced with initial evidence of widespread, progressive, catastrophic brain damage among its former players, the NFL might have taken steps to find out what's happening, or at least how to address it. This is not what happened. Recognizing the challenge posed by CTE to the NFL's incredibly lucrative business, the league instead challenged the *science* behind football-related CTE every step of the way. Adopting the playbook designed and implemented by Big Tobacco over half a century ago, the league denied and defended. That this insidious strategy was exposed over a half century ago didn't discourage the NFL from trying it again. America's most popular sports league hired conflicted scientists who could be counted on to produce studies that minimized the risk of brain damage among football players while also attacking studies done by independent scientists that assert what is now widely accepted as truth: the brains of many, many football players have been irreparably damaged by the hits they took (and take) on the field.

If Big Tobacco couldn't get away with its obfuscations fifty years ago, back in the relative dark ages of media, how did the NFL believe it could do so recently, when everyone has exponentially more tools for finding and disseminating the facts of any case? It is the common, knee-jerk response of most wealthy industries when they find themselves on the wrong side of science. In the short term it buys some time and saves some profits; in the long run, it's doomed to fail. Unfortunately for the NFL, its business enjoys a far higher profile than any of the others I discuss in these pages. Foundry workers are not on TV every Saturday (college) and Sunday (NFL) for five months out of every year. Many of the league's fans are parents of school kids who play football. The old news adage about trauma and reporting goes, *if it bleeds, it leads.* The brain doesn't openly bleed, but the concussion story was nevertheless destined to lead the news.

This history of obfuscation and duplicity by the NFL begins in the early 1990s, when the initial signs of a coming epidemic of brain damage first came to light. For decades, as the defensive players had gotten bigger, stronger, and faster, and their hits on the offense harder and harder, more and more players were slower and slower getting up after collisions, or they had to be helped off, occasionally with the support of teammates or on carts. The evidence was anecdotal, but reporters focused on the jump in the rate of concussions occurring every Sunday, on the increase in the number of well-known players, especially quarterbacks, who couldn't continue to play. Their symptoms didn't disappear with time. They got worse.

At a public forum in New York City in 1994, journalist David Halberstam questioned Paul Tagliabue, then the NFL's commissioner, about the mounting toll of concussions among the league's players. Halberstam was not just any journalist: He had been awarded a Pulitzer Prize in 1964 for his coverage in the *New York Times* of America's involvement in Vietnam. His subsequent book, *The Best and the Brightest*, was one of the most important ever published on the subject of the war. So he and his question could not be easily dismissed by Tagliabue or anyone else. But of course the commissioner did try. *Sports Illustrated* described the encounter: "Calling the matter a 'pack journalism issue,' [Tagliabue] waved away concern, saying that the NFL has 'one concussion every three or four games.' After a few more calculations, Tagliabue pronounced a figure of 2.5 concussions for every '22,000 players engaged.' His response raised echoes for Halberstam.... 'I feel I'm back in Vietnam hearing McNamara give statistics,' he said."[3]

Ironically, Junior Seau is mentioned in the very next paragraph of the *Sports Illustrated* article. The previous Sunday, the hard-hitting linebacker had knocked New York Jets' quarterback Boomer Esiason "senseless." Tagliabue tried to be dismissive, but this tactic was never going to work, not in the face of such high-profile questions and reporting. This concussion story was becoming a massive PR problem, with the league facing pressure from players, the press, and, perhaps most consequentially, from the fans and from parents wondering if they should stop their kids from playing football. If sizable numbers of parents did take this route, and if more boys followed their sisters to the soccer fields, the long-term fan base of the league would be endangered. Clearly, the NFL had to do *something*.

Soon after his public skewering, Tagliabue announced the formation of the Mild Traumatic Brain Injuries (MTBI) Committee, charging it "to scientifically investigate concussion and means to reduce injury risks in football." To staff this committee, he could have turned to independent physicians or renowned brain researchers. He did not do that. Instead, the commissioner turned to people he knew and could trust, some with profound conflicts of interest: representatives from the NFL Team Physicians Society, the NFL Athletic Trainers Society (now called the Professional Football Athletic Trainers Society), and NFL equipment managers. These committee members had financial ties to the league and to specific teams, and certainly had some incentive to *not* acknowledge that football was damaging the brains of their players. Almost all would be inclined toward other conclusions.

The MTBI's published papers included the reassuring statement that "none of the Committee members has a financial or business relationship posing a conflict of interest to the research conducted on MTBI in professional football."[4] (Author's note: Yes, they did.) The chair of the committee, Elliot Pellman, was a rheumatologist with no particular expertise in neurology or brain trauma. He was, however, Tagliabue's personal physician, and he and others on the committee were clinical consultants to various teams. In that capacity, they were personally responsible for determining whether concussed players were too damaged to return. Consciously or not, they were not likely to welcome the idea that sending players who had been knocked woozy right back onto the field might contribute to their risk of long-term brain damage. Independent they were not.

Then there's the name of the committee—*Mild* Traumatic Brain Injuries—which itself implies that the MTBI Committee was preordained *not* to find severe effects from the collisions inherent in the game. Before any data were collected, the injuries were labeled "mild." No one was surprised that this is exactly what the MTBI found. Eventually. For the first eight years—that's right, *years*—the committee found out nothing. Between 1994 and 2002, it published nothing. But when questioned, the league could point to the committee as proof that it was working on the problem. Then, in the following three years, between 2003 and 2006, the MTBI committee published 13 papers, all in the same journal: *Neurosurgery*.

One after another, these papers presented conclusions that minimized or denied the existence of any long-term effects of head trauma from playing football. They gave the league and the team owners the results they wanted: pro football simply wasn't that dangerous. The decisions made by the teams' physicians were the right ones. The rare concussion was treated appropriately. The game did not need to be reformed. The two MTBI co-chairs, Pellman and David Viano, a biomechanical engineer, authored a paper that summarized the MTBI committee's research and recommendations. Here are a handful of the assertions in this summary, all of which turned out to be misleading or erroneous:

- "Because a significant percentage of players returned to play in the same game and the overwhelming majority of players with concussions were kept out of football-related activities for less than 1 week, it can be concluded that mild TBIs in professional football are not serious injuries."
- "There have been reports in which researchers have concluded that there may be an increased risk of repeated concussive injuries, and there may be a slower recovery of neurological function after repeated concussions in those who have a history of previous ones. The results of this study in professional football players do not support that conclusion."
- "This 6-year study indicates that no NFL player experienced second-impact syndrome, chronic cumulative injury, or chronic traumatic encephalopathy from repeated injuries."
- "The results of this study indicate no evidence of worsening injury or chronic cumulative effects of multiple mild TBIs in NFL players."
- "There were concerns based on the results of the earlier studies of mild TBI that perhaps some players were being returned to play too soon after injury, thus resulting in more prolonged post-concussion syndrome and perhaps creating the risk of more severe brain injury....The NFL experience thus supports the suggestion that players who become asymptomatic and have normal results on examinations performed at any time after injury, while the game is still in progress, have been and can continue to be safely returned to play on that day."[5]

In teaching my students how to review epidemiologic studies, I often tell them, "what the results giveth, the methods taketh away." Some of the methodologic flaws in these studies, including ones that would guarantee that fewer neurological effects would be found than actually exist, were obvious. Others were more subtle. But there were *lots*. Selection bias, where the participants in the study are not representative of the universe of people who should have been included, is just one of these flaws. One study, for example, included only players who were identified as having an MTBI and who then voluntarily participated in neurological testing. In all, only 22 percent of concussed players who were eligible to participate actually did. And these players represented only

16 percent of the concussions. In this relatively small group of players (143), the neuropsychological function of those who stayed off the field for more than a week after the injury was compared with those who returned to the field more quickly. No one was tested for their brain function more than ten days after the concussive event.

Not surprisingly, many of the flaws in these MTBI papers were spotted easily by the peer reviewers (experts who volunteer to review studies like these before they get published), and *Neurosurgery* published these cautionary reviews in tandem with each paper. This was unusual. With most journals, editors who receive reviews that identify fundamental methodologic flaws generally just reject the paper, or at the least send it back to the authors and request major revisions. Why did *Neurosurgery* publish the MTBI papers, flaws and all? I note only that the editor of that journal at that time was Michael L. J. Apuzzo, who also was a medical consultant to the New York Giants, and later to the NFL commissioner's office as well. Some researchers eventually nicknamed *Neurosurgery* the "Journal of No NFL Concussions," although it did subsequently publish the controversial first report of CTE found in the brain of a deceased football player.[6]

The limitations in these "no harm, no foul" papers, tacitly admitted by the journal that published them, did not stop the NFL's medical experts from suggesting that the football players that make it all the way to the pros have brains that are resistant to brain damage:

> [T]here may be a natural selection of athletes that make it to the NFL because players more prone to concussion may have been weeded out during high school and college play. Brain responses shown here may represent those of players who are most resistant to the damaging effects of neural deformation during head impact.[7]

This is a remarkable statement. The NFL was claiming that the new standards and concussion protocols that had already been implemented in many colleges and high schools were less necessary in the pros, *because natural selection made professional brains more* resistant to brain injury. This would represent a new wrinkle on the "survival of the fittest" doctrine.

Did anyone actually believe this? Whether he believed it or not, Tom Brady at least carried water for the statement. In late 2018, the Patriots' quarterback remarked in an interview, "Your body gets used to the hits. The brain understands the position that you are putting your body into, and my brain is wired for contact. I would say in some ways it has become callous to some of the hits."[8] The Pellman and Viano summary agreed: "[M]any NFL players can be safely allowed to return to play on the day of the injury after sustaining a mild TBI [traumatic brain injury]. These players had to be asymptomatic, with normal results on clinical and neurological examinations, and be cleared by a knowledge-able team physician. There were no adverse effects, and the results once again are in sharp contrast to the recommendations in published guide-lines and the standard of practice of most college and high school foot-ball team physicians."[5]

While the NFL was purveying its own seriously compromised, dis-honest "research," it simultaneously challenged other reports whose conclusions it didn't like. A 2009 study from the Institute for Social Research at the University of Michigan reported that former NFL play-ers aged 30 to 49 were nineteen times more likely to develop neurolog-ical disorders than nonplayers the same age.[9] The NFL paid for the study, but when it was released, its spokesperson dismissed its results, claiming "there are thousands of retired players who do not have memory problems."[10]

Given the NFL's deep pockets—and access to a journal that seemed willing to publish just about anything submitted by a certain group—the MTBI researchers might have been able to maintain the charade for a long time. But then, inevitably, football players with CTE started to die.

———

Autopsies are more difficult to challenge than epidemiological studies. The damage in the CTE-diseased brains of NFL players is revealed and then reported for all to understand. The earliest prominent case of CTE in an NFL player was Mike Webster, the legendary center for Terry Bradshaw and the Pittsburgh Steelers in the 1970s. "Iron Mike" played 15 seasons with the Steelers, helping lead the team to four Super Bowl victories in the late 1970s and in 1980, before finishing up his career with two seasons with the Kansas City Chiefs. He was one of the great-est centers to play the game and was named to the NFL's 75th Anniversary All-Time Team. In 2002, Webster died young, at age 50, from a heart attack, and his brain was autopsied by neuropathologist Bennet Omalu. Omalu's involvement was not planned; as the most junior pathologist in the Allegheny County coroner's office, he was working the Saturday that Webster's battered body arrived. He was assigned the autopsy that turned him into a national figure. Three years later, in 2005, Omalu used that autopsy as the basis for a study co-authored with colleagues at the University of Pittsburgh and published in *Neurosurgery*. This was the first published case of CTE in a professional football player.[11]

In retrospect, the finding that Webster's brain was damaged should not have been a surprise. As the center, Webster was the core of his team's offense. On play after play after play for seventeen seasons, he took hit after hit after hit. He was Iron Mike in spirit and dedication, but his skull and brain were made of softer, more fragile stuff. Even before his retirement in 1990, Webster had started exhibiting troubling and often dangerous behavior. In a profile published in 1997, the *Pittsburgh Post-Gazette* reported that this former football great was "homeless, unemployed, deep in debt, beset with medical ailments, lacking health insurance, in the midst of divorce, in the care of a psychiatrist and on medication, and involved in a complex lawsuit over real estate investments." The story added, "After waging war on the gridiron and routinely flattening the enemy, Iron Mike was finally dented, dinged and damaged by forces that he simply could not wrestle to the ground."[12]

Note that Omalu's study was not an accusation against the NFL; it did not assert the causal relationship between football and CTE. It simply raised an alarm and called for more research. Omalu naively believed his nonjudgmental work would be welcomed by the owners. Instead, they responded the same way they responded to any cautionary note whatsoever on the subject of severe brain disease among football players: deny and defend. Specifically, three MTBI committee members—Ira Casson, who would become the leading medical spokesperson for the NFL once Pellman became sufficiently radioactive, along with Pellman and Viano, wrote a lengthy letter to *Neurosurgery* challenging Omalu's diagnosis. Casson is a neurologist, but neither he nor the other two were pathologists, nor were they experts in examining brain tissue. Rather than stating that these striking abnormalities in Webster's brain were of concern and should trigger additional research among football players, they insisted there was insufficient evidence to link the abnormalities to football, or even to label them CTE. These three men, all of whom were in the NFL payroll, called on Omalu and his colleagues to retract their report.[13]

The Omalu team did not comply. Instead, the following year, the pathologist and his colleagues published a second paper, also in *Neurosurgery*, this time studying the brain of Terry Long, offensive lineman for the Steelers from 1984 to 1991, playing alongside Webster for five of those years. Long's career was only half as long as Webster's but more than enough to cause irreparable damage. As a lineman, he had also taken hit after hit on play after play. In 1991, he attempted suicide following a failed steroids test. In 2005, he took his life by drinking antifreeze.[14] In November 2006, the same month that Omalu published his findings on Long's brain, Andrew Watson, who had played with the Philadelphia Eagles, committed suicide; Omalu would find CTE in his brain as well. And then there was a fourth suicide, and a fifth—eventually more than a dozen among former pro football players. In each case, the brains Omalu studied looked like those seen in professional boxers, who when they are autopsied are often decades older than these former football players were at the time of their deaths. Under the microscope, the tissue shocked the pathologists. It became clear that the cause of this damage wasn't just the concussions. It must have been the basic pounding, play after play, especially dangerous for the interior linemen who experience the most impact.

In the face of mounting evidence and publicity, the MTBI committee kept churning out studies exonerating head impacts. In one, researchers tapped rats on their tiny heads to simulate the hits in a professional football game played by men weighing several hundred pounds.[15] It's almost laughable, except that it's not laughable at all.

With Big Tobacco, the industry's research charade had bought four decades of unimpeded profits before Congressman Henry Waxman (D-CA) finally dragged the CEOs of the tobacco companies to testify in 1994. Under oath, these executives asserted they did not believe that cigarette smoking caused cancer. With the NFL, the increasingly infamous MTBI committee had also bought the league some time—about a decade—but this CTE story was not going to die. An ever-growing body of research suggested a literally fatal flaw at the heart of America's most popular sport, and the league's reaction to this research brought into question the integrity of one of our most powerful and prominent institutions. In 2009, a congressional committee chaired by John Conyers (D-MI) summoned the new NFL commissioner, Roger Goodell, who had replaced Paul Tagliabue in 2006. When Goodell refused to acknowledge a link between football and brain damage among players, Representative Linda Sánchez (D-CA) made the obvious comparison with tobacco industry's denial of the link between cigarettes and lung cancer. A national uproar ensued.

Within a few weeks, Goodell was motivated to dissolve the discredited MTBI committee and launch a new research initiative with a new name: NFL Head, Neck, and Spine (HNS) Committee. The old guard was out. The league's new flagship investigation was stocked with actual neurologists and brain surgeons. Members of the new committee would not be paid by the NFL (although they would have their expenses covered and they would receive free Super Bowl tickets). Overnight, the whole line of questionable research the league had been promoting for over a decade was summarily swept under the rug. The league could no longer simply assert that research by conflicted scientists was adequate to understand the relationship of football and brain damage. Why not? The research was untenable. It was embarrassing. It was wrong. The league and its experts were getting pilloried in the press and pressure from the public and the players union was mounting. Firms that sell a product directly to consumers, as the NFL does, are more sensitive to public opinion than, say, makers of asbestos or pesticides or textile dyes.

Pressure continued to mount on the league. In 2011, former players filed a class action lawsuit, accusing the NFL of waging a "concerted effort of deception and denial" in order to "conceal the extent of the concussion and brain trauma problem."[16] Eventually 5,000 former players joined the suit, and, after much controversy, the owners agreed to pay out a settlement of approximately $1 billion. This sounds like a lot of money, but for the league it represents only a tiny percentage of its revenue in a single year. And for the players, the amount appears to not come close to adequately compensating the plaintiffs who joined the suit and the many more who will become disabled by CTE in coming years. The NFL estimates that perhaps 6,000, or 30 percent of all former players, could develop Alzheimer's disease or moderate dementia and be eligible for compensation.[17] Pressure also came from the NFL Players Association, led by their newly elected president De-Maurice Smith, who demanded the league agree to implement a comprehensive concussion protocol, including the enlistment of sideline experts, improved diagnosis and treatment, and a mechanism to jointly enforce the agreement.

The NFL needed to change its image. Goodell announced that the league was donating $30 million to the National Institutes of Health, the umbrella organization (consisting of 27 institutes and centers) that stewards much of the U.S. government's biomedical research. The money would launch a new Sports and Health Research Program, to involve the nation's premier medical research organization in investigating, among other topics, CTE in football players. The NFL's press release announcing the gift reads, "National Football League Grants $30 million in Unrestricted Funding to the Foundation for the National Institutes of Health for Medical Research."[18] Note the adjective "unrestricted." The agreement between the NFL and the NIH said clearly that the NIH would be the arbiter of who receives the funding. The NFL was obliged to provide the promised $30 million, paid over several years, even if the agreement covering management and direction of the program was terminated.

Following its normal protocols, the NIH issued a request for scientists to submit proposals for a longitudinal study of CTE among football players. The proposals were evaluated through a peer-review process, the results of which would inform the NIH's decision of where the funding would be awarded. The academic researchers who were part of the NFL's HNS Committee were among many that applied. But the winners of the competition were the researchers associated with Boston University, led by Robert Stern, the director of clinical research at the university's CTE Center and an expert in neurodegenerative diseases. Stern was not a stranger to the NFL. His group had done extensive research on brain disease among football players and had become the leading institution for examining the brains of deceased players. In the class action lawsuit players had brought against the NFL, Stern had filed an affidavit opposing the settlement, asserting that the proposed settlement would result in players with brain damage not receiving adequate compensation.

The NFL now balked. Various officials, including Pellman, who served as the league's medical director, complained to the NIH on three grounds: Stern had a conflict of interest, having filed that affidavit; the group was unqualified (their expertise was in neuropathology, not in conducting the longitudinal study they were chosen to undertake); and their project plan did not meet objectives of the overall initiative. The league requested that the funding go to the applicant group that included three investigators from its own Head, Neck, and Spine committee, one of whom was participating in the negotiations with NIH around the grant.[19]

Clearly the NFL had a different understanding of the meaning of "unrestricted" funding. The league was challenging a longstanding NIH policy that donors are explicitly prohibited from involvement in the grant-selection process, and the NIH proceeded without heeding the concerns the NFL had raised about Stern and his group. The government agency held that the Boston team was well qualified and that the proposed study met the project's objectives. To the NFL's allegations of Stern's conflict of interest, NIH policy was also clear: authoring a scientific paper (or an affidavit) is not the same as having an employment relationship. Stern did not have an employment relationship with NFL players or the league itself, and accordingly he had no conflict of interest.

The subsequent congressional inquiry into this disagreement found that while the NIH did engage in negotiations with the NFL and attempted to address some of the league's concerns, "NIH leadership maintained the integrity of the process and thus ensured that the best applicants received the grant." Nevertheless, the NFL, accustomed to getting what it wants and unhappy with the outcome of the NIH's peer-review process, pulled its support from the endeavor, falling about $18 million short of their initial promise of $30 million in unrestricted funds. The league was willing to brave the bad publicity, likely in the hope that the public's attention had shifted elsewhere.[20]

In 2015, Hollywood took up the players' cause—sort of. The movie *Concussion* dramatized the work of Omalu in investigating the Mike Webster tragedy and the NFL's attempts to subvert his findings. Will Smith played the starring role of Omalu. The NFL fought back on this front as well. As reported in the *New York Times*, "In dozens of studio emails unearthed by hackers, Sony executives, the director, Peter Landesman, and representatives of Mr. Smith discussed how to avoid antagonizing the NFL by altering the script and marketing the film more as a whistle-blower story, rather than a condemnation of football or the league.... Dwight Caines, the president of domestic marketing at Sony Pictures, wrote in an email on August 6, 2014, to three top studio executives about how to position the movie. 'We'll develop messaging with the help of NFL consultant to ensure that we are telling a dramatic story and not kicking the hornet's nest.'"[21]

The following year, the flaws in the bogus research of the MTBI committee were topped by a new revelation in the *New York Times*: the committee's concussion database, meant to catalog all concussions diagnosed by league medical staffs between 1996 and 2001 and the backbone of the league's claims around concussions during that period and beyond, was incomplete. This was discovered by reporter Alan Schwartz, who obtained a copy and compared cases in the database to the league's publicly disclosed weekly injury reports. It was easy to break the anonymity of the cases, since the database has plenty of identifying information about each listed episode, including the date of each concussion. The *Times* study showed that at least 10 percent (or 100 cases) of the 1,000 head injuries diagnosed by team doctors and reported to the league were missing from the research. This included all the pertinent injuries suffered by members of the Dallas Cowboys, one of the league's iconic (and wealthiest) teams. Other journalists published findings that challenged the league's studies on other grounds and exposed the prevarications. That bibliography is a long one. The work of the journalists had a huge impact, promoting the important findings of Omalu and others in the academic literature—and exposing the tainted academic studies that were published in peer-reviewed journals alongside them.

––––––

"Professional football is more dangerous than almost any other job in America. Why don't you do something about it?" For seven-plus years at OSHA, I entertained that question too many times to count. My answer was disappointing to some who thought OSHA could be the savior here: if I wanted to make this federal agency the enemy of the majority of Americans, the easiest way to do so would be to announce that we were going to mandate changes in their favorite professional sport in order to make that sport's workers much less susceptible to injury—especially one specific injury. Besides, OSHA had far more pressing issues to address, including protecting workers who had no voice at all in their workplace but who were exposed daily to hazards that could destroy their lungs or cut off their fingers.

OSHA may not provide the solution to the perils faced by football players, but the tide is turning as public awareness increases. On this subject, at least, fans do want to know the truth—although they may not want to think about what that truth should entail in terms of changes to the game.

Football isn't alone, of course. The scrutiny into the harms of football extended quickly to North America's other popular and violent sport, hockey, and its billion-dollar National Hockey League (NHL). Alas, the world's largest hockey league could do no better than its football brethren in demonstrating the usual knee-jerk reaction: announce that the problem isn't real and attack independent scientists who claim otherwise. When former hockey players filed their own class-action suit, the hockey league demanded the Boston University CTE Center, which was not a party to the suit, hand over large quantities of records and materials, so the NHL could "probe the scientific basis for published conclusions" and "confirm the accuracy of published findings."[22]

In 2016, Senator Richard Blumenthal (D-CT) asked NHL Commissioner Gary Bettman, "Do you believe there is a link between CTE and hockey?" Bettman's response was a 24-page letter that delivered his characterization of the scientific evidence to date: "The relationship between concussions and the asserted clinical symptoms of CTE remains unknown."[23]

5

A Spirited Denial

"PLEASE DRINK RESPONSIBLY" is the standard fine print accompanying alcohol advertising in the United States. And while we could reasonably debate the alcohol manufacturers' sincerity in saying it, it's undeniably good advice: alcohol is a causal factor in more than 5 percent of all deaths worldwide, which amounts to about 3 million deaths a year. Alcohol hits the young hardest: globally, 13.5 percent of deaths among people between the ages of 20 and 39 are alcohol-related.[1]

With this knowledge, one might well wonder how these drinks ever achieved their popularity in the first place. One might even sympathize with popular demands for their prohibition. But alcohol is different, of course. For many of us, a drink or two does relieve stress and increase our enjoyment of social situations. A glass or two of wine with dinner is lovely. We believe that the litany of ill effects pertains only to excessive drinking by people who have drinking problems. By drinking in moderation, we believe that we will be spared some of the undesired outcomes, like cirrhosis, and we'll most certainly avoid alcohol-related deaths from driving.

"Drink responsibly" is a fabulous and useful marketing pitch, but it is also dishonest. I hate to be the bearer of bad news (again), but even when consumed in moderation, wine, beer, and hard (distilled) liquors shorten more lives than they extend. I'm not trying to frighten everyone into abstaining from their nightly beer or glass of wine or snifter of brandy. After digging into the research in depth, and even as I better understand the science and concede the risk, I personally have no intention of forgoing a beer after work. On the danger scale, alcohol in moderation is no match for, say, cigarette smoke, which on average cuts ten years off the life of every smoker.[2] But in following the alcohol industry's money as it works with unflagging zeal to sow doubt and uncertainty in the face of the best science concerning even moderate drinking, there is a lot going on. When it comes to the manipulation of the epidemiology and basic science pertinent to its products, Big Booze belongs in the same class and the same book with Big Tobacco as well as Big Pharma and Big Sugar, both of which will figure prominently in later chapters.

In keeping with the product defense model that was developed by the tobacco industry, much of the money from the alcohol industry is channeled through a trade organization with a misleading name: the Alcoholic Beverage Medical Research Foundation (ABMRF, more recently called ABMRF/The Foundation for Alcohol Research). And to their credit, this group funds some serious medical research. But what it also does is challenge *others'* medical research and epidemiology, using all of the classic methods of the product defense industry.

ABMRF was launched in 1982 by beer and malt beverage producers in the United States and Canada. Its first president, Thomas B. Turner, was a former dean of the Johns Hopkins University Medical School, an affiliation that brought great prestige and credibility to the new organization. His first board of directors mixed well-known scientists with titans of the brewing industry whose names alone suffice for identification: August A. Busch III, William K. Coors, and Peter Stroh.

According to the history written by Turner himself in 1993, "[B]y the middle of the twentieth century, a new effort at prohibiting all alcoholic drinks was in the making." As historical narratives go, this was wildly alarmist. In the many decades that followed the demise of Prohibition in 1933, there has been no serious movement in that direction. It wasn't going to happen—but higher taxes and stricter controls on labeling and advertising might. Turner also expressed concern that the National Institute on Alcohol Abuse and Alcoholism (NIAAA) was focused on "the clinical and biochemical basis of the more dire results of alcohol consumption and treatment." In other words, the government's research focused on the effects of heavy consumption. Of course, the industry knew better than to attempt to defend that stigmatized behavior. It would be happy to study "those factors that lead or permit a minority of individuals to go beyond the limits of sensible drinking." And the new organization would go one important step further; it would step into the breach left by NIAAA and support research into *the whole range of consumption levels*. It would prove what Turner and the brewers believed: if we drink in moderation, "no deleterious health effects would be observed."[3]

According to Turner and the ABMRF, alcohol is not just safe when enjoyed in moderation. It is positively beneficial, particularly when it comes to life expectancy. For decades, industry scientists have promoted (and still are promoting) the idea that alcohol's effects on overall life expectancy could be best represented in a J-shaped curve (Figure 5.1)

The horizontal axis plots alcohol consumption in number of drinks per day; the farther right on this scale, the more drinking. The vertical axis plots mortality rates; the higher on this scale, the greater the risk of dying.

The message of the J curve: Nondrinkers—those to the far left of the horizontal scale—have a somewhat *higher* mortality risk than the moderate drinkers at the bottom of the curve. The bottom of the curve—lowest mortality risk at a few drinks per day—is where we all ought to be!

If correct, this graph would be the ultimate proof of the industry's basic claim that drinking in moderation is positively beneficial. And at first glance, it is a reasonable proposition. Many studies, some as far back as the 1920s (i.e., pre-Prohibition), *do* show higher death rates among both nondrinkers (the left edge of scale) and heavy drinkers

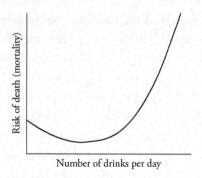

FIGURE 5.1 The J-Shaped Curve

(the right edge) than those in the middle—the people who drink "moderately."

But the first glance doesn't hold up under greater scrutiny. The problem is what epidemiologists call *selection bias*. Very different types of people inhabit different parts of the curve, and these differences are more—much more—than just how much alcohol they drink.

The heavy drinkers on the far right include people with other characteristics that go along with heavy drinking, including smoking and poor diet, most prominently. Their greatly elevated risk of dying early is therefore driven by a *combination* of factors, all of which must be taken into account in a truly rigorous study.

Back on the left side of the curve, the epidemiological challenge is perhaps even more daunting. These nondrinkers include people who have made the choice not to drink, perhaps for religious reasons (many Seventh Day Adventists, for example). The great majority of these teetotalers will also abstain from smoking. Some of them also avoid eating meat. As a group, these nondrinkers have a very healthy profile comprising a combination of healthful factors. And just like the unhealthful factors in the high-risk category, all of them need to be considered. But this left edge of the curve is also inhabited by individuals who may avoid alcohol consumption for one of many reasons, including ill health. In many studies, it includes *former* drinkers. Another complicating factor. Any given study needs to be careful dealing with all this. Many are not.

This essential nuance does the alcohol industry no favors, of course. The industry has invested millions to make the case for the J-curve—and every other manifestation of the claim—that alcohol in moderation is beneficial. Much of the funding goes to sympathetic scientists who are happy to be the beneficiaries of the manufacturers' largesse. A year before ABMRF was officially founded with Turner as its first director, he had been the lead author of the key paper that would subsequently frame the industry's PR campaign over the next several decades. The title was "Beneficial Side of Moderate Alcohol Use," produced with the financial support of the brewers and published in Johns Hopkins' own publication, the *Johns Hopkins Medical Journal*. The paper's product defense message was straightforward: "(A)ccumulating data indicate that the moderate use of alcoholic beverages by adults may reduce

the risk of myocardial infarction, improve the quality of life of the eld-
erly, relieve stress, and contribute to nutrition."[4]

One question: what is "moderate"? Turner and his team reviewed
studies of health conditions recognized at the time as alcohol-related,
and they concluded that, for an average-size man, moderate drinking
was anything less than 80 grams of alcohol—a little less than six drinks
a day, or five drinks three days in a row. These were the levels "below
which adverse effects on health are rarely observed." (Turner eventually
decided that the numbers for women should be a little lower.) The notable exceptions—that is, factors that *could* be affected by fewer than
five or six drinks a day—were the risk of traffic accidents and fetal alcohol syndrome, although in both cases Turner claimed the evidence was
not at all definitive. No other illnesses or adverse events were caused by
moderate drinking, according to Turner.[5]

ABMRF used its Johns Hopkins link to great advantage in touting
any other study it funded that supported the industry's positions.
Immediately after publication of a suitable study, the Johns Hopkins
press office would issue a press release, lending the study greater cre-
dence and strengthening the link between the two bodies. Over time,
however, the industry's fervent advocacy of "moderate" drinking became
too much for the prestigious university. The culminating episode was
publication of a study by a Canadian researcher long associated with
ABMRF, which the *New York Times* summarized under a headline that
read "Less Illness Found in Beer Drinkers."[6]

Such findings would have been a boon for bartenders everywhere, but
alas, it didn't hold up. Unaffiliated outside experts decided to take a closer
look at the methodology that had produced this delightful conclusion,
and it didn't survive under scrutiny. It turned out that the researchers had
used responses collected in door-to-door surveys, which for fairly obvious
reasons aren't reliable: survey subjects voluntarily reporting to a stranger
at their front door might have felt strongly inclined to understate their
consumption. Or how often they got sick. Or maybe both. Or maybe the
opposite. Who knows? As science, it is laughable, because there's no way
of validating how these thousands of people portrayed themselves while
standing at their door and talking to someone with a clipboard.

The study was titled "Alcohol Consumption and Morbidity in the
Canada Health Survey: Inter-Beverage Difference," which sounds

authoritative.[7] Adding to its authority was the press release issued by Johns Hopkins, which didn't include any explanation of the methods employed in the study. From there, a veteran science writer for the *Times* simply summarized the press release. And that's illustrative of how a successful PR campaign works.

So the dissemination of questionable science just coincidentally happened to yield stunningly good news for the companies that paid for the study? The ensuing scandal (within the field, at least) was too much for Johns Hopkins, which used this episode as the rationale for severing its relationship with ABMRF, even though the organization was still directed by the former dean of its medical school.[3]

For ABMRF, the work goes on. Today, most of the money we know about (and there is likely plenty we don't) flows through three entities: ABMRF, the European Foundation for Alcohol Research, and the *Institut de Recherches Scientifiques sur Les Boissons* (the Institute for Scientific Research on Drinks). This model for funding industry-favorable research is the same used extensively by the tobacco industry and quite a few others. The scientists on the boards of these organizations are by definition conflicted, since they are selected by and paid by the industry, often because they have published studies that align with the industry's positions. These research bodies are unlikely to fund research that opposes the needs of the industry.

The alcohol industry's research foundations have of course funded hundreds of scientists whose work has potential to suit the industry's interests. For the most part these grants are quite small, and the funding is a tiny proportion of the total alcohol research funding flowing from U.S. and EU government agencies. These industry grants are important, however. By offering small amounts of funding (ABMRF has capped awards at $50,000 per year but generally provides less) to junior faculty who would otherwise have difficulty gaining financial support, the grants help shape the careers of these researchers, focusing them on issues and methods the industry supports and tying them into the industry network.[8]

Of course, as ever, product defense research is of little value if it isn't accompanied by public relations. The industry has gone well beyond simply funding researchers and putting out press releases. It has become sophisticated in its promotion of the message that alcohol drinking in moderation is beneficial to health, and alcohol manufacturers have formed literally dozens of national and transnational organizations that public health advocates label "social aspects and public relations organizations," or SAPROs. Ostensibly set up to provide a social good— education and warning about the harms of excessive drinking—the SAPROs appear to be exemplars of corporate social responsibility, fulfilling a public good. But while warning us that we shouldn't drink and drive, and that designated drivers are the best way to get home, these same organizations use these platforms to subtly, and not so subtly, promote the positive aspects of alcohol consumption.[9]

One particularly impressive effort came out of a 2006 conference, "The Harms and Benefits of Moderate Drinking," jointly sponsored by a SAPRO called the International Center for Alcohol Policy (ICAP, now renamed the International Alliance for Responsible Drinking), and the industry-funded Boston University Institute on Lifestyle and Health. While this conference in Cambridge, Massachusetts, included researchers who disagreed on the validity of the J-curve, the abstract of the official conference summary (the only element that many physicians and reporters would read) perfectly presented the intended takeaway:

> [M]oderate drinking when defined as excluding any binge drinking, has been shown to have predominantly beneficial effects on health....the consensus of the conference was that the total scientific evidence strongly supports an inverse association between moderate alcohol consumption and the risk of cardiovascular diseases, and possibly diabetes, cognitive decline, and total mortality.[10]

This report on the meeting gave the impression of being authoritative, although it never went through peer review and was simply a report of the opinions of the conference organizers, paid by the alcohol industry, which also paid the scientific journal *Annals of Epidemiology* to publish all the papers in a special supplement. To juice the impact of the summary touting the J-curve, the industry bankrolled the printing of thousands of copies of the summary and distributed them free to the 66,000 subscribers to the *American Journal of Medicine* and the *American Journal of Cardiology*[9] This end-run infuriated several of the conference participants, who objected to this alcohol marketing effort, asserting that the widely promoted summary "did not convey the degree to which there was debate at the symposium regarding apparent protective effects for alcohol on coronary heart disease and the opinion regarding the matter was highly polarized."[11]

More than a decade later, with extensive evidence pointing in the opposite direction, the industry is still recommending the summary, including its perfect abstract, to all comers.[12]

———

In the classroom, when talking with students about the common mistakes made by epidemiologists, including those manifested in numerous alcohol industry studies in support of the J-curve, I always introduce a different but equally unfortunate analysis involving another popular beverage. By coincidence, it's a study that was overseen by Brian MacMahon, a former ABMRF board member and the longtime chair of the department of epidemiology of the Harvard School of Public Health.

MacMahon was the lead author of a 1981 paper that reported an association between pancreatic cancer and…coffee.[13] You may remember the headlines. They were numerous, and understandably big. This was a finding that hit home. In an interview on the widely watched *Today Show*, MacMahon told the host, "I will tell you that I myself have stopped drinking coffee"—no doubt alarming the millions who require some caffeine in the morning in order to get going.[14] MacMahon's study was deeply flawed, beginning with the choice of its control subjects. In selecting these subjects, he chose people with noncancerous diseases of the digestive system, many of whom had likely stopped drinking coffee *because of their conditions.* So instead of demonstrating that coffee causes pancreatic cancer, MacMahon's study came closer to demonstrating only that digestive illnesses cause people to give up coffee. (Multiple subsequent studies have exonerated coffee as causing pancreatic cancer.)

Similarly, the overall benefit in life expectancy from moderate drinking—the J-curve effect—almost disappears in analyses that limit comparisons to people who are pure abstainers (i.e., not those who are forced to abstain because of a health condition) versus those who drink occasionally.[15]

Some may also recall a major to-do in 1991 stemming from a *60 Minutes* piece extolling the "French Paradox": how despite a diet rich in fats and cholesterol, the incidence of coronary heart disease in France was 40 percent less than in the United States. Why? As the story goes, it was the wine; more specifically, red wine; more specifically still, *French* red wine.[16] As in the coffee example, there was more to the story than meets the eye, but nevertheless there remains pretty convincing evidence that alcohol (but not red wine specifically) may well provide a small but real protective effect on heart attacks. One huge recent study looking at cardiovascular disease, combining 83 studies involving 600,000 current drinkers, found a slightly (6 percent) lower risk for heart attacks among people who consumed up to seven drinks a week, or one per day on average.[17]

My reading of the very extensive literature on what the alcohol industry terms "moderate" drinking: the benefits of *very* moderate intake are probably real, but limited only to the small decrease in heart attack risk. However, that benefit is outweighed by increases in deaths from other causes, and as a result the J-curve is illusory. The reality is that even one drink a day, on average, results in a small increase in overall mortality risk. More than one drink, but still in the range of "moderate" consumption, results in greater risk of both cardiovascular disease and cancer. Heavier drinking, even if only occasional, has other associated risks.[18] Add it all up and alcohol becomes the third-highest cause of death and disability caused by disease worldwide. (It accounts for about 18 percent of deaths from violence, including car wrecks, of course.)[1]This doesn't mean we should stop all alcohol consumption immediately. But we need to be aware of the risks and trade-offs, even at low levels of consumption.

The science of "observational epidemiology" on display in each of these studies has its limits (as does all science), but it is also the basis of much of what we know about the relationships between diet (including alcohol) and disease. The best studies attempt to differentiate among the subjects' risk factors (including their environmental exposures—food, drink, work) and then correlate each factor with health or disease status. The challenges are great, and there always remain some uncertainties.

Given these limits, the only really convincing way to demonstrate that truly moderate drinking improves health would be with volunteers assigned to different groups and given different "treatments"—in other words, a randomized clinical trial exactly like the ones used to determine a potential prescription drug's effectiveness and side-effects in treating a targeted medical condition. These randomized trials are the gold standard, and the alcoholic beverage industry has long wanted to support one—with one unspoken stipulation. The industry would have to be sure that the study would produce the desired results about the benefits of moderation.

But how could the industry make this happen? Specifically, what levers could they pull to ensure a study that was sweeping in scope and convenient in findings?

It's not surprising that the industry's recent attempt to do so begins with Washington's revolving doors between public and private work. The examples that get the most attention are political appointees who leave high-paying corporate jobs to spend a few years regulating their old industries, only to return to even higher-paying jobs in those same industries later, this time with insider knowledge about how to best avoid regulation.

Less well known, but probably more common, is the migration of career staffers from within the federal agencies. After twenty or more years in federal service, employees become vested in their pensions, at which point many of these civil servants change sides and join the businesses they formerly worked with or regulated—and at a much higher salary. The National Institutes of Health (NIH) isn't immune to these influences. Neither is the National Institute on Alcohol Abuse and Alcoholism (NIAAA), one of its 27 specialized institutes and centers, and the one responsible for researching the effects of consuming alcoholic beverages. NIAAA's current director, George Koob, was an academic scientist before coming to the institute, and in that capacity he was a recipient of research funds from ABMRF, the industry's main trade group. He also served on AMBRF's medical advisory board.[19] In 2012, shortly after Samir Zakhari retired as director of the NIAAA's Division of Metabolism and Health Effects (a career spanning 25 years), he joined the Distilled Spirits Council of the U.S. (DISCUS) as its Senior Vice President for Scientific Affairs.

In 2013, a small group of NIAAA professional staff, researchers who had mostly become administrators, had bought into the need for a randomized clinical trial and engaged executives from across the alcoholic beverage industry about funding the once-and-for-all study that would show the positive impact of moderate drinking. To succeed, this trial would have to be large and therefore expensive, likely more than a hundred million dollars. NIAAA could never fund this with taxpayer money. The only potential source for financial support was the industry itself. And to make that happen, the federal staffers no doubt also realized that the methodology for the study would have to be acceptable to the industry. A compliant methodology would make the industry pretty confident about the results.

Recall that in 1993, ABMRF had disparaged the NIAAA for historically being too interested in the harmful effects of alcohol, which the industry considered an issue only with excessive consumption. These executives must have been only too delighted to learn of the institute's sudden interest in moderate consumption. And thus was born the Moderate Alcohol and Cardiovascular Health trial (MACH). Between 2013 and 2014, NIAAA staffers secretly met numerous times with representatives of the liquor industry and the academic scientists that the NIAAA staff had pre-selected to run the study. The federal staffers hid these activities from higher-ups at NIAAA (which at the time was undergoing a transition to its new director, Koob) and, of course, the media and therefore the public.[20]

One of the leaders of the effort was Harvard's Kenneth Mukamal, who had written a paper calling for a trial like the one eventually planned. According to documents obtained by the *New York Times*, in 2013 and 2014, Mukamal traveled to meetings and discussed the study designs with members of the alcohol industry. Also present was Ken Warren, whose retirement as acting director of NIAAA gave way to Koob—and who was now serving as an advisor to Anheuser-Busch InBev, the world's largest brewing company and parent company of Anheuser-Busch.[21] (There's that revolving door we were talking about.)

During this period, the collaborators designed a study that called for 8,000 volunteers age 50 or older, who by definition were at increased risk for cardiovascular disease or diabetes because of their age. The 8,000 would be randomized into two groups: one group would agree to drink one drink per day (they could choose from wine, beer, or distilled liquor); the other would not drink alcohol at all. It is noteworthy that the first group of participants would be allowed to choose their beverage; if the results of the study were positive, then the data would not promote one beverage over another. The time period would be six years—long enough to observe development of heart disease or diabetes, but not new cases of cancer.

Excluded from consideration would be heavy drinkers and people with history of drug or alcohol abuse, liver or kidney disease, and some types of cancer. Women with close relatives with breast cancer were also not eligible to participate, since they were presumably at higher risk for alcohol-related breast cancer.[22] Researchers at 16 medical centers in the United States, Europe, South America, and Africa would track the participants, counting the number of deaths, as well as heart attacks, strokes, and other events. Members of the groups assigned to drink would be given some reimbursement for their alcohol purchases.[20]

Mukamal's slide presentation to the NIAAA staffers and the alcohol executives promoted the study as "a unique opportunity to show that moderate alcohol consumption is safe and lowers risk of common diseases."[23] An NIAAA staff member also sent an email to an industry source, noting that "one of the important findings will be showing that moderate drinking is safe." These are virtually admissions that the MACH team—government and academic researchers working together in solicitation of industry money—were going into the study believing it would give them and the industry the finding the industry had long coveted. For their part, the industry saw it as such. One email from the leadership of SpiritsEUROPE, representing that continent's largest liquor manufacturers, gloated about "the possibility of clinical trials to show the J-curve in all its glory."[20]

Given the potential PR value of a randomized clinical study under federal auspices that yielded bulletproof results, it is not surprising that AB InBev, Heineken, Diageo, Pernod Ricard, and Carlsberg pledged $67.7 million toward what was shaping up as a $100 million budget. The industry's money would be routed through the NIH Foundation, the institutes' vehicle for receiving private-sector funds for NIH-funded studies (necessary because, by law, private parties are not permitted to voluntarily contribute to government agencies for specific activities).

Following the revelations by the *New York Times* in 2018, NIAAA director Koob got out in front of any public notion of conflict of interest, declaring that MACH would be an unbiased test of whether alcohol "in moderation" protects against heart disease. "The money from the Foundation for the NIH has no strings attached," he told the *New York Times*, whose reporter Roni Caryn Rabin also noted that Koob was raising his voice during the interview. "Whoever donates to that fund has no leverage whatsoever—no contribution to the study, no input to the study, no say whatsoever."[19]

No input? The industry participated in the planning and design of the MACH study from day one. Details about that collusion (I use the term advisedly) continued to trickle out through Freedom of Information Act requests lodged by Rabin and the *Times*. As more details leaked to the press, national outrage increased, and NIH Director Francis Collins appointed an advisory committee of senior scientists to examine the origin and development of the MACH trial. This group concluded the study had been rigged to find beneficial effect, but not negative outcomes. One quote: "Interactions among several NIAAA senior staff members and industry appear to intentionally bias the framing of the scientific premise in the direction of demonstrating a beneficial health effect of moderate alcohol consumption."[20]

There are two specific elements of the MACH methodology that would yield results that could be easily misinterpreted (no doubt with the help the industry's marketing teams) to show the moderation benefits, with no negative effect on cancer risk, cirrhosis, auto crashes, family violence, or any of the other outcomes of alcohol consumption:

- The study population was limited to one subgroup—adults age 50 or higher who are at increased risk for cardiovascular disease or diabetes but who were otherwise pretty healthy—people who might quite well benefit from the one-drink-a-day regimen (just like those people from France who were featured on 60 Minutes). The candidate group excluded younger people, at greatly increased risk for alcohol-related violence.
- Six years duration is sufficient for many studies, but it's woefully, clearly insufficient for detecting increased risk of cancer—even though there is no doubt that increased cancer risk associated with alcohol is far higher than the presumed decrease in heart attacks these investigators expected to see.

The committee's investigation found that the MACH study was also rigged in another way: the selection of its principal investigator. The PI in such studies is not a figurehead; he or she runs the show. Mukamal, the Harvard physician-scientist who helped promote and set up the study with industry representatives (long before it was ever announced to the public), clearly wanted the job. The team at NIAAA went to great lengths to assist him in preparing his application but provided no similar help, and in fact made it difficult, for other scientists who might want to apply. In the end, the choice of PI was easy; Mukamal was the only applicant.

Not that his selection turned out to mean anything. The MACH study died the death it richly deserved. The NIH advisory committee's report to Francis Collins was damning and useful, but the basic facts had already doomed the initiative long before Collins killed it. No doubt wanting to avoid further damage to its reputation, Anheuser-Busch InBev, which had pledged $15.4 million, pulled its funding.

Did the alcoholic beverage industry call the shots here? Yes, and in league with loyal partners in Washington. The MACH scandal is a particularly dramatic example of "industry capture" of the federal agency in charge of regulating it, or at least of a sizable number of its staff. The emails and documents uncovered in the investigation make clear that the NIAAA staff and the industry were on the same page, all firmly believing in the J-curve, with the federal staffers eager to convince the beverage manufacturers to pony up.

———

Most people know that cirrhosis of the liver, which often leads to liver cancer, is strongly linked with heavy alcohol consumption. What's less known is how the link between alcohol and other cancers is also an established fact. Cancer may not be as well-known a consequence of alcohol consumption as, say, traffic deaths or intimate partner violence, but it certainly isn't *unimportant*. In 1987, the International Agency for Research on Cancer (IARC, part of the World Health Organization, and mentioned in many other chapters here) conducted a review of the literature to date and classified alcohol consumption as a human carcinogen, linking it with increased risk of cancers of the mouth, larynx, pharynx, esophagus, and liver.[24] Other studies continued to accumulate. In

2000, the U.S. National Toxicology Program conducted its own in-depth review and seconded IARC's conclusion.[25] In 2007, IARC convened a fresh panel of experts to review all the new work, and then again in 2009. With each review, the panels reported strengthened human and animal evidence: alcohol as a causal factor in all of the cancers identified in 1987, plus colorectal and female breast cancers, two of the most common.[26] (With breast cancer: the higher the consumption, the greater the risk, particularly for women already at increased risk. But even one drink a day provides a small but statistically significant increase in risk.)[27]

According to the World Health Organization, in 2016 (the most recent year statistics were available), alcohol was responsible for 4.2 percent of all cancer deaths worldwide.[1] This causal relationship between alcohol and cancer is powerful but not well-known. A national poll in the United States, commissioned by the 40,000-member American Society of Clinical Oncology, found that only 30 percent of Americans know that drinking alcohol is a risk factor for cancer.[28] In England the numbers are even lower. One survey found only 13 percent of English adults so informed.[29] The alcoholic beverage industry would like for those numbers to stay right there or, preferably, go down. Its uncertainty campaign focuses on two claims: the risk is very low to begin with, and extremely low with moderate consumption. The industry's PR flacks will acknowledge that heavy drinking or "binging" will increase risk of cancer and heart disease as well, but they go to great lengths to reassure their customers that drinking in moderation simply isn't dangerous.

Here I need to point out that one generally accepted component of our understanding of cancer causation is that there is no threshold below which a human carcinogen does not increase cancer risk. Very low exposures increase your individual risk by a very low amount, and low exposure to a population of millions will likely still result in quite a few cases, with no possibility of identifying which cases would not have occurred without that exposure. At least theoretically, therefore, every exposure increases risk. The increase in risk associated with each sip of wine is so infinitesimally small as to be almost meaningless, but the glass of wine every evening for twenty years is not quite so meaningless. And this is what the epidemiological evidence confirms. I also note that, as far as we can tell, there probably isn't a better or worse form of alcohol. Wine, beer, spirits—all increase your risk of cancer some small amount.

That basic fact about cancer causation directly contradicts the industry's message that "moderate" drinking is actually good for you, and it has been a challenge for the industry since the early twentieth century, when a French pathologist published the first paper linking absinthe consumption to esophageal cancer. In 1989, immediately following IARC's headline-earning designation of alcohol consumption as a human carcinogen, Thomas Turner (the same doctor who went from being dean of Johns Hopkins' medical school to the first president of ABMRF, the industry's main research arm) and several ABMRF-affiliated scientists, including Harvard's Brian MacMahon, a former board member, conducted their own "critical review" of the literature and concluded that "there is not adequate and consistent scientific evidence that the moderate use of alcohol is associated with enhanced risk" of any of the cancer types identified by IARC. ABMRF and other industry groups had been diligent for decades in questioning the findings of studies that implicate alcohol in cancer causation. In fact, Turner and his colleagues were so confident that "the weight of the evidence that alcohol is at most a minor factor in cancer causation," they ensured that the ABMRF provided little support to research that might question that conclusion.[3]

In the 1980s, with the increasing study of breast cancer as a possible repercussion of alcohol use, the Distilled Spirits Council of the United States (DISCUS) hired H. Daniel Roth, one of the product defense veterans going all the way back to the tobacco wars that began in the 1970s. He provided much of the "evidence" the tobacco industry used to oppose OSHA's effort to issue a standard to reduce workplace exposure to cigarette smoke. He attempted to accomplish for alcohol what he had for cigarettes: review the scientific literature and reject the existence of a causal link seen in so many studies.[30] With both environmental tobacco smoke and alcohol consumption, he opined that there were too many biases and confounders to allow sound conclusions. In both cases, just sow doubt and uncertainty, early and often.

To this day, the industry feels that it has to defend the claim that light or moderate drinking is actually beneficial. Its minions across the globe never sleep. Much of the information they provide is misleading;

some is simply wrong. Samir Zakhari (mentioned above as one of the many federal researchers and administrators who take advantage of the revolving door in Washington, moving between government and industry) has been a key figure downplaying the link between alcohol and cancer, always citing his career at the NIAAA to give credibility to his position. Following a well-publicized alcohol and cancer symposium in Wellington, New Zealand, Zakhari wrote in an op-ed in Wellington's daily newspaper: "Attributing cancer to social moderate drinking is simply incorrect and is not supported by the body of scientific literature."[31] In 2017, responding to yet another review of the evidence reaching the same conclusion as the IARC panels,[32] the DISCUS rebuttal quoted Zakhari laying out the organization's basic position: "Based on my own 40-year career as a biomedical scientist, including 26 years at the National Institute of Alcohol Abuse and Alcoholism, the science regarding cancer and alcohol consumption is far from settled. In fact, the existing epidemiological studies do not demonstrate causation, nor do they account for the multitude of confounding factors.... This is particularly true for moderate consumption. For example, there are some studies that suggest an association between moderate alcohol consumption and an increased risk of breast cancer. However, there also are numerous studies that show no association."[33]

Such statements perturb many in the public health community, and they mobilize to counter them. In January 2018, the first statement issued by the American Society of Clinical Oncologists on "Alcohol and Cancer" acknowledged that the "importance of alcohol drinking to the overall burden of cancer is often underappreciated" and that "even modest use of alcohol may increase cancer risk." The statement called for more public education about the risks of alcohol consumption. In 2018, the journal *Drug and Alcohol Review* published an extensive review of the claims made by 27 of the industry's favorite SAPROs (these "social aspects and public relations organizations" introduced earlier) concerning the link between alcohol and cancer. This review was led by Mark Petticrew of the London School of Hygiene and Tropical Medicine, and included Elisabete Weiderpass, who became director of IARC in 2019. Their work identified three classic product defense strategies through which the evidence for the link was misrepresented, and provided examples of each:[34]

- Denial/omission: Applying brute force to the PR problem with any connivance at hand. An example from the International Alliance for Responsible Drinking: "Recent research suggests that light to moderate drinking is not significantly associated with an increased risk for total cancer in either men or women." This statement is simply false.
- Distortion: Misrepresenting the risk. An example from the Wine Information Council: "All the studies show that the knowledge about the causes of breast cancer is still very incomplete, and as scientists from the National Institute on Alcohol Abuse and Alcoholism in the USA recently pointed out, some other (possible confounding) factors have not been considered in the research relating the consumption of alcoholic beverages to breast cancer." When is knowledge not "incomplete"? On breast cancer risk, incomplete knowledge has not stopped the NIAAA from issuing this warning: "Women who have about one drink per day also have an increased chance of developing breast cancer compared to women who do not drink at all."[35]
- Distraction: Avoiding discussion of the *independent* effects of alcohol on common cancers and focusing instead on other causes. Breast cancer and colorectal cancer appear to be a particular focus for this misrepresentation. An excellent example from Drinkaware in the UK: "The fact that you are female is a risk factor in developing breast cancer. We also know breast cancer is age-related so you're more likely to develop it as you get older and that you're more prone to breast cancer if it is part of your family history. These are all factors beyond our control. We also know that risk is related to the 'hormone environment' that women experience during the course of early pregnancy, childbirth and breastfeeding which all exert a protective effect." This is all true, but irrelevant to the issue of alcohol's causation, which is real and independent of the other risk factors.

This all is very troubling. These advocacy groups may provide some useful information, but when paired with denials and misdirection, to what end? Their policy advocacy is shaped by the needs of the industry, not by a commitment to public health. They actively oppose policies like warning labels and excise taxes, aimed at reducing alcohol consumption across the board. Instead, they promote policy solutions that sound good but do little to actually decrease drinking.

The alcoholic beverage industry should support studies on the effectiveness of public education and policy, but not if they shape those efforts to privilege sales over public health. Many questions on the alcohol-and-cancer causation remain, but we can't leave it to industry-affiliated scientists to answer them, or even to pose them. With alcohol, as with all other products that cause harm, industry should be required to pay for the research, but the structure of this research—setting the agenda, selecting the researchers who get funded—must be independent, or the studies will be conflicted, with all credibility forfeited.

6

The Deal with Diesel

DIESEL ENGINES DON'T quit. An old truck, even one that is slow to start and then makes an infernal racket, can still rack up hundreds of thousands of miles, even with minimal maintenance. Diesels are also more efficient and economical than gasoline engines, and far less flammable. Basic accounting therefore dictates that most of our high-mileage modes of conveyance—trucks, buses, railroad engines, and mining, farm, excavation and construction equipment—are powered by old, loud diesel machines.

So why doesn't the United States have more diesels on the road? For those of us over 40, say, the problem with the old diesel engines has always been self-evident: that cloud of black smoke spewing from the exhaust pipes. Younger generations have gotten a bit of a break, because the latest technology is much cleaner-burning (and quieter), but the trade-off of diesels has always been their stubborn indestructibility in exchange for fouling the air and promoting smog in cities across the globe.

Although knowledge of the health problems associated with diesel exhaust has informed the United States' auto policy for decades, the industry's product defense enablers are *also* still on the job, working hard—even after decades of ever-increasing scientific understanding—to convince the public that the black smoke is harmless to our health: saying in effect, *who you gonna believe—us or your lying eyes?*

People should believe their eyes, although sometimes diesel exhaust emissions can be invisible and still dangerous. Diesel emissions are a complex stew of gases and particles composed of thousands of chemicals, and none of the stuff is good for us. Inhaled in sufficient quantity, long-term exposure is associated with increased risk of stroke, ischemic heart disease, chronic obstructive pulmonary disease, and lung cancer. The gases in this engine exhaust include carbon monoxide, sulfur dioxide, and a collection of nitrogen oxide compounds referred to as NOx (pronounced "knocks"). The nitrogen molecules are important air pollutants by themselves, causing lung and cardiovascular disease while also reacting in the atmosphere to form ozone, more particulates, smog, and acid rain. They also reduce crop yield and play a major role in climate change (this despite for every mile driven, diesels emit *less* carbon dioxide—a major greenhouse gas—than gas engines). George Washington University scientist Susan Anenberg estimates that in 2015, diesel emissions were responsible for about 175,000 premature deaths globally, including 40,000 in Europe, 39,000 in China, 36,000 in India, and 11,000 in the United States.[1]

For decades, the U.S. Environmental Protection Agency has joined regulators in many countries with smog-bound cities to push the engine industry to design new diesels that put out less NOx emissions, use low-sulfur fuel—sulfur is a contributor to the smog problem—and filter out particulates. The results have been dramatic, but not dramatic enough. Thanks to all the trusty old engines still chugging away on roads and rails, there is still too much diesel-related pollution, and its effects are enormous.

It's worth noting here that diesel engines are also unevenly distributed around the world. The United States has stronger diesel regulations than much of Europe, and Americans have healthier lungs as a direct result. The Global South, where older diesel engines predominate and regulations are much weaker, is where air pollution is most predictably deadly.

The black element in the smoky clouds that billow from exhaust pipes on diesel engines is a particulate matter called DEP, short for diesel exhaust particulates. (A *particulate* is what it sounds like: a particle floating in and transferred by a larger cloud or liquid.) Extended inhalation of diesel exhaust emissions increases humans' likelihood of developing lung cancer. Thanks to experiments with rats, we know the culprit is the particulates in the emissions, not the diesel-exhaust gases. Expose rats to diesel exhaust and they get cancer; filter out the particulates and expose the rats to what's left, and they do not.

Many of these particulates are tiny—less than one micrometer ($1\mu m$) in diameter and able to penetrate deep into the lung tissue. They are primarily but not exclusively carbon, and it isn't clear exactly which of the many chemicals in this particulate soup are responsible for the lung cancer. Until we know that answer, and until the identified chemicals are controlled by the engine technology, regulators correctly focus on reducing exposure to any diesel particulate small enough to breathe, and to the lowest possible level. One important reason for this is that a range of toxic chemicals stick to the small particles and are carried with them deep into the lungs.

Of all the health hazards posed by diesel exhaust, the particulates have been the subject of the most comprehensive disease research. It almost goes without saying that this research has been the target of industry's intense pushback. Attack, manipulate, re-analyze, delay, delay some more, repeat; it's been going on for decades. And since the mid-2000s, Volkswagen and other German automakers have led a concerted push to sell a new generation of diesel-powered cars to consumers, a campaign that turns out to have been premised on bogus claims of lower pollution. (That story is the subject of Chapter 10.) This chapter focuses on those cancer-causing particulates in diesel exhaust, which remain the subject of obstruction in dramatic and amazing fashion.

This science of particulate health impacts isn't easy. Every air-breathing creature on this planet is exposed to diesel particulates—along with lots of other stuff. Precisely attributing the percentage of an increased cancer risk to the particulates, or any other cause, is challenging for plenty of reasons. With urban residents especially, it is exceedingly hard for scientists to accurately reconstruct 30 or more years of environmental exposure, and then to compensate for other causes of lung cancer, including smoking and asbestos. One approach is to follow specific groups of people who are exposed to diesel exhaust as an occupational hazard over a period of many years: truck drivers, railroad employees, bus mechanics, and underground miners are the classic subjects. Compare their risk of lung cancer with the risk demonstrated by the rest of us who experience less exposure, then try to factor in at least some of the variations inherent within population exposure levels—for example, comparing residents who live near streets and highways (and their soot-belching trucks) with residents of the same city who live at a greater distance from the main emission sources. The results of these intricate comparisons can then be used to estimate increased risk of lung cancer posed to the general public by diesel emissions.

For much of the twentieth century, scientists harbored concerns that DEP increased cancer risk,[2] but in the absence of hard data there was little to be done about it. Then, in the 1980s and continuing in the 1990s, several studies of diesel-exposed workers reported increased risk of lung cancer in the range of 30 to 50 percent. This may seem like a small increase, but from a public health perspective it was seismic. A 30 to 50 percent increase meant thousands more cases annually, many of them resulting in death.

By 1988, the WHO's International Agency for Research on Cancer (IARC) had seen enough of the accumulated evidence to classify diesel exhaust as "probably carcinogenic" to humans. That same year, the U.S. National Institute for Occupational Safety and Health (NIOSH), created in 1970 by the same legislation that created OSHA, signed by President Richard Nixon, also recommended that DEP be considered a potential occupational carcinogen. Shortly thereafter, the Mine Safety and Health Administration (MSHA, created in 1977) formally requested that NIOSH perform a risk assessment for exposure to diesel particulates to serve as the basis for a new standard.

About the same time, NIOSH and the National Cancer Institute (NCI) decided it would be worthwhile to study the effects of particulate exposure on one of the most heavily exposed populations, underground miners, who had the highest exposure to diesel emissions of any occupational group. But designing the study was rife with complications. For the purposes of this study, coal and metal mines were excluded, as were any other mines where asbestos, silica, radon, or other carcinogens where present and therefore might confound the results. In underground coal mines, it's also difficult to distinguish between the respiratory effects of diesel-related particulates and coal dust. Moreover, these mines require forceful ventilation regardless, because any build-up of methane from the coal dust is potentially explosive. Headlines and funerals periodically remind everyone of this fact.

So for once, this was a mining story that was *not* about coal miners. It focused on the thousands of other miners working in limestone, salt, and other non-coal mines whose exposure to noxious emissions was "just part of the job." This non-coal non-metal mining population was sufficiently large (more than 10,000 people), and the emissions exposure levels were very high: giant diesel engines powered underground mining equipment, and environmental measurements had been made over decades that enabled the researchers to more accurately estimate actual exposure levels. Moreover, smoking history could be obtained from these workers (or, in the cases of those who had died, family members), so the scientists could control for use of tobacco, another lung carcinogen. Overall, it was an excellent cohort to analyze, and the researchers picked eight mines for the minutest examination: one limestone, one salt, three potash (a potassium-rich salt used for fertilizer), and three trona (a "non-marine evaporite mineral" and the primary source of calcium carbonate in the United States).

Under the best of circumstances, several years are required to conceptualize such a study, lay out in detail how it will proceed, gather the data, and then proceed to final results and interpretation. With the Diesel Miners Study, it took a few years before NIOSH and NCI even had the protocol ready to go. In 1995, they dutifully sent the study protocol out for external review. The mining and diesel equipment industries, both of which had been following developments with the planned study and the circulation of the final protocol, kicked their opposition into high gear. There were no results yet, not even any data collection, but the mere dissemination of the protocol marked a significant step forward for any of the regulatory agencies charged with examining the risks posed by diesel particulates.

The industry pushback was waged by a group of companies working under the auspices of the Methane Awareness Research Group Diesel Coalition (MARG), later repurposed as the Mining Awareness Research Group Diesel Coalition (still MARG—maybe wanting to save the money required for new stationery). MARG embarked on a multiyear campaign to at least delay the study's progress, if not kill it completely. It's a familiar first strike in instances where human health interests threaten bottom-line profitability: even quality science is treated with contempt and antagonism. MARG waged an unprecedented, full-court-press legal and political campaign to stop the study of the underground miners. Leading the obstruction was Henry Chajet, an attorney with what was, at the time, one of the main law and lobbying firms in Washington, Patton Boggs. What followed was long and ugly, and it was carefully explored and written up by my former student and then colleague at George Washington University, Celeste Monforton, in an *American Journal of Public Health* article aptly titled, "Weight of the Evidence or Wait for the Evidence? Protecting Underground Miners from Diesel Particulate Matter."[3]

One notable, in fact pioneering, feature of MARG's campaign is how the mining corporations (along with Navistar International, the heavy equipment and truck manufacturer formerly known as International Harvester) enlisted congressional committees to do the dirty work they could not do on their own. This strategy has been embraced by other industries eager to devalue the science showing the dangerous nature of their products. When there was a Republican majority, the U.S. House of Representatives' Science Committee (and I use the term "science" advisedly, since most of its Republican members seem to have little regard for the scientific enterprise) led a series of attacks on research that industry didn't like, scientists that industry didn't agree with, and scientific agencies and organizations whose pronouncements and reports implicate the products.

In 1998, the Diesel Miners Study was not ready—not even close, as we will see—but the United Mine Workers of America petitioned MSHA for a new standard, pointing out that most earlier studies had found higher cancer risk among diesel-exposed workers, so the health-advocating federal officials at MSHA decided to move ahead and officially propose strengthening the standard protections afforded to underground miners. In response, the mining industry and Navistar International enlisted a slew of product defense experts who could be counted on to highlight and challenge every iota of the existing studies. This was their first tactic in rebuffing and delaying federal action, and it was effective. Some of the methodological flaws they alleged in the earlier studies were arguably fair—but that didn't mean that the studies' results and conclusions were wrong. The studies cited by MSHA were unquestionably the most advanced that had been performed to date, and by citing them they were upholding the law as written by Congress at the time of the agency's creation. The Federal Mine Safety and Health Act of 1977, succinctly known as the Mine Act, requires federal overseers to protect the health and safety of miners and instructs MSHA to consider the "best available evidence" in setting standards.[4] The agency had identified 47 scientific studies, 41 of which found some degree of association between lung cancer and occupational exposure to diesel particulates. Were these perfect studies? No. But as French Enlightenment writer Voltaire rightly pointed out, the perfect is the enemy of the good.

The product defense industry seemingly does not care for Voltaire. One of their basic strategies is to demand perfection from all research (or at least all research whose findings they don't like), ignoring the fact that imperfect studies are still useful—and often they are all we have. In 1998, as MSHA sought to strengthen protections for mine workers, the weight of the scientific evidence held that exposure to the exhaust emissions from diesel engines is likely to increase risk of lung cancer. Industry interests held that worker health should take a back seat to a cultural pursuit of more perfect science.

The industries' product defense teams also took another tack, arguing that the upcoming Diesel Miners Study was a good reason to delay any new MSHA standards for the underground mines. This took nerve: they were *praising* the value of the study they were in fact trying to sabotage at every opportunity. But the product defense industry has always had plenty of nerve. In this instance, industry argued that the underground mining study "has the potential to fill in many knowledge gaps... [and would] offer definitive data on the actual mining population... not a biased view of various academic studies." The campaign was even able to insert the following language in the report that accompanied the 1999 House Appropriations Bill: "The [congressional] Committee believes that the promulgation of a proposed rule on diesel exhaust should be informed by the ongoing NIOSH/NCI study of Lung Cancer and Diesel Exhaust among Non-Metal Miners." By praising a study that would be completed in the distant future (at which point they'd continue trying to kill it), mining and diesel equipment companies got Congress to parrot the industry talking points that called for a stay on any new protections for mine workers. (MARG's success in the halls of Congress shouldn't surprise us. I don't know what the group was spending in the 1990s, but in 2011 alone the group spent $120,000 on lobbying federal lawmakers.[5])

To top it off, the trolling obstructionists of MARG even stated in public hearings and in writing that they were *cooperating* with the NIOSH and NCI researchers and, along with the rest of us, eagerly awaiting the results. As Monforton wrote in her closely researched take-down, "These public remarks and written comments neglected to mention their relentless efforts to halt the study."[3]

On one front, MARG lobbied congressional committees to stifle the study. On a second, it touted the same study as a great reason to delay new regulations. On a third, it took the offending agencies to federal court with a blizzard of technical claims. And the only claim that eventually succeeded at the U.S. Court of Appeals was a nitpicking one: that NIOSH had failed to file their Board of Scientific Counselors' charter with the appropriate congressional oversight committee. Of course, this point was wholly irrelevant from a scientific perspective, but it demonstrates that no gambit was too irrelevant or trivial to push to the limit. The appellate court instructed the district court "to determine an appropriate remedy" for the filing error—a *pro forma* ruling, but one that gave the then-chairman of the House Education and Workforce Committee, William Goodling (R-VA), the opportunity he needed to intervene on behalf of his seemingly favored constituents. Since Goodling's Committee had jurisdiction over NIOSH, Goodling asked the judge to require NIOSH to provide all data and drafts from the Diesel Miners Study to his committee for review.

In 2000—four years after the initial circulation of the Diesel Miners Study protocol, and a full decade after the study had been first proposed—MARG went venue shopping and found a sympathetic judge who instructed NIOSH to give to the committee "all draft reports, publications, and draft results or risk notification materials prepared in connection with the Diesel Study, for review and approval prior to finalization and release and/or publication and distribution of such materials." To be clear: a team of government scientists was told to submit its work, midstream, to a team of elected nonscientist politicians so that the politicians could make sure it was all to their liking. As it happened, I had spent a year working as a Robert Wood Johnson Foundation Health Policy Fellow on that same congressional committee a few years earlier, and I can attest from personal experience that the committee staff had absolutely no ability to understand, let alone evaluate, the material Goodling was able to acquire. But a good-faith review had never been the point of this request; the point was to give the material to those at the mining companies, who could in turn gain some leverage to further delay the research.

On January 19, 2001, the day before President George W. Bush was inaugurated and still many years before the mining study would be completed, the Clinton-era MSHA issued new federal regulations requiring a gradual lowering of the permissible level of diesel particulates in all underground mines, metal, nonmetal, and coal. Estimated compliance cost per mine: $128,000 per year. For any reasonably profitable mining company, that is not a budget buster. For many, it's barely a budget consideration. Nevertheless, and as is typically the case whenever the government issues new health standards, the various impacted industries raised all possible objections in the "public comment" period leading up to the rule's implementation. And of course, once the regulations were issued, these same industries took the agency to court over them. In this case, the mining industry also received serious relief from the incoming Bush administration—so much so that the ink was not dry on the first legal petition before MSHA delayed enforcement of the exposure limit for one year.[6]

When that new date passed in 2002, the federal regulators again backed away from enforcement. The following year it issued a new set of exemptions and weakened standards. And in November 2003, the industries caught an even bigger break when NIOSH and the National Cancer Institute held a public meeting to discuss where things stood with their long-awaited study of diesel in underground mines.

With MARG and other industry representatives present in full force, NIOSH and NCI announced that data collection for the Miners Study was nearly complete and that analyses were already under way. Industry reps proceeded to request copies of the government's PowerPoint presentations, which were provided as a matter of courtesy—one that would backfire.

Despite the fact that the slides provided by government scientists clearly noted that the depicted data sets and analyses were incomplete—with no information whatsoever about duration of exposure, level of exposure, and other key factors—they were ripe for cherry-picking in the hands of MARG. And that's exactly what MARG's hired gun, an epidemiologist named Gerald Chase, did. His subsequent interpretation claimed that the data from the shared PowerPoint "demonstrates that the initial review of data from the NIOSH study...does not show any excess lung cancers above the expected rate for the general population."

In its incomplete state, the PowerPoint presentation—*a summary of the aspects of the study, not the study itself*—demonstrated no such thing, but MARG used the conclusion to argue that the new MSHA standards must be revisited. Not surprisingly, President Bush's appointees at MSHA complied, establishing a 45-day public comment period on Chase's MARG-funded report. Scientists at NIOSH were handcuffed by the earlier legislation requiring their communications be submitted first to the House of Representatives for review: in fact, a standing order issued by the federal judge dictated that all public remarks from NIOSH had to be submitted to the House *90 days* in advance. As Monforton wrote in her summary of the process, "The government scientists most capable of responding to the MARG-sponsored report were excluded from the process."[3]

Even the most cursory reading of this story demonstrates that the industry's campaign to kill the regulation, even after they'd first taken the teeth out of it, was skillfully orchestrated by Washington lobbyists well acquainted with the ways of both Congress and federal agencies. The business of delaying the key study during the late 1990s was masterfully executed. In the years that followed, the industry had cultivated new friendships in the Department of Labor, which oversees MSHA and OSHA, both regulatory agencies. In contrast, NIOSH and NCI, as scientific research agencies, have traditionally been shielded from interference by political appointees. So, yes, I'm prepared to believe that MSHA knew that NIOSH could not legally defend its own work. I *know* that as a result of all these lobbyist "sound science" shenanigans, top-drawer legal and lobbying work, and good electoral fortune, an alliance of mining firms, led by the MARG Diesel Coalition, successfully used the courts and Congress to game the regulatory system for a decade. Other industries can boast about uncertainty campaigns that have lasted much longer, but MARG certainly deserves dishonorable mention.

But put a big asterisk on the prize, because all that obstruction not-withstanding, new modified standards did nevertheless go into effect over the next few years, under the auspices of the Bush administration. An agency can delay only so long; if the Bush administration's MSHA had wanted to kill the diesel rule, it would have had to go through the same standard-setting process as the agency did to enact the rule in the first place. The new legal limits on diesel particulates were still too high to eliminate cancer risk, but they did reduce the permissible exposure levels by about 80 percent. Michael Wright, head of health and safety for the United Steelworkers, which represents many miners in metal mines, characterized the improvement cannily: "It used to be like working in the tail pipe of a bus; now it's like working four or five feet behind the bus."

So in the end, MARG failed to stop the new MSHA standards, and it also failed to stop the Diesel Miners Study. In 2010, a somewhat unbe-lievable twenty years after planning for the underground-mining study began, the first results were in, and a series of papers was finally pub-lished.[7] (One of the lead scientists estimated that the industry's delay-ing tactics accounted for five of those years.) Once again, the pertinent industries and their prominent product defense consultants geared up for the fight. The initial published papers aimed only to report on the methods employed in the study; MARG's experts, of course, judged them to be all wrong and incomplete.[8] The mining lobbyists headed to court, and a federal district judge in Louisiana gave them (and the House Committee on Education and the Workforce) the right to a 90-day review of the study's results before any publication. The Justice Department appealed, and the Court of Appeals in the Fifth Circuit stayed the order. But by then the 90 days had passed, and MARG could no longer turn to the court for help. More importantly, the Democrats had gained control of the House of Representatives and were eager to see the studies published.

That didn't stop the mining companies, though. Their attorney, the aforementioned Chajet from Patton Boggs, made a last-ditch effort to slow publication of any future reports. Since he evidently didn't know in which publication the studies were going to be published, he sent a threatening note to the editors of at least four scientific journals, warning against "publication or other distribution" of data and draft documents, threatening unspecified "consequences" if they failed to comply.[9]

This attempt to exert prior restraint, reminiscent of Richard Nixon's ill-fated efforts to stop the Pentagon Papers, received widespread coverage within the field and went over badly with the scientific community. The journal *Science* quoted Trevor Ogden, editor of the journal *Annals of Occupational Hygiene*: "Despite our attempts to be neutral on various controversies, this journal has more frequently been accused of being on the employers' side. However, I am disgusted by the many actions being taken to delay [the Diesel Miners Study] publications and prevent their being open to public examination."[10]

No one should be surprised to learn that the published research confirmed the link between exposure to diesel particulates and risk of lung cancer. Overall, covered miners in the subject period were about 25 percent more likely to develop lung cancer than non-miners living in the same state, and the most heavily exposed miners, those who had worked underground for longer periods, were three times more likely to get lung cancer than the least exposed.[7] I don't imagine the industry and its lawyers and consultants were surprised, either. The earlier studies showing the association may not have been as methodologically strong as the Diesel Miners Study, but nor were they fly-by-night jobs.

While the mining industry took the lead in opposing the research, they weren't the only industry with a financial stake in the results of the Diesel Miners Study. The diesel engine manufacturers had been closely following developments, too. Even before the findings were published, this industry, led by Navistar International, had commissioned product defense scientists to produce a series of "weight of the evidence" literature reviews.[11] Again, to no one's surprise, these studies added no new evidence, but they criticized the studies others had done, and they all pretty much reached the same set of conclusions: *There isn't sufficient evidence linking particulates with lung cancer in humans. The studies that found increased cancer in diesel-exposed workers were flawed. Cancer in lab animals exposed to diesel particulates? The rats developed cancer because their lungs were overloaded with dust, not because particulates cause cancer, because they don't.* Keep moving. Nothing to see here.

The publication of the state-of-the-art Diesel Miners Study results was a big setback for such an argument. There had been problems in the earlier research, but this much more authoritative study was a game changer. Moreover, in the same time frame as this study, the National Institutes of Health initiated funding of a study of a different cohort of workers with occupational exposure to diesel emissions: the trucking industry, whose drivers and mechanics were subjected to lower emissions levels than the underground miners, but still significant exposure. And this was a much larger group of workers; the study focused on 30,000 of them. It was designed and run by a team of public health scientists from Harvard, Tufts, and the University of California–Berkeley. Their results also found increased risk associated with cumulative exposure to diesel particulates.[12]

Both reports were major news items, or at least as major as occupational epidemiological studies ever are. The twin results also prompted a reclassification of diesel particulates by the World Health Organization's cancer-study wing, the International Agency for Research on Cancer (IARC). Instead of "probably carcinogenic to humans," diesel exhaust particulates were now designated as a full-blown human carcinogen.[13] This change would trigger additional regulation and likely opened the engine manufacturers to lawsuits. The announcement shook the industry and prompted a wave of industry-sponsored studies meant to produce different conclusions. (One of them, by Volkswagen, is part of the Dieselgate scandal detailed in Chapter 10.)

On top of all that bad news, there was more coming out of OSHA (which I was at that point leading on behalf of the Obama administration). Once the Diesel Miners Study was finished, it was OSHA's job to use those results to try to reduce workplace exposures, even though we had no exposure standard we required employers to meet. And our concern wasn't limited to just cancer risk; as noted earlier in this discussion, diesel emissions had been linked to numerous other diseases and conditions as well. Collaborating with our sister agency MSHA, we issued a hazard alert that advised workers and employers that prolonged exposure to diesel exhaust emissions can increase the risk of cardiovascular, cardiopulmonary, and respiratory disease, as well as lung cancer.[14]

Now facing these federal challenges to their existing ways of business, the vehicle and engine manufacturers took over from the mining industry as the leaders in challenging the emissions science. Responding to IARC's "carcinogenic" classification, the manufacturers made two arguments. One was valid and understandable but not relevant; the other, in my view, was simply wrong.

The legitimate point was made by the title of one of the industry's publications: "Evaluation of carcinogenic hazard of diesel engine exhaust needs to consider revolutionary changes in diesel technology."[15] For more than a decade, while downplaying the health problems, the engine industry *had* been making remarkable progress in improving diesel technology, lowering the potency of the emissions and therefore the dangers resulting from extensive exposures to both particulates and the nitrogen oxides. Each generation of diesel engine, especially the large ones designed for trucks and trains and heavy equipment, has been less-polluting than the previous one. The advances had reduced particulate exposures by 98 percent in just three decades, and therefore reducing the carcinogenic potential of the exposures as well. The EPA, along with the State of California (a force to reckon with, powerful enough to issue *and enforce* its own anti-pollution rules) and European regulators had all insisted on improvements. The industry now argued that the Diesel Miners Study—and all of the earlier ones, for that matter—that had prompted the IARC's new designation and MSHA's new standards had studied only workers exposed to the old technology. True enough, but the refutation was simple: Those old, dirty diesel machines didn't just disappear. The outmoded engines giving off particulate emissions were (and are) in use everywhere, spewing soot and, according to the best available evidence, causing cancer. And as I discuss later in this chapter, the rat studies launched at least in part to counter the IARC classification don't provide the reassurance the industry proclaims.

The engine manufacturers' second argument was the default, all-purpose objection we have seen time and again: the studies were weak science that yielded wrong results. The trade association representing diesel polluters insisted on access to the raw data for the studies on truckers and underground miners, essentially asserting that the researchers who did all the work—designing the study and collecting and analyzing the data—got the results wrong. By employing this tactic, industry aimed to do more than just criticize or rework the data analysis

performed by government scientists: it also aimed to remove the observational studies of health effects of air pollution from consideration in
regulatory settings. Game, set, match. Should the data be delivered, the
industry insists on the prerogative of commissioning one or more re-
analyses by outside parties, which is to say their own scientists and
consultants who specialize in product defense, and manufacturing uncertainty, under the guise of "sound science."

Eventually the diesel industry did bring their own re-analysis team,
as we will see, but first the researchers involved in both studies agreed
to share their materials with the Health Effects Institute (HEI). This is
a unique institution, chartered by Congress in 1980, that receives half
of its funding from the EPA and half from industry (including the
engine manufacturers). The institute does science while steering clear of
policy pronouncements. And it generally conducts its studies with rigor
and transparency.

In its relatively short history, HEI has been no stranger to arbitrating
differences between public and industry interests, particularly as they
relate to air pollution. The landmark Six Cities Study, conducted by
scientists at the Harvard School of Public Health, found that residents
in Steubenville, Ohio, the city in the study with the most air pollution,
had a 25 percent higher "all-cause" (overall) mortality risk than residents of the study's least polluted city: Portage, Wisconsin. The study
found that air pollution particularly increased the likelihood of dying
from lung cancer or cardiopulmonary disease.[16] In 2000, HEI confirmed the Harvard scientists' findings, and in turn the EPA used the
study as the basis for regulations under the Clean Air Act aimed at reducing health effects associated with air pollution. Initial projections
estimated that the new rule would prevent 15,000 premature deaths,
250,000 asthma attacks, 60,000 cases of bronchitis, and 9,000 hospital
admissions every year.[17]

As was the case with the Six Cities Study, HEI's rigorous, independent re-analysis confirmed the findings of the Diesel Miners Study,
asserting it "provided results and data that provide a useful basis for
quantitative risk assessment of exposure in particular to older diesel
engine exhaust."[18]

That should have ended the controversy, but, of course, it didn't. The
offended industries still wanted the raw data and could obtain them

thanks to Senator Richard Shelby (R-AL). The sordid history of this episode came to a head with a mere four lines of text, no more, cleverly attached by Senator Shelby to the 920-page omnibus appropriation bill for fiscal year 1999. Called the Data Access Act, it is also known as the Shelby Amendment (I always like to give credit where credit is due.) This amendment guarantees public access, by way of the Freedom of Information Act (FOIA), to "all data produced" by federally funded research scientists employed by nonprofit institutions. The Shelby Amendment was an open invitation for anyone to use the Freedom of Information Act to harass scientists, question their work, muddy the waters, delay action, and perhaps even steal intellectual property. The idea was to institutionalize these strategies—to construct bureaucratic mechanisms with which corporate interests can question the science underlying not just regulation but virtually any "'information'" disseminated by federal agencies as well. It would be the very triumph of uncertainty.

Even more galling: the disclosure stipulation does *not* pertain to private studies paid for by corporations. According to the logic of this legislation, industry should be free to dredge and manipulate the data of government-funded work, but federal agencies and outside groups should not be free to reanalyze industry-sponsored research submitted to the government agencies during the regulatory process. Agencies are legally required to consider these critiques in regulatory proceedings, essentially weighting the scale to favor one set of analyses over the other. Do we require better evidence of the hidden agenda behind the Shelby Amendment?

According to published accounts at the time, the motive behind the Shelby scheme was the displeasure of the corporations most responsible for air pollution—mainly oil companies and coal-burning electric utilities—that did not have access to the raw data at the heart of the otherwise bulletproof Six Cities Study, science that now possessed the seal of approval from HEI. That was the reporting at the time, but it should not come as a complete surprise that recent research using the documents discovered through a certain high-profile court case has pinpointed the actual origins of the Data Access Act. Hint: they were *not* the usual air-pollution suspects. No, the Shelby Amendment was dreamed up by an industry so besmirched in the public eye that few legislators would support anything it sponsored—an industry that needed other industries to front for it. That's right: Big Tobacco used air pollution controversy as a cover to advance its own agenda, having realized long before that reanalyzing a study's raw data in order to change its conclusion was a particularly effective way to neutralize dangerous science.[19] This discovery about tobacco's culpability didn't surprise me. The cigarette manufacturers are often lurking in the background in the campaign to manufacture doubt.

One final updating note: The Shelby Amendment did not turn out to be a complete victory for industry. After receiving thousands of comments and complaints from scientists, research institutions, and public policy experts, the Clinton-era Office of Management and Budget (OMB) interpreted the famous four lines rather narrowly, "limiting requested data to published or cited research used by the federal government in developing legally binding agency actions." This gave government-funded scientists, including the ones at NCI and NIOSH, the ability to limit data sharing so re-analyses could be accomplished without jeopardizing the confidentiality of study subjects.[20] This may have been only a temporary setback; polluting industries want far more— and have been unrelenting in their efforts (as I detail in Chapter 13).

Even though they had signed on to the process, the diesel exhaust industry (the engine makers, trucking companies, auto and truck manufacturers, and the petroleum industry) rejected the findings of the HEI evaluation of the Diesel Miners Study. Roger McClellan, one of the industry's long-time consultants and coauthor of numerous negative reviews of emissions science, issued a new report disputing HEI's conclusion about the mining study's validity. He was commissioned by the industry, specifically a trade organization called the Industrial Minerals Association–North America, but McClellan was paid through its law firm, Crowell and Moring.[21] (This legal maneuver was perfected back in the early days of Big Tobacco. When money flows through a law firm, all communications between the parties can be protected from discovery in a lawsuit.)

Thanks to the Shelby Amendment, the diesel industry was also able to work out a limited data-sharing arrangement with the NIOSH and

NCI researchers, obtaining their raw data but pledging to maintain the confidentiality of the individual study subjects. For the re-analysis job, industry hired Exponent, one of the leading product defense firms, along with several other scientists who had done similar works for other industries that wanted to defend their dangerous products. And the diesel exhaust industry got exactly what it wanted: a group of new papers re-analyzing the mining study (with no new data, of course) and exonerating the diesel particulates of any crimes against human health.[22]

As should be clear by now, I am always suspicious of these *post hoc* analyses, or re-analyses, undertaken by investigators who already know the study's results. When studies are first proposed, the investigator must lay out the data analysis plans in advance. But once you know a study's results, it is easy to design a re-analysis to make those results—if they are positive—go away. Change some parameters, select new cut-off points between categories, and statistically significant differences suddenly disappear, estimates of risk are suddenly reduced. Such alchemy (known in the trade as data dredging) is rather easily accomplished by a competent (if unethical) statistics craftsman, whereas the opposite—turning insignificance into significance—is far more difficult.

As I write these words in late 2019, seven years after the findings of the Diesel Miners Study were finally published, the industries' effort to re-analyze the investigation is still going strong. We now stand at five critiques and counting. This work doesn't come cheap. I'm not privy to the hard numbers, but these papers no doubt cost hundreds of thousands of dollars at a minimum. But how is this a problem, since the work is supported by many of the world's largest and most powerful corporations? Here is the funding acknowledgment for just one of the five studies:

> A coalition of trade organizations working through the Truck and Engine Manufacturers Association (EMA):
> American Petroleum Institute (API)
> European Automobile Manufacturers Association (ACEA)
> American Trucking Association (ATA)
> International Organization of Motor Vehicle Manufacturers (OICA)
> Alliance of Automobile Manufacturers (Alliance)
> European Research Group on Environment and Health in the Transport Sector (EUGT)

Association of Equipment Manufacturers (AEM)
Association of American Railroads (AAR)
European Association of Internal Combustion Engine Manufacturers (EUROMOT)[23]

Where will all this reanalysis and revisionist "sound science" lead? I'm confident what to expect because we've seen this drama before—multiple times and with many of the same actors. First, the product defense consultants will continue to produce impressive-looking (at least to nonexperts) studies exonerating diesel emissions. I had to laugh when I read one paper from 2012 concluding that "the weight of evidence is considered inadequate to confirm the diesel–lung cancer hypothesis." That paper's lead author was John F. Gamble, who discloses that his work was supported by "CONCAWE (CONservation of Clean Air and Water in Europe), a European trade association of oil companies working on environmental, health, and safety issues in refining and distribution."[24] In 1998, Gamble, an Exxon employee at the time, published a similar critique of the Six Cities Study of air pollution, asserting that "the weight of evidence suggests there is no substantive basis for concluding that a cause-effect relationship exists between long-term ambient $PM_{2.5}$ [very small particulates] and increased mortality."[25] In fact, *hundreds* of studies have since demonstrated that Gamble was mistaken about the deadly impact of $PM_{2.5}$ exposure but he is still carrying water for the oil industry.

So, first is the inevitable parade of mercenary studies and re-analyses, but while the hired guns are reanalyzing the benchmark Diesel Miners Study for the umpteenth time, new scientists are publishing new studies, involving new cohorts in different parts of the globe, linking this exhaust with lung cancer. Four years after the IARC classification of diesel emissions as a carcinogen, two European panels, the Nordic Expert Group for Criteria Documentation of Health Risks from Chemicals and the Dutch Expert Committee on Occupational Safety together, issued a document reviewing hundreds of studies on the effects of exposure to diesel. This group had the advantage of a few extra years of new research and access to the concerns and commentaries published by industry experts. Their conclusion: "There is extensive epidemiological evidence for an association between occupational exposure to diesel exhaust and lung cancer."[26]

Second, and only a few years from now, I predict, the industry will simply give up and acknowledge that emissions from their old engines cause lung cancer, and probably bladder cancer as well.[27] All those expensive, disingenuous studies will be seen the same way we look at the tobacco industry's sponsored studies of decades ago: attempts by dirty industry to sow scientific confusion. That impressive list of trade associations is fighting a rear-guard action, destined to lose. My guess is that the firms will persevere for as long as possible in an attempt to limit legal liability, since, after all, thousands of individuals have likely been sickened by the diesel exhaust from the many old engines still in use on our roads and in underground mines.

The good news: diesel engines keep getting cleaner and cleaner, remarkably so. They put out fewer emissions, and all our lungs are better for it. Some engine companies, like Cummins Engine, are not only developing methods to dramatically reduce emissions, they have embraced the public health regulations that EPA and other agencies have issued that require reduced emissions. This has been a good business decision for them, and I don't say that cynically. They recognize that they can do well by doing good, and they are playing a very positive role in cleaning the air.

As much as we would like to, we can't yet conclude that the soot coming out of the new engines doesn't cause cancer. It would take years to conduct the epidemiologic studies on the long-term effects of exposure to new diesel engines, of course. Cancer from environmental exposures doesn't appear until decades after first exposure, and the new engines haven't been around for very long, so any cancer seen now would be unlikely to have been caused by exhaust from the new engines.

So, for the moment, the best we can do is animal studies, and while the results are promising, they are not the exoneration the industry is claiming. Even before IARC concluded diesel particulates were a human carcinogen, HEI and the industry had been conducting research on the subject, contracting with the Lovelace Respiratory Research Institute (which comes up again in Chapter 10), a private nonprofit laboratory in New Mexico. These were among the earlier studies showing that exposure to high levels of DEP gave rats lung cancer.[28] The scientists at Lovelace built exposure chambers in which rats would breathe exhaust from new heavy-duty diesel engines. The exposed rats were no more likely to develop cancer than ones who just breathed filtered air. While this is certainly good news, I don't think it is the proof the industry claims it is. To understand why, you need some background in how these studies are designed.

The operating theory underlying animal cancer studies is that if a chemical causes cancer in animals, it is likely to cause it in humans as well. When toxicologists set up animal studies, they try to give the animals as high a dose as possible that won't cause acute or immediate effects, because they can't perform a study large enough to detect the effect of a smaller dose. Let's say a component of air pollution causes cancer in one in every thousand people exposed at the level most of us are breathing it. That would be considered a public health disaster and eliminating that substance would save countless lives. But to prove that exposure level caused cancer in lab animals, you'd need a study involving thousands of animals. Instead, toxicologists generally give very high doses to a far smaller number of animals and compare the rate of cases with that found in a group of unexposed animals. If the difference is statistically significant (and you still need a pretty sizable group to find statistical significance) then you can say the material is an animal carcinogen.

The fatal flaw with the Lovelace studies of the new technology engine exhaust is that the particulate exposure level tested was very low. The old engines put out 100 times more soot than the new ones; the rats in the new engine studies were exposed at low levels, and, happily, didn't develop cancer. From a public health perspective, however, the Lovelace investigators asked the wrong question, or at least used the wrong exposure levels. We aren't interested in the effects of exposure to the exhaust from a single engine, since no one is exposed to only one engine. We want to know if the accumulation of particles from thousands of engines in our environment increases cancer risk, in other words, do higher levels of new engine diesel particulates cause cancer. And even if the particulate levels in our urban air are lower than in the past, partially because these new engines are much improved, it is still necessary to expose the rats to higher amounts of emissions, or use many, many more rats to rule out a small but important increased risk of cancer. So, while the Lovelace study shows that the engines are safer than the old ones, they don't prove what is coming out of these cleaner engines is truly safe.

The improvements in new diesel engines should not deter federal agencies like EPA, MSHA, OSHA, and the other regulators from continuing to push for cleaner air. MSHA, for one, hasn't given up trying to increase protection for underground miners, or at least it didn't under the Obama administration. In July 2016, the agency reopened its rule-making process—asking stakeholders to provide information on a range of subjects necessary for it to update its 15-year-old standard. The response from the mining industry was vociferous and not surprising: Don't do it. An attorney from the aforementioned Crowell and Moring, representing Murray Energy (the same firm responsible for the Crandall Canyon mine disaster, where six miners and three rescuers were killed[29]) and the Bituminous Coal Operators' Association, wrote: "the Companies want to state categorically that they believe the current MSHA diesel-exhaust related rules are more than amply protective of the health of their employees. There is no need to engage in a new rulemaking on this issue for underground coal mines."[30]

The coal operators can relax. David Zatezalo, former coal company CEO and the Trump administration's appointee to head MSHA, essentially put the whole process into deep freeze, extending the information-collection period (remember, it opened in July 2016) to March 26, 2019. That ridiculous delay guarantees that no new standard will even be proposed until after the 2020 presidential election.

At the EPA, an unbelievable development in 2018 put much of America's cleaner-air progress in jeopardy. This story began in 2010, when the latest EPA diesel emissions standards took full effect. In order to skirt the new rules, a small number of diesel truck dealers came up with the idea of buying *engineless* tractor truck bodies from the various manufacturers, installing rebuilt engines from the bad old days, then claiming that these "gliders" predated the latest EPA emissions standards and should therefore be exempt from those standards. (A few such trucks that had been retrofitted with rebuilt diesels had been around for years—they were a good way to take advantage of an engine that could be salvaged after a crash had ruined the rest of the truck—but after 2010 they offered a very tempting way to get around the new emissions standards.) Business started booming, from fewer than 1,000 gliders sold in 2010 to 10,000 five years later. EPA investigators became alarmed by the shape of the curve on that graph—it would seriously imperil the nation's atmosphere—and announced that henceforth no manufacturer could produce more than 300 gliders annually. With such a restriction in place, total annual production would be limited to a small fraction of the quarter-million trucks sold each year in the United States—if the businesses survived at all.

In 2015, House Representative Diane Black (R-TN) introduced legislation to annul the Obama administration's limit and expand the loophole for as many gliders as the market would bear. That legislation went nowhere, but in 2017, following the election of President Trump, Black went straight to Scott Pruitt, the new head of the EPA, and requested that he overrule his professional staff and allow unlimited glider production.

And this is where the story gets really good. Black attached to her request a 2016 study produced by Tennessee Technological University concluding that the rebuilt old engines were as clean-burning as the very latest diesels. Soon enough it was discovered that this study had been funded by the Fitzgerald family business in Tennessee, which also promised to build a new research center at Tennessee Tech. Various Fitzgerald interests also contributed at least $225,000 to Black's unsuccessful campaign for governor. (During his own campaign, Donald Trump visited one of the Fitzgerald dealerships, which sells baseball caps emblazoned with the slogan "Make Trucks Great Again.")

In November 2017, EPA chief Pruitt announced that he was proposing an exemption to the 300-unit limit for three manufacturers, one each in Indiana, Iowa, and Tennessee (Fitzgerald Glider Kits, the largest manufacturer).[31] He noted it was in response to a request from Fitzgerald, who also provided a copy of a letter from the president of Tennessee Tech, touting the results of the Tennessee Tech report (although never mentioning that Fitzgerald made payments to the University).[32] Only days later, professional EPA staff produced an analysis that challenged any conclusion that the gliders are no more polluting than the new systems. Quoting *New York Times* reporter Eric Lipton whose work revealed much of this subterfuge, "The analysis said EPA tests found that the Fitzgerald trucks emitted nitrogen oxide levels during highway operations that were 43 times as high as those from trucks with modern emissions control systems. The air pollution from these glider trucks was so bad that one year's worth of truck sales was estimated to release 13 times as much nitrogen oxide as all of the Volkswagen diesel cars with fraudulent emissions controls, a scheme that resulted in a criminal case against the company and more than $4 billion in fines."[33] The EPA report noted that its testing equipment broke down in urban traffic. "The filters were overloaded with particulate matter," the report stated. In the accompanying photo, a filter that had been white when new was solid black. Chet France, former director of assessment and standards at the EPA's Office of Transportation and Air Quality, noted that there are enough indestructible diesel engines in salvage yards to support a prosperous glider market for decades.

As the story unfolded in 2018, a study published in the *Journal of the American Medical Association* (*JAMA*) found that repealing the "glider" restrictions would yield 41,000 premature deaths over a decade and 900,000 cases of cases of respiratory ailments.[34] Some of the faculty at Tennessee Tech were concerned that the questionable report, which had gained national notoriety, reflected badly on them and their school. The interim dean of the College of Engineering wrote that the report had been primarily the work of a graduate student. His letter continued, "No qualified, credentialed engineering faculty member (1) oversaw the testing, (2) verified the data or calculations of the graduate student, (3) wrote or reviewed the final report submitted to Fitzgerald, or (4) wrote or reviewed the letter submitted to Diane Black with the far-fetched, scientifically implausible claim, that remanufactured truck engines met or exceeded the performance of modern, pollution-controlled engines with regards to emissions."

Within days, the university's president advised the EPA that "experts within the university have questioned the methodology and accuracy" of the study and advised the agency not to take the report under consideration. The EPA replied that the glider decision "only noted the existence of the study" but did not rely on it. Pruitt claimed it did not have the authority to regulate the production of the rebuilt gliders. That was patently false, as demonstrated by the eventual decision of his successor to reverse Pruitt's decision without taking any public input.[35]

Putting aside the health and environmental impacts of deregulating gliders, the surprising aspect of this story is how Pruitt, with the support of the Trump White House, was willing to go against the wishes of some major players in the U.S. economy: trucking companies and engine manufacturers, both of which lost out as "new" gliders used junkyard engines rather than expensive new engines. Anti-regulatory zealots, like self-proclaimed junkman Steven Milloy (so called because he's the proprietor of junkscience.com and author of a book titled *Green Hell: How Environmentalists Plan to Control Your Life*), who long advocated for Big Tobacco, seemed to be more able to advance their positions than large corporations. I attribute that to what I saw as President Trump's desire to reverse anything the Obama administration did—if Obama supported it, Trump would do the opposite, no matter what the consequences.

Once Pruitt was forced to step down because of multiple ethical scandals, the glider deregulation could no longer survive. Tennessee Tech sent another letter to the EPA reporting that it had conducted an internal investigation that found that the key statements in that first letter were inaccurate. Andrew Wheeler, a former corporate lobbyist and a more traditional Republican operative who replaced Pruitt, killed the initiative. Did the embarrassment of using phony results from a study paid for by the firm that stood most to benefit influence Wheeler's decision? I think not, since they have embraced many other studies, equally bogus. I suspect the large firms that make and use new, cleaner diesel engines pointed out to him that not only would all these new gliders pollute the air and kill many Americans, it hurt their bottom lines. While the first argument should have swayed him, it is far more likely the latter did. Either way, he made the right decision, and killed the glider deregulation.

7

On Opioids

DIFFERENT CULTURES AND countries take different approaches to the burdens of physical pain. Almost universally, the excruciating physical tolls of diseases like cancer and sickle-cell anemia are treated aggressively with prescription painkillers. In the United States, this sort of treatment has been extended more broadly, with the same pain medications employed for chronic pain also provided to individuals experiencing musculoskeletal injuries, dental work, and surgical recoveries.

Why have so many U.S. doctors prescribed powerful opioids to so many patients at such high doses? It is now recognized that the change in medical practice contributed to the opioid epidemic that is manifesting with tragic consequences now and, inevitably, well into the future. The dynamic of the epidemic is changing, and the proximate cause of most of the overdoses is heroin and black market fentanyl. But many individuals have been first sucked into the opioid cycle by the array of choices produced *legally* by some of the most successful and profitable pharmaceutical manufacturers in the United States—companies whose financial growth have been enabled by persuading physicians with a particular kind of scientific campaign.

I am not suggesting that these companies are solely responsible for the opioid crisis. Powerful social and economic factors contribute to this complex epidemic. Starting in the 1990s, the increased use of opioids for pain brought reduced suffering and welcome relief to many. But there is no question that if the prescription opioids had not been available in virtually unlimited quantities beginning in the 1990s, either taken as legally prescribed or diverted to the illicit market, this epidemic would not be nearly as extensive. Many individuals who have died by overdose would be alive today. This chapter focuses on the producers of these drugs, because the ensuing epidemic is rooted in their abuse of the science.

Human brains have a remarkable mechanism for controlling pain. When we are injured or hurt, our bodies produce their own chemical opioids, which bind to receptors in the brain and nerves, reducing (or, ideally, blocking) the pain. In many instances, this natural mechanism isn't strong enough to handle the pain, and for centuries products made from opium, and later chemically derived morphine, have been used for pain relief. These medications work for many. With a catch, of course: Their addictive properties have been well recognized and have always been a concern.

Synthetic opioids, as well as semi-synthetic ones derived from natural opioids, were first developed in the lab a century ago. They achieved marginal medicinal use beginning in the 1960s, then widespread use in the 1990s. These days, two of the most well-known synthetics are oxycodone, the main active ingredient in the brand-name product OxyContin, and fentanyl. Fentanyl, a synthetic opioid, one of the more potent, is 50 times stronger than heroin. The term "opioids" is therefore a broad category of natural and synthetic products, all of which bind with specific receptors in the brain that block pain while also producing, to one degree or another, a euphoria that can sometimes be craved by users. Those individuals who begin to seek out opioids to the exclusion of other goals, no matter the harmful consequences in their lives, have developed an addiction.

The recent opioid epidemic dates to 1995, when Purdue Pharma, a privately owned company based in Stamford, Connecticut, introduced OxyContin, the brand-name of a new formulation of oxycodone. This new product featured a much larger dose than earlier versions of oxycodone-based pain killers like Percocet and Percodan, and also promised longer-lasting pain relief (12 hours, as opposed to just four). In order to get approval for this formulation from the Food and Drug Administration (FDA), Purdue Pharma convinced the agency that while OxyContin was more potent than earlier formulations, the "longer-acting" attribute would make this opioid less likely to cause addiction. Their logic was based on the claim that a more controlled release of oxycodone would be less likely to cause euphoria and craving than short-acting forms.

In time for the medication's launch, the FDA bought this argument—and permitted the company to claim the medication was less likely to be addictive on its label. Reality soon proved otherwise, however, and patients who became addicted soon realized the pills could be crushed and then snorted or even injected. Meanwhile, the FDA medical officer in charge of the review was hired by Purdue Pharma.[1]

The drug industry, in particular Purdue with its newly obtained FDA approval, endeavored to convince physicians that pain was undertreated in our society (arguably true), that the new painkillers were a safe way to treat pain because they were virtually nonaddictive (very untrue), and they could not easily be abused (outrageously untrue).

How did they do it? The first step was finding and using material from the existing medical literature that would serve as cover for inventing a whole new world of "facts" to mask the addictive properties of the drugs they were marketing. In the early 1990s, there was very limited evidence either way as to the addictiveness of opioids prescribed. The companies found a few small studies (if you even call them studies) that appeared to say what they needed—that opioids were safe and nonaddictive—and then trumpeted the results. When we look at those "studies" now we can see their limitations in design and scope, but in these early years of extensive opioid use, at least a decade before the full-blown epidemic began, the hard numbers were not yet in evidence—tens of thousands of users had grown addicted. The presiding naiveté made it a little easier to believe, or to pretend to believe, the charade.

One key industry exhibit utilized by pharmaceutical companies was a five-sentence letter to the editor in the *New England Journal of Medicine,* published in 1980. It carried the title "Addiction rare in patients treated with narcotics." This is the complete text:

Recently, we examined our current files to determine the incidence of narcotic addiction in 39,946 hospitalized medical patients who were monitored consecutively. Although there were 11,882 patients who received at least one narcotic preparation, there were only four cases of reasonably well-documented addiction in patients who had no history of addiction. The addiction was considered major in only one instance. The drugs implicated were meperidine in two patients, Percodan in one, and hydromorphone in one. We conclude that despite widespread use of narcotic drugs in hospitals, the development of addiction is rare in medical patients with no history of addiction.[2]

As a letter (not an actual paper), it never went through peer review— the academic process whereby other experts weigh in on a document's claims and methods to endorse, or more often trash, its suitability for publication. In other words, citing this letter was the 1990s equivalent of citing a very thoughtful online comment. Nevertheless, it became a *cornerstone* of the industry's later campaign promise that opioids carry a low risk of addiction when prescribed for chronic pain. The letter was certainly impressive. The title's message seemed definitive; one of its authors was Hershel Jick, the respected director of the Boston Collaborative Drug Surveillance Program; and it was published in one of the nation's most prestigious medical journals, so it saw a sizable increase in references after Purdue introduced OxyContin to the market fifteen years later.[3] For the next quarter-century it would be cited hundreds of times in the medical literature and completely misrepresented in the popular press, likely with the help of Big Pharma's PR flacks. In 2001, *Time* magazine even described it as a "landmark study," assuring readers that any concerns that patients would become addicted to opioids was "basically unwarranted."[4] Eventually, in 2017 the editor of the journal issued an unprecedented warning that the "letter has been 'heavily and uncritically cited' as evidence that addiction is rare with opioid therapy" and Jick later pointed out that the letter, whose misuse he had no responsibility for, had many limitations, including that it only addressed use of opioids in inpatient hospital settings and there was no follow-up after patients were discharged.[5]

The episode with the *New England Journal of Medicine*'s five-sentence letter may have been the most flagrant example of the industry's misleading physicians and regulators, but there were plenty of other examples in which the industry promoted short-term studies of people prescribed opioids for pain following surgery, burns, or some other acute event. The studies were often paid for by the opioid industry, written either by the doctors on Pharma's payroll or industry ghostwriters.[6] There was rarely any follow-up. It turned out to be pretty easy to make the case that these drugs were not addictive if you cherry-pick the studies and then misinterpret the findings.

It was even surprisingly easy to invent a whole new diagnosis: *pseudoaddiction*. The idea here was that a craving for opioids accompanied by behavior aimed at obtaining the drugs—*addiction*, in common understanding—was in fact driven by the *still unrelieved pain* for which the patient had been prescribed the opioid in the first place—pseudoaddiction. The actual term and the initial description originated with one study describing one (one!) patient. Despite the fact that there really is no hard (or even soft) evidence supporting the concept, it took off. The manufacturers sponsored publications like "Responsible Opioid Prescribing," informing physicians that signs of pseudoaddiction (rather than true addiction) include requesting drugs by name, demanding or manipulative behavior, seeing more than one doctor to obtain opioids, and hoarding.[7] And the best way to treat pseudoaddiction? More opioids, of course. A 2015 review of the literature unearthed a grand total of six papers challenging the concept. All were written by physicians *not* paid by the manufacturers.[8] Overwhelming their well-intentioned output were hundreds of articles discussing pseudoaddiction while making no attempt whatsoever to empirically validate the concept. It was not a fair fight, and the results were predictable. The bogus, well-moneyed work overwhelmed the serious science.

Now recall the fundamental claim for OxyContin: twelve continuous hours of pain relief at a sustained, lower release is better than many competitors' four hours, and also less enticing for problematic users who crave the quicker hit offered by the older, more immediate drugs. An investigation by the *Los Angeles Times* (using documents uncovered in litigation as well as studies submitted to the FDA) revealed that Purdue's own studies found that OxyContin tablets release approximately 40 percent of their active ingredients immediately, after which release slows. As a result, the drug wears off in less than 12 hours for most patients, leaving the patient desperate for more. For some patients, it wears off in less than six hours. The result is a double hit: the underlying pain has returned, and the patient begins acute withdrawal from the medication. Together, these compel the individual to seek more medication, often at a higher dose. Evidently Purdue knew all this but continued to market the drug as effective for 12 hours, driving up usage and addiction—and profits.[9]

Certain manufacturers developed new formulations that purported to make the drugs less easy to misuse. In 2012, for example, Endo Pharmaceutical marketed Opana ER, which it claimed to be "crush-resistant" compared with its original Opana formulation. (Crush-resistant would make it unsuitable for snorting.) Promoting the drug to pharmacy benefit managers, the company failed to point out that studies it performed, but never published, showed that the new product could be ground with a coffee grinder, or just chewed to release the drug.

Along with these workarounds for those driven to use the drugs illicitly, the crush-resistant pills reconfigured the marketplace for the Endo product: injection replaced snorting among people misusing Opana. In 2015, disaster: a rural Indiana county that had never had more than five new HIV cases a year reported more than 100 new cases in less than three months, the disease spread by syringe-sharing around injection of Opana ER.[10] The outbreak was finally halted when, after much delay and pleading from public health officials, then-governor Mike Pence agreed to a short term needle exchange program, limited to the county where the outbreak occurred.[11] Two years later—and too late—the FDA finally ordered Endo to stop selling the reformulated drug entirely, the first and only time that the agency had removed an opioid pain medication from the market due to the concerns of misuse and addiction.[12]

The evidence is simply overwhelming: opioid producers suppressed some studies, misrepresented and elevated others, claimed their drugs were neither addictive nor easily abused, and claimed that the most effective approach to addressing patient pain was to continuously increase dose of the drug. But not to worry! These drugs are not particularly addictive. *You don't believe us?* Just ask our PR campaign. As demonstrated in other industries and going back to the heyday of tobacco, a company or industry's uncertainty and misinformation campaign about a given product's harmful impacts needs to unite questionable science with a full-court press of multi-sector public relations. The opioid producers' three-front campaign targeting regulators, physicians, and the public followed the well-established formula perfected over the decades by Big Tobacco: Perpetrate ad-hoc "sound science" (i.e., paid-for science with beneficial conclusions) and the motivated manipulation of existing science; hire "key opinion leaders" to promote the products; invent and enrich front groups to advocate the importance of unfettered sales.

In the case of opioids, manufacturers started with physicians who specialized in pain management, likely believed that pain was under-treated in our healthcare system, and that opioids should be used more widely for that purpose. The firms then hired them as "influencers": physicians who could attract the attention of other physicians—the ones who actually write the scripts—and advance the industry narrative in professional circles. These key opinion leaders were quite well paid for their services.

I've mentioned the study that helped get the ball rolling on pseudo-addiction—the one with only one subject. One of the authors of that groundbreaking paper, physician and dentist J. David Haddox, became one of Purdue Pharma's paid speakers before becoming, eventually, the company's vice president for health policy. Another star influencer was Russell Portenoy, a pain medicine specialist at Beth Israel Medical Center in New York. Portenoy was highly visible in the field, serving as editor in chief of the *Journal of Pain and Symptom Management* and editor of the journal *Pain*. He and his program received millions of dollars in funding from the opioid manufacturers. The gospel he preached was not just for physicians but for the public as well, and centered on destigmatizing opioid use. Appearing on *Good Morning America* in 2010, Portenoy asserted, "Addiction, when treating pain, is distinctly uncommon. If a person does not have a history, a personal history, of substance abuse, and does not have a history in the family of substance abuse, and does not have a very major psychiatric disorder, most doctors can feel very assured that that person is not going to become addicted." Portenoy eventually recanted in 2012, admitting to the *Wall Street Journal* that he "gave innumerable lectures in the late 1980s and nineties about addiction that weren't true." He added, "Did I teach about pain management, specifically about opioid therapy, in a way that reflects misinformation? Well...I guess I did."[13]

Drug makers paid out millions of dollars to physicians who would make a similar case to their peers, giving direct payments and also bringing the doctors to conferences at luxury resorts and fancy dinners where the companies could promote their products.[14] Hundreds of physicians received six figure payments, and thousands of others were paid more than $25,000 each.[15] This was in addition to the huge, heavily incentivized sales force (600 reps at Purdue alone) employed to meet with physicians at their offices. The system worked. The physicians prescribed larger and larger numbers of pills. The drug companies, the salespeople, the overprescribing physicians—they all got very rich.

The other key component of the opioid industry's marketing effort were groups with names that sounded like objective, professional societies or patient-advocacy organizations. Many of these well-funded organizations were really just operatives for promoting the producers' lies. According to the 2017 lawsuit filed by then–Ohio attorney general Mike DeWine, these groups generated treatment guidelines and programs that encouraged long-term use of opioids. They also did Pharma's dirty work "by responding to negative articles, by advocating against regulatory changes that would limit opioid prescribing in accordance with the scientific evidence, and by conducting outreach to vulnerable patient populations." The fancily named American Pain Foundation, for example, produced educational materials for patients, reporters, and policymakers that promoted the benefits of opioids for chronic pain and minimized the risk of addiction. It targeted pain medication for veterans and ran multimedia campaigns to inform patients of their "right" to pain treatment. The organization was so singularly dependent on the manufacturers that in 2012, when the Senate Finance Committee began an investigation into the links between it and the manufacturers, the American Pain Foundation's board of directors (which included the aforementioned Richard Portenoy and other prominent physicians) promptly dissolved the organization.[7]

The FDA requires that drug-company advertising be truthful and labels have to be approved by the agency. However, advertising that doesn't promote a *specific* product name or brand but mentions only diseases or those that mention only drugs (without linking the two) are not required to provide warning information or even to reflect the accompanying risks in a fair and balanced way. The opioid industry took full advantage of this loophole, following FDA rules when promoting their own products but broadcasting very different messages in the less specific, unbranded versions. The advertisements for Endo's Opana ER, for example, included this FDA-approved statement: "All patients treated with opioids require careful monitoring for signs of abuse and addiction, since use of opioid analgesic products carries the risk of addiction even under appropriate medical use." In contrast, an Endo campaign promoting opioids in general only stated: "People who take opioids as prescribed usually do not become addicted." [7]

Totally legal.

––––––

In considering the origins and history of industry misinformation campaigns, the gold standard for effectiveness was designed by Hill and Knowlton, the global public relations firm that worked with cigarette companies following the cancer revelations of the 1950s.

The Sackler family, owners of Purdue Pharma, was involved in public relations, advertising, and marketing drugs long before they were manufacturing opioids. They were brilliant at advertising. In fact, their revenues from that first business had provided them the capital to purchase Purdue Pharma in the first place. The OxyContin PR campaign alone, working with a budget of $200 million, was in terms of profit one of the most successful campaigns in the history of contemporary society. At the time of the Sacklers' Purdue acquisition, advertising and marketing had already made them multimillionaires; one drug later made them billionaires. Within a few short years of OxyContin's introduction, annual sales reached $1 billion. By 2010, it was a $3 billion drug, even though it never represented more than a small percentage of the share of opioid prescriptions.[16] According to Forbes, the Sacklers are now the nineteenth richest family in the country, wealthier than the Rockefellers. (That's down a few places from 2015, as the campaign to limit opioid addiction has become more widespread and successful.[17]) Of course the wealth generated by opioids isn't limited just to Purdue and its interests. Some of the biggest Big Pharma companies, including Johnson & Johnson (whose subsidiary Janssen Pharmaceuticals sells opioids), Teva, and Allergan, have profited from the massive growth in opioid sales.[7]

On one side of the ledger, phenomenal profits; on the other side, tragic consequences. The toll hardly needs summarizing here, beyond the cold fact that opioids have killed tens of thousands and destroyed the lives of thousands more, have decimated families and whole communities, and are responsible for the first drop in U.S. life expectancy in more than two decades. The largest killers are now illicit fentanyl and heroin, replacing the legally manufactured opioids that helped launch the epidemic. In the United States, overdoses involving opioids, licit and illicit, killed 42,000 people in 2016. That number jumped to almost 48,000 people in 2017, similar to the annual number of HIV/AIDS deaths at the height of its epidemic.[18]

In my seven years overseeing the U.S. Occupational Safety and Health Association (OSHA), I saw one component of the opioid epidemic up close—the relationship of workplace injuries, pain, and addiction. The stories were heartbreaking. Coal miners and construction workers, injured on the job, take pain pills in order to get back to work—and get paid again. It saddened but didn't surprise me to see the high rates of overdoses in areas around the coal fields in West Virginia and Kentucky, knowing how the miners would do everything in their power, including self-medication, to keep working. The linkages between the opioid epidemic and work injuries were first documented by Gary Franklin, medical director of the Washington State Department of Labor and Industries, the agency that runs the state's OSHA program. Workers are eager to get back to work, and physicians who treat injured workers, especially when the employer chooses the physician, often push injured workers off workers' compensation (known for decades as "workman's comp"). Franklin demonstrated that workers with back injuries who were given opioids were more likely to become addicted to the drug and ended up being disabled and out of work *longer* than workers not given opioids. He documented how the number of opioid-overdose deaths among injured workers in Washington shot up shortly after treatment guidelines were changed in the late 1990s to recommend the liberalized use of opioids.[19] Those guidelines were strongly influenced by physicians, including Richard Portenoy, and organizations like the American Academy of Pain Medicine, one of the front groups bankrolled by drug manufacturers. It was a perfect storm: the short-term need of getting employees back to work quickly, combined with the drug industry's false advertising that denied the addictive capacity of these powerful drugs, resulted in the addiction, disability, and subsequent overdose deaths of many workers injured on the job.

Lost amid the rightful public attention to opioid use and misuse is the enormous number of children who are for all intents and purposes orphaned by their parents' diminished capacity for parenting, or in some cases deaths.[20] Before 2012, the number of children placed into the foster care system nationally was dropping each year; it has since then started to rise, with greater increases in states where more overdoses are occurring.[21] In West Virginia, the foster care rate increased by 42 percent from 2014 to 2018.[22] And whereas during the AIDS epidemic, there was a mathematical model I created that estimated the number of children who would lose their mothers to the disease (and with it, how much funding was needed to support orphaned children), no such model exists for opioids.[23] But given the large numbers of young adults dying of overdoses, I have no doubt that the number of children orphaned by opioids is already surpassing that from HIV/AIDS.

As revealed in journalist Barry Meier's 2003 book *Pain Killer*, documents collected by the U.S. government in its criminal prosecution against Purdue reveal that company executives, including members of the Sackler family, were receiving numerous reports of misuse of their drug as early as 1997, less than two years after the drug hit the market (and then the streets). By 2003, seven years after OxyContin was introduced, thousands of patients who claimed they had become addicted to the drug had joined lawsuits against the manufacturer. One settled in New York for $75 million. Three years later, the Department of Justice began the first criminal case against Purdue, through which many of the documents and reports publicly available have surfaced. This was during the George W. Bush administration, and Purdue hired a team of well-connected attorneys, including former New York City mayor and soon to be Republican presidential candidate Rudy Giuliani, to try to work out a deal. According to Meier's *Pain Killer*, even before criminal indictments could be issued, high-level DOJ officials pressured the prosecutors to back off and accept a plea deal. Purdue pled guilty to a felony charge of illegally misbranding OxyContin in an effort to mislead physicians and consumers into believing that the drug was less addictive and less subject to misuse.[1]

Corporations can't go to jail, but executives can. The deal with the government allowed three executives (but no members of the Sackler family) to plead guilty to misdemeanors and avoid prison; the company and its executives also agreed to pay fines totaling $634 million. That sounds like a lot, but it is still just a smidgen of the revenue that OxyContin continued to generate. The settlement did lead to some changes in warning labels and marketing policies, but physician prescribing patterns had already been set, and many patients were already dependent on the drugs, so the changes had only modest impact on either opioid sales or the devastating growth of the epidemic.

Some states also filed suits against Purdue, and these cases typically settled for relatively small sums. More importantly, the files in all of these cases were sealed, so no outside parties could see the secret documents uncovered in discovery. New cases could not build off previous cases and changes in opioid control policies that might have helped stem the epidemic were delayed. The failure to effectively corral opioid companies has led to new legal strategies to change the behavior of the manufacturers in meaningful ways (following the example of tobacco, where states sued cigarette manufacturers for the costs of providing medical care to smokers with cancer or lung disease). With the opioid manufacturers, increasing numbers of states, counties, cities, Native American tribes, and unions have filed lawsuits against Purdue, Johnson & Johnson, Teva, Endo, Allergan, as well as drug distribution firms, alleging they have driven up the costs of the medical care and social services borne by the plaintiffs. The litigation was initiated by a bipartisan group of state attorneys general and based on materials gathered through investigative subpoenas and document requests. As these suits have produced more incriminating documents, members of the Sackler family, and others who served on Purdue Pharma's board of directors, have been sued as well.[24]

The papers filed by the states contain a particularly damning indictment of the marketing practices of Purdue and the other manufacturers. Complaints from Kentucky, Tennessee, and Ohio, states that have been decimated by the epidemic, detail how these companies cynically marketed their products to maximize their profits, ignoring the obvious catastrophic impact of their work. They figured out what they needed to claim to get FDA approval and to convince physicians to prescribe their drugs.

By fall of 2019, the legal system was beginning to catch up with these outrages. In a historic decision, Johnson & Johnson was found by an Oklahoma judge to have helped fuel the opioid epidemic in that state and fined $465 million. That firm, Purdue Pharma, and the rest of the industry now recognize they will have to pay some price for selling a product that has caused such enormous devastation across the country, and they are inexorably moving in the direction of settling the many lawsuits they are facing.

———

Opioid sales and prescriptions have been dropping since 2012, but the companies are still selling far more pain-killing pills than needed. The work of Washington State's Gary Franklin and others has helped reduce the almost automatic prescribing of opioids to injured workers who report pain. But the successful indoctrination of the medical profession by the opioid industry is hard to overcome. For example, most people don't need narcotics to control the pain of a sprained ankle. Nevertheless, from 2011 to 2015, 25 percent of insured people who appeared at emergency rooms across the country following an ankle sprain and who had never taken opioids (and so were presumably not angling for the drugs) were given opioids.[25]

Some legislative progress has occurred. In October 2014, the U.S. Drug Enforcement Administration tightened controls on physicians' ability to prescribe drugs containing hydrocodone, prohibiting prescription refills. Compared with the 12 months before rescheduling, dispensed hydrocodone combination product prescriptions dropped by 22 percent.[26] But the epidemic had been seeded before this policy change; less access to legal products has resulted in more use of illegal products, and heroin and illicit fentanyl are less expensive than legal pills diverted to the black market.

Looking back on the origins of the opioid epidemic, it's clear what could have been done to stop it before it was so entrenched. Certainly the FDA could have refused to agree to language on drug labels about the purported safety and effectiveness of long-acting opioids that was not supported by evidence. Academic researchers could have steered clear of funding from the industry and called out the practice of anecdotal observations misleadingly presented as studies (recall that five-sentence letter to the editor of the *New England Journal of Medicine*). Companies like Purdue should have sounded the alarm on misuse much faster, rather than keeping evidence of growing addiction under wraps.

Public disclosure of the enormous special-interest payments to physicians might have made the public at least somewhat skeptical of the claims of safety and effectiveness. (The United States made some progress in this area with the Affordable Care Act, also known as Obamacare, which required drug manufacturers to disclose their payments to physicians and hospitals and publish those data on the web. This could change, or cease, if the Affordable Care Act is repealed or substantially weakened.)

As of the publication of this book, the secret funding of front groups remains legal in the United States. Corporations continue to fund "AstroTurf" organizations—groups that operate under the guise of being grassroots but are actually mercenary political actors employed to convince legislators, regulators, and the public that there is real popular support for an industry's product.

The smoking guns—the documents that tell us the truth about OxyContin and some of the other drugs, as well as the truth about outrageous and deceitful marketing campaigns—were coughed up by the drug makers in the lawsuits and federal prosecution of Purdue. Yet under the terms of these settlements, Purdue was allowed to seal the record and none of those documents were made public. We have them now, a full decade later, only because state attorneys general have initiated a new round of suits. Fear of reputational damage is a powerful motivator of good behavior; had these documents surfaced earlier, or during the actual lawsuit, it is likely that Purdue, Johnson & Johnson, and the other firms would have been compelled to voluntarily stop some of their marketing ploys, and far fewer of these lethal pills would have been sold.

8

Deadly Dust

IN DECEMBER 2009, eleven months after President Obama was inaugurated for his first term, I took up my new duties as assistant secretary of labor for the Occupational Safety and Health Administration, or OSHA. I'd been nominated for the position four months earlier. With the Democrats in control of the Senate at the time, I expected eventual confirmation. I also expected some opposition, if only token, from corporations I'd criticized in an earlier book, *Doubt Is Their Product*, for sponsoring counterfeit science. But to my great surprise, these interests stayed on the sidelines. The actual attacks came from a totally unexpected group: gun rights advocates. Some members of some pro-gun groups got very worked up about a blog post I had written about gun control following the Virginia Tech massacre in 2007.[1] As one headline on the website *Outdoor Life* asked, "Can Obama's Anti-Gun OSHA Pick Be Stopped?" That question was meant as a rallying cry to Second Amendment hardliners, warning them of the threat posed by what was termed a "subtle" OSHA appointment: "David Michaels...has made past attempts to frame guns in terms of public health. Exploiting it to further citizen disarmament is something the academic left, from which Michaels hails, has been pursuing for years."[2]

I had spent much of my professional life dealing with issues of workers' health and safety, and the notion that guns could come under OSHA's purview had never occurred to me. I had to ask the agency's top attorney, and I was equally surprised by his response: "Yes, they can." It seems that a few years earlier, oil company ConocoPhillips had tried to prohibit workers from bringing loaded guns onto their refinery grounds in Oklahoma. When leaders of the National Rifle Association got wind of this initiative, they instructed the Oklahoma legislature to ban employers from banning guns. And when the legislature complied, the oil refineries pointed out that a federal OSHA regulation would preempt state law.

I believed then, as I do now, that banning loaded weapons from oil refineries is a reasonable safety rule. But I was also not about to invite a Second Amendment fight that the agency didn't need and politically couldn't win. There were bigger health hazards to address. So I met with staff from the Republican senators on the committee overseeing my confirmation, and I firmly promised that OSHA, under my leadership, would not issue any regulations banning guns in workplaces.

If the product defense lobby had spurred the Second Amendment lobby into taking up the cudgels against me (which I believe they did), then the strategy backfired. The Republicans on the confirmation committee focused almost solely on guns, because those were the lobbyists and constituents they were hearing from. Once they had my promise on the subject, the challenges to industry that I'd outlined in the book went mostly unchallenged. About nine months after the White House called to ask if I wanted the position—and that may seem like a long time to wait for confirmation, but it was actually pretty quick by DC standards—I sailed through unanimously and took up residence in OSHA headquarters within the Department of Labor's big gray building on the National Mall.

From the day of my nomination, I knew that OSHA's number one priority in the area of health protection would be strengthening the standard of allowable exposure to silica in the workplace. That may sound like a series of very technical terms; it is. But it's important. Exposure to silica takes people's breath away—literally. It is especially true for the millions of workers across the United States (not to mention the world) who are regularly exposed to these tiny crystalline particles in the course of their employment. The majority are in the building trades, where silica is ever present. That cloud of dust enveloping a worker operating a jack hammer on a roadway? Silica. Or the worker cutting bricks with a saw? Silica. Or the worker shaking the sand out of a mold in the foul air of a steel foundry? Silica. In gas and oilfield fracking operations, silica is used to keep the fissures in the shale open for the oil or gas to flow out. Granite countertops are composed of silica, and many of the new kitchen surfaces that appear to be marble are fabricated from "artificial stone," a manufactured silica composite.

The minuscule size of the silica particles is what makes them "respirable," that is, easy to breathe into the lungs, where scar tissue forms around the inhaled particles and makes breathing increasingly difficult. The damage can happen slowly over many years, or much more quickly if the exposure is greater. The ancient Romans, famous for their stonework, recognized that rock mining was causing a progressive, disabling, and often fatal disease. Today, that disease has a name—*silicosis*—and we know that it subtracts about 11 years from the life expectancy of afflicted workers. At any given time, dozens of workers are awaiting lung transplants, because their own lungs have been destroyed. Inhaled silica has also been shown to cause lung cancer and kidney disease.

But silica is only dangerous if it is inhaled. And inhalation can be prevented by vacuuming or wetting silica dust as it is released; both interventions are relatively easy and cheap. So why was strengthening the federal standard for a dangerous substance a challenge? It's because OSHA and most federal regulatory agencies must fulfill steep requirements before they can issue new or improved standards, and because the agencies lack the endless resources of the product defense industry that bombards them with uncertainty campaigns at every step.

A word first about OSHA. Most of the agency's health standards for workplace exposures to toxic substances were set in the early 1970s, when the agency was established by Congress during the presidency of Richard Nixon. The enacting legislation gave the agency permission to adopt any of industry's voluntary PELs ("permissible exposure limits") existing at the time, and that's what the agency did: they made rules to protect workers exposed to chemicals based on information provided by the chemical industry. Almost half a century later, OSHA still has PELs for relatively few chemicals—altogether about 500, compared to the many thousands that are used in commerce. And among those 500, OSHA has updated or issued new standards for 27. Yes, just 27. The agency has greatly improved the PELs for some of the important toxic substances (asbestos, benzene, formaldehyde, lead), but for the remaining 95 percent the ancient standards set up by the industries are still in effect—too inadequate, weak, and in most instances totally unreflective of the accumulating science.

Understandably, because OSHA represents the U.S. federal government in keeping workplaces safe and healthy, many responsible employers and workers think that meeting OSHA standards equates to having safe workplaces. Alas, this is incorrect. As the agency's administrator, I tried to be honest about this shortcoming, even though it was not the approach that had been taken by my predecessors. (The instinct of most agency leaders is to defend their regulations, since they are usually under attack by forces that want them to be weakened.) In speeches and interviews, I advised employers who wanted to assure the health of their employees to reduce exposure levels below OSHA's standards, because OSHA standards are not a guarantee of safety. In fact, most old OSHA standards are so weak that workers can be made sick even if they are exposed at levels permitted by the standard. One example is the chemical n-hexane, a common solvent used as a cleaning agent in the printing, textile, furniture, and shoemaking industries. For many years, it was a component of glues and rubber cement; inhale enough of it and you get high, hence the popularity of glue-sniffing. The high is in fact a toxic neurological effect, and it can cause long-term damage. OSHA's workplace exposure standard is 500 parts per million (ppm), even though the medical literature is filled with cases of symptomatic workers who were exposed at levels far *below* that standard. What's more, research from the National Institute for Occupational Safety and Health (or NIOSH, OSHA's sister agency, also created in 1971 to conduct research in workplace health and safety, but nested in the Department of Health and Human Services) has recommended that OSHA reduce its n-hexane standard by 90 percent, to 50 ppm. That the agency hasn't been able to address these shortcomings speaks to the profound lack of resources—both in funding and regulatory authority—that any OSHA administrator faces. And many workers are paying the price for our country's failure to make workplace safety and health a priority.

The 27 standards issued since 1971 are nonetheless success stories. They have no doubt saved thousands of lives, just as many thousands more could be saved by updating other standards. But OSHA cannot just look at the scientific literature and set a new standard by fiat, no matter how overwhelming the evidence. The rulemaking process is painstakingly detailed and complex. OSHA has to prove that exposure levels legal under the old standard pose a significant risk to employees and that the new standard eliminates or reduces that risk. The agency must simultaneously demonstrate that meeting a new requirement is economically and technologically feasible for most employers. Accordingly, most of the several hundred ancient PELs are going to wait a long, long time for any binding update. In my communications as the head of OSHA, I therefore advised responsible employers to voluntarily forget those old standards and look to others instead (NIOSH's, for example, or the enforceable standards set by California OSHA, since state OSHA programs can issue regulations stronger than federal ones). Online, we published an annotated list comparing OSHA standards to the stronger recommendations.[3]

The response to this transparent approach was fascinating. Many health and safety professionals thought (incorrectly) I was being courageous, imagining it was difficult to acknowledge your agency was not doing something well. It wasn't difficult at all, in fact, since the status quo was so clearly a failure. Even the chemical industry welcomed the new approach, and for good reason. The large chemical manufacturers are often sued when workers working for smaller employers are sickened by exposure to chemicals manufactured by the large companies. They benefit when exposures are better controlled by the smaller employers. Presumably a stronger OSHA standard would result in fewer workers getting sick, and therefore fewer workers filing suit against chemical manufacturers.

Talking plainly about OSHA's shortcomings was useful and probably saved some lives, but it still did nothing to solve the underlying problem that persists today: the OSHA standard-setting process is broken and desperately needs to be fixed. As far back as 1974, NIOSH (which issues recommendations but has no power to regulate) had informed OSHA that the federal silica exposure standards were out of date and needed to be strengthened. The mere existence of a PEL—the level of silica exposure that was legally permissible—wasn't enough. An effective standard would have to include requirements for engineering controls, medical surveillance, education and training, and other provisions proven to be essential in preventing work-related disease. But it wasn't until 1997, almost 25 years later, that the agency finally started work on a new standard. That embarrassing, literally injurious delay primarily reflected OSHA's lack of resources. Then an additional dozen years passed before my arrival at OSHA—another embarrassing, injurious delay that reflects the realities at OSHA during those years, the last eight of which were the George W. Bush administration. Under Bush, my immediate predecessor Ed Foulke and his boss, Secretary of Labor Elaine Chao (later the Secretary of Transportation under Donald Trump), had embraced the administration's anti-regulatory fervor and halted OSHA's work on new standards that would have protected workers from toxic exposures. During those purgatorial eight years, the agency issued exactly one health standard—for hexavalent chromium, a powerful lung carcinogen—and only because a federal court ordered it to get moving.

So by 2009, the year I was confirmed and 35 years after NIOSH told OSHA to strengthen it, the silica standard was *still* waiting for an update. It stood out as the undisputed hazard requiring immediate action by an administration that actually cared about protecting worker health. More workers are exposed to silica on the job than almost any other toxic substance, and the associated standards for it were confusing and out-of-date. (There are high levels of silica dust in mines as well, but miners are covered by a different agency—MSHA, the Mine Safety and Health Administration. MSHA's silica standard for mines was out of date as well, but colleagues there were waiting on OSHA to take the lead before beginning the difficult political work of changing the mine standard.)

————

Fortunately, the work on the OSHA silica standard did not have to wait until after I was sworn in. Not long after he was inaugurated, President Obama appointed Jordan Barab to be Deputy Assistant Secretary of Labor, and Barab ran the agency until I arrived. Barab had worked at OSHA under President Clinton and knew how much time and effort it would take to update the silica standard, so he immediately instructed the staff to open the files and start working again on the rule.

Most federal standards are deeply convoluted or oddly framed. In the case of the silica standard, its strangeness resided partly in the fact that there were *two* silica standards with *two* exposure limits: 100 micrograms per cubic meter ($\mu g/m^3$) for general industry; 250 $\mu g/m^3$ for construction work. Both numbers were based on 50-year-old scientific evidence, and the different regulations reflected an early, pre-OSHA attempt to regulate construction safety (albeit using measurement techniques that are no longer in use). Standards should not be different for different industries; inhalation is inhalation, and a construction worker can get just as sick as a foundry worker or hard-rock miner. The challenge therefore was to produce one new standard suitable for all industries. What that number would be, exactly, was a much more complicated issue.

While we've known anecdotally for centuries that silica causes silicosis, the scientific *evidence* for these health effects has grown substantially in recent years, and we now recognize that levels of exposure much lower than 250 $\mu g/m^3$, and in fact lower even than 100 $\mu g/m^3$, can cause the disease. In addition, it has become clear that silica exposure increases the risk of lung cancer. With carcinogens, there is no safe level of exposure; risk declines as worker exposure gets lower, but it probably never hits zero. If silica is a human carcinogen, then it follows that the OSHA standard should be set at the lowest feasible level.

That said, there is inherent challenge in establishing lung cancer risk in working populations. Blue-collar workers are generally more likely to be smokers than the general population, and in some cases may be exposed to other lung carcinogens, like asbestos. It took some time for the scientific literature to deal with these complications and mature. As this body of work solidified, and as more studies began to find high rates of lung cancer in silica-exposed workers, the industries with a financial stake in silica mobilized. A new entity calling itself the "Silica Coalition" swung into action to limit the perceived damage that would be inherent to new regulation. And in research conducted by historians Gerald Markowitz and David Rosner, it seems that the Silica Coalition's very reason for existence was to oppose OSHA's strengthening of the silica standard. Markowitz and Rosner revealed the group described itself as a "diverse coalition of trade associations and companies involved in the mining, processing, production, and use of silica and silica-containing materials," established in 1997 in anticipation of "OSHA rulemaking to control worker exposure to crystalline silica dust in the not-too-distant future."[4]

Operating with the financial backing of the Silica Coalition, the strategy rolled out by product defense scientists and the other usual suspects was the standard one: disparage the results of any study finding health effects associated with exposure to airborne silica. The first claim was that there really was no excess cancer risk, because older studies hadn't detected it. This was false. In science, older is generally not better, but even in the older studies there were indications of the increased lung cancer risk. (Meta-analyses, which combined data from several studies, showed the increased risk more clearly, as did evidence in animals.) On the basis of this evidence, the World Health Organization's International Agency for Research on Cancer (IARC) concluded in 1996 that inhalation of crystalline silica "is carcinogenic to humans."[5] (Three years later, the U.S. National Toxicology Program [NTP] would agree and follow suit.[6]) IARC is a premier organization referred to numerous times in these pages, and its listing of silica as a carcinogen was particularly alarming for the coalition, which promptly commissioned a paper to attempt to poke holes in IARC's methodology.[7] This was followed by a second paper, with the same lead author but who was now identified as working for the venerable product defense firm Exponent. The Exponent-authored paper claimed that IARC's science did not adequately consider the effects of smoking.[8] (In a typical-of-the-industry attempt to reduce transparency, the acknowledgment of both papers stated they were paid for by the Silica Coalition with no further explanation or identification of that organization, defeating the purpose of the disclosure requirements.)

Another industry tactic: float a more moderate conclusion. In this case, industry operatives conceded that workers exposed to silica were at increased risk of lung cancer—those studies were too convincing to deny—but claimed that the excess cancer risk was only seen among workers who had first developed silicosis (which is generally caused by much higher levels of exposure). In other words, silica exposure didn't cause cancer unless it first caused silicosis. Industry only needed to lower exposure to levels sufficient to prevent silicosis, and cancer prevention would necessarily follow.

This argument, if true, would get around the fact that carcinogens have no safe level of exposure. A key study was completed by a group of Chinese researchers plus Kyle Steenland, a distinguished epidemiologist at

Emory University. This enormous study (34,000 workers) was performed in China and found increased risk of lung cancer among nonsmoking silica-exposed workers who did *not* have silicosis.[9] This study, plus the IARC and NTP designations, should have ended the debate over silica and lung cancer. It didn't, of course. Industry still submitted the same arguments they had submitted again and again. The advantage we had at OSHA was that their rote arguments had become very easy to refute.

In preparing the proposed new rule, I testified at an oversight hearing held by the House Education and the Workforce Committee. (This is pretty standard stuff. Part of the performance of being on an oversight committee is holding hearings to let everyone know you're overseeing.) One member of the committee, Representative Larry Buschon (R-IN), a cardiothoracic surgeon, questioned me about silica and cancer relationship:

> I'm a thoracic surgeon, so I want to focus a little bit on what you said earlier as it relates to silica dust. I'm curious about your comment about silica-dust-related lung cancer, because I've been a thoracic surgeon for 15 years and I've done a lot of lung cancer surgery, and I haven't seen one patient that's got it from silica dust....I don't like it when people use buzz words that try to get people's attention, and cancer is one of those....Do you have scientific data to show the increase of lung cancer is...caused by silica dust exposure?[10]

Epidemiologists regularly have to explain to physicians, especially surgeons, that personal observations are rarely useful for understanding disease causation. But this was an extreme case. I reminded the physician congressman that simply looking at a tumor reveals nothing about its cause. When I told him about the NTP and IARC designations, he skeptically asked for more information: "Can you submit the best study that you know to the Committee so I can review that? Because I'd be interested to see that. Because again, if you look at the American Cancer Society, it's not on the top of their list."[11] As if to answer Representative Buschon, some months later the American Cancer Society's magazine aimed at physicians like the congressman (its tagline reads "A Cancer Journal for Clinicians") published a cover story titled "Silica: A Lung Carcinogen."[12]

By early 2011, OSHA's health scientists had completed a 437-page assessment of silica's health effects, going through study after study to justify many times over the case for a new PEL of 50 µg/m³. When I questioned why the review needed to include such a deep dive into the details rather than simply a reference to the various studies, the standards writers predicted (correctly) that the new standard would be challenged in court. Opponents of *any* new standard would manufacture scientific uncertainty—pull apart each cited study, attempt to magnify any inconsistencies and limitations, and claim that because each was flawed in some way, they failed in aggregate to provide evidence that the standard needed strengthening.

By discussing each study up front and in detail, the OSHA experts would be able to demonstrate that the agency understood any limitations and had accounted for them in the overall analysis. It would still not be enough to keep us out of court, because nothing would keep us out of court. That's just the way it is.

In March 2011 we submitted the first draft of the proposed new standard to the White House for review by their regulatory staff—which, no matter the administration, is always sensitive to industries' claims that regulations are overly burdensome.[13] The White House also sent the proposal out for the required interagency review, the point of which is to assure consistency: one federal agency can't issue rules that contradict those issued by another federal agency. Moreover, different agencies have different, often opposing interests that have to be reconciled. This is a strictly internal process, with officials forbidden to publicly reveal any details. I expected that our progress on the proposal would now slow down with the addition of these many more cooks in the kitchen. What happened instead was much worse: it simply stopped. It sat with the White House for a year and a half. Regularly asked by reporters about the status of the silica proposal, I generally replied that it was a lengthy and complex proposal and the review was not yet completed. This was true enough, but I couldn't divulge what was actually going on. The 2012 election was coming soon, and the election of any Republican would mean President Obama's two major first-term legislative achievements—healthcare reform (the Affordable Care Act) and financial market reform (commonly known as Dodd-Frank)—would likely be overturned. Many agency actions that were potentially controversial were put on hold until after the election. I wasn't happy, but I understood the caution. Not only did I want to protect those two major policy achievements, but I knew that if the president was not reelected, the silica proposal would be dead anyway.

After President Obama's successful reelection in November 2012, we were back in business. I received word that the president had received a full briefing concerning the 50 µg/m³ standard, including the requirement that employers use engineering controls to maintain that level, chief among them vacuuming or wetting devices on power tools and machinery. Only if these engineering controls weren't adequate could they require workers to wear respirators in addition to the engineering controls.

The president listened to the briefing and asked a reasonable question: why couldn't we just go straight to the respirators? Wouldn't they be the easiest, cheapest fix? To answer that question, I was summoned for a meeting at the White House to explain (or defend, really) our proposal. I did not expect this, but I should have. Old-timers at OSHA staff told me that White House staff working for every president since OSHA's early days had tried to push the agency into using respirators over engineering controls. (When President Carter's Council of Economic Advisors directed OSHA to prioritize respirators to prevent brown lung disease in cotton mills, Secretary of Labor Ray Marshall and Assistant Secretary for OSHA Eula Bingham threatened to resign in protest. The economists backed off.)

At my silica meeting with the White House Chief of Staff and officials from the Office of Management and Budget, I explained what we call the "hierarchy of controls," which are the bedrock of industrial hygiene and of OSHA policy and practice. The basic principle is to modify the work environment rather than the worker; the hierarchy prioritizes engineering controls over less effective personal protective equipment like respirators. All of OSHA's newer chemical standards, as well as voluntary industry consensus standards, require installation of feasible engineering controls before reliance on respirators.

I then pulled out a respirator I brought with me in a bag. I was pretty sure few if any of the White House staff had ever seen one up close. I offered any of them the opportunity to put it on—and to wear it, preferably all day—but my offer was declined. While it was sitting on the table in plain view of all participants, I presented the myriad of reasons why respirators are the last choice, not the first. First of all (and, to many outsiders, surprisingly), respirators are not nearly as effective as using vacuum or wetting devices to control dust exposure. They are hot and unpleasant, particularly if you are doing heavy work and sweating. When you are wearing a respirator, you can't talk, so communication is difficult, which is a safety hazard. Workers with serious heart or lung problems can't wear respirators safely, so OSHA requires every worker to be given a physical exam before being allowed to wear one. Some who flunked those exams would then likely be fired, unable to do the required work. And since facial hair breaks a respirator's seal, workers must be clean shaven. I didn't want OSHA to be blamed every time a worker was told by an employer, "If you want this job, you need to shave your beard."

Soon afterwards, the White House cleared our proposed rule limiting silica exposures to 50 $\mu g/m^3$ in all industry sectors. This new limit would cut the current standard for general industry (100 $\mu g/m^3$) in half and cut the construction industry's 250 $\mu g/m^3$ by a whopping 80 percent. Other proposed requirements included exposure assessment, dust control methods, respiratory protection, medical surveillance, education and training, and record-keeping.

OSHA risk assessment experts estimated that the new standard would prevent about 700 silica-related deaths and 1,600 cases of lung disease per year. The associated cost to affected industries would be around $637 million each year. This sounds like a lot of money, but for the individual employers that make up the nation's construction industry, the average annual cost would be about $1,200, and $550 for firms with fewer than 20 employees. To make the cost more palatable, OSHA staff had to get creative in developing ways for small employers to meet the proposed requirements as easily as possible. This meant first researching the exposure levels associated with different construction tasks (like cutting with a masonry saw or using a jack hammer), then putting together a matrix that told them how best to control its resulting silica exposures. Following the listed precautions would assure that the workers' exposures would be under the new PEL and therefore safe. There was precedent that indicated these new requirements would work and would not be too onerous: California has had many of the same rules in effect since 2008, including requirements for dust suppression through wetting or vacuuming when using power tools on silica-containing building materials, and many thousands of homes had been built in California with no acute hardships on the affected contractors.

By law, OSHA is not supposed to make decisions by weighing costs against benefits—which really amounts to pitting employers' costs against workers' lives lost and lungs destroyed. The reality is that no agency can issue a standard without making such a calculation, because a standard that costs more than the value of its benefits would have an extremely difficult time getting through White House review. But how do you compare dollars to lives? It is a tricky and unpleasant process. To make the calculation work, economists convert lives lost and lungs destroyed into dollars, using guidance issued and updated by the White House. At the time of the silica rule, a life was considered to be worth $9 million (in 2012 dollars); the dollar value of the prevention measures is the "benefit" in the cost-benefit analysis. As ever, the benefit needs to outweigh the cost—ideally by a steep margin.

The other unpleasant part of the process is a concept called "discounting." Because current resources can be invested and will grow with time, one dollar now is worth more than one dollar in the future; today's dollar brings the promise of three decades of compounding interest. Since lives are turned into money in this system of calculations, a life saved 30 years from now is therefore worth significantly *less* than a life saved today. But at the same time, the dollar value of life increases over time as income rises and because of inflation. This is another abstract and stark exercise for which the White House sets the parameters and conversion rates. Depending which conversions you use, the 2019 value of preventing silica from killing someone 30 years from now is between $1.2 million and $3.7 million.

In some ways, President Trump made such calculations easier by declaring that his White House is primarily interested in deregulation, which eliminates rules that are costly to industry no matter their benefits. As one of his first acts in office, Trump issued an executive order declaring that an agency wanting to issue a new rule must withdraw two existing rules whose costs had to exceed those of the new rule, no matter how many lives the old ones saved.

Working under the old system, however, President Obama's OSHA had to make a case not only for the cost-benefit, but also that the new requirements were technologically feasible and that the costs would not cause significant financial harm to any of the affected industries. Developing the evidence and documentation to meet these requirements are among the reasons it takes so long for OSHA to issue health standards. Working on the silica standard, our staff spent years doing site visits, observing how employers currently controlled silica exposure and calculating the cost of these controls. There was no moving forward to propose our new standard without a deep understanding of these issues. More than a dozen staff, plus contractors, worked for at least five years on this effort. I write this with a great deal of pride; I don't think we could have produced a more carefully conceived and executed proposal.

Applying a dollar value to the diseases prevented and the lives saved, OSHA's economists estimated the annualized benefits of the new rule to be about $5.2 billion. Matching that number against the $650 million in estimated annual costs yields a net benefit of about $4.5 billion each year.

That was a powerful, convincing number, one we believed was solid and backed by strong evidence. But we also knew that our new rule, however beneficial on paper, would entail taking on a big chunk of American industry in all 50 states. More than 2 million workers were potentially exposed to silica, and more than 85 percent of them worked in construction industries. Their working conditions would have to change. This new regulation in the workplace would be a significant new requirement on OSHA's part, I had to admit.

So in August 2013, we had our official, White House–vetted proposal for the new standard, and we braced for the next challenge: the laborious and contentious process of requesting and considering public input. OSHA has a remarkable standard-setting process that takes pains to consider both the *evidence in the record* and the public input. Any stakeholder who disagrees with the evidence in our proposed rule—our assertion that exposure to silica increases lung cancer risk, say, or our estimate of the cost of a device to keep the dust down—can challenge it at a public hearing or by submission of written comments (which will also end up in the public record). Stakeholders also have multiple opportunities to present their own evidence and arguments, and the burden is on them to do so if they want OSHA to weaken or strengthen the rule. The interested parties generally have three months to send in evidence (referred to as "comments") prior to the first official public hearing.

When I teach students in public health, I urge them to make the time to attend an OSHA standards hearing, which is the Halley's Comet of our field: it doesn't come around often (once or twice a decade), but when it does, it's something to experience. Anyone, no matter what their background or expertise, who signs up to testify at the hearing is given five minutes to speak, and then is questioned by the OSHA staffers who are writing the regulation. Any of those speakers, sitting in the audience before or after they testify, can ask questions of any other speaker, which means that you can see industry experts cross-examining those representing unions, and vice versa.

After the public hearing—which for larger standards can last for weeks—there are two additional periods in which stakeholders can submit additional data or comment on anything presented in the hearings to that point. This is followed by a long period in which OSHA staff analyze the testimony and all the comments and prepare to respond to them in the final proposal.

If everyone in the room had the same objective—truth—I would describe the process as Socratic. But everyone doesn't have the same objective. Still, anyone with a point to make can make it. With silica, we held fourteen days of hearings and kept the comment period open for almost a year. By the time all was said and done we had received more than 2,000 comments for a total of 34,000 pages of materials.

The hearings were fascinating, and sometimes dramatic. (I attended only the opening and closing sessions. OSHA's attorneys decided that I should not be present at the others, since I was the ultimate decider. If I made a comment or answered a question, this might suggest I was making decisions before all the evidence was in.)

Workers with silicosis testified about their illnesses and how it impacts their lives and those of their families. One of them was Alan White, a foundry worker from Buffalo, New York, whose lungs were so shot he couldn't walk the mile between his home and the job without stopping time and again to catch his breath. White was 47 years old. At foundries, molten metals are poured into molds lined with sand, which is then knocked off when the metal cools into the desired shape. The air at White's copper and brass plant was fouled with silica dust. He and his coworkers were offered respirators, but they rarely used them. "You didn't wear masks," White said. "You either took the heat and the dust, or you didn't work there."[14]

Not long before the hearing, White's union, the United Steelworkers, flew him to Washington to visit OSHA's offices. He was a human reminder to all of us working on the silica standard of what I tell epidemiology students: statistics are people with the tears wiped away. Working in public health, studying and writing about diseases in the comforts of an office, it is easy to forget that the effort is about trying to protect real people from workplace hazards that threaten their lives. Alan White made sure none of us forgot that lesson. We escorted him to meet the boss, Secretary of Labor Tom Perez, who had recently replaced Hilda Solis as the new secretary.

Tom Perez proudly tells any visitor to his office that he hails from Buffalo, and the two men immediately bonded over stories of their hometown, including their shared affection for the Buffalo Bills football team. Alan White's story turned Secretary Perez into our greatest proponent in the administration. "There are three things on my agenda for OSHA," he told us frequently. "Silica, silica, and silica."

After the hearings, White subsequently returned to Washington again and met with staff at the White House. After meeting him, I rarely spoke publicly about the proposed silica rule without including a reference to this gentleman from Buffalo and his silica-destroyed lungs. His story eloquently and powerfully explained the need for our standard.

Also supporting the OSHA proposal at the hearings were all manner of public health professionals, including some of the nation's experts in occupational lung disease working for NIOSH or leading academic medical centers. They testified about the scientific literature linking silica with lung disease and cancer. Labor, led by the AFL-CIO and the unions representing construction workers, brought in industrial hygienists to show how many employers were already successfully applying the measures OSHA was proposing to require. For the first time in the agency's history, non-English-speaking workers testified about the conditions under which they work, and the particular hazards facing vulnerable workers who have little voice in their workplaces.

As for industry, some employers and employer organizations (like the National Asphalt Pavement Association, which represents firms that do road construction) testified that they *welcomed* the standard. Many were already working to keep silica exposures below the proposed standard, and they didn't enjoy being at a financial disadvantage when competing with employers who put their profits above the health of their employees.

But the major players proceeded as they always do. Their campaign kicked off before the first hearing, with a *Wall Street Journal* editorial announcing that the proposed standard was unnecessary, technologically infeasible, and would cost many times the OSHA estimate.[15] At the hearings and in the submitted comments, we heard from product defense scientists who regularly defend asbestos, benzene, diesel exhaust, and a host of other toxic exposures. All asserted that only the highest levels of exposure to silica increase risk of silicosis; exposures below the old standard were completely safe; studies linking exposure and lung cancer were flawed—silica is not a carcinogen—and failed to acknowledge that only people with silicosis develop lung cancer. These hired guns were careful to avoid talking about the human costs of silica exposure.

Louis Anthony (Tony) Cox, a risk analyst and one of industry's most reliable product defense experts, spoke on behalf of the American Chemistry Council, the trade organization representing American chemical manufacturers. Cox delivered a diatribe alleging the uncertainty of all of OSHA's calculations and estimates, which is standard fare for someone working in a capacity like his. But Cox also alleged that OSHA hadn't demonstrated that exposure to silica causes silicosis—a disease that *by definition* is caused only by silica exposure.[16] Incredulous, NIOSH epidemiologist Robert Park replied, "We're not stupid," pointing out that it was "ludicrous" to question this relationship, since there are numerous studies showing that silica causes silicosis.[17] (Later, under President Trump, Cox was appointed to chair the EPA's Clean Air Scientific Advisory Committee, which helps EPA assess

the science underpinning the nation's most important standards protecting our lungs.[18])

Also present on behalf of the American Chemistry Council (ACC)
was an economist who, 10 years earlier, had questioned the assumptions
and data in OSHA's chromium standard (as well as several EPA standards) as part of a larger argument that OSHA had dramatically under-
estimated the costs of meeting the standard. This ACC contribution
ignored the benefits of a strengthened silica standard altogether—probably realizing that it was distasteful for some of the nation's largest corporations to argue over how many workers their product would kill—
while also claiming that the standard would cost not OSHA's $637
million, but more than $8.6 *billion* annually, with dire consequences
for the U.S. economy.[19]

In lobbying against new regulation, exaggerated claims about the
regulation's costs, while ignoring the benefits, has long been a cottage
industry. In fact, almost every new OSHA standard ends up costing far
less than industry's hysterically inflated estimates. The standards generally end up costing even less than OSHA's own estimates because new
regulations drive technological innovation, which agency economists
are not allowed to factor into their cost estimates.[20]

Every health standard OSHA has proposed over the past half-century
has been met with identical claims that it was unnecessary, infeasible,
and would cost more than estimated. None of those claims has proved
true. At the height of the AIDS epidemic, for example, OSHA issued
its blood-borne pathogen standard, aimed at protecting healthcare
workers from exposure to HIV, hepatitis B, and other blood-borne
diseases. The standard required, among other things, hepatitis B vacci-
nations for healthcare workers, "sharps" disposal containers, self-
sheathing needles, and the use of personal protective equipment like
latex gloves. The negative response from much of the healthcare
industry was vociferous. Dentists claimed they would not be able to
continue to practice dentistry if required to wear gloves and masks.
Now, the standard's requirements are old news and self-evidently good
practice. There are sharps containers in every hospital room. All dental
personnel wear gloves and masks. (Who would go to a dentist who
didn't wear gloves?) And no one remembers that the OSHA standard is
the reason.

Throughout the silica hearings, as with every new workplace exposure standard put forward by OSHA, the question of an exposure "threshold"—a level below which exposure doesn't cause disease—was key. For industry, finding such a threshold is the holy grail of standard-setting. They always manage to find one, and it is always somewhere *above* the current standard, which in turn supports their argument that there is never any reason to lower the standard or make it more protective. With silica, one threshold study proffered by the industry's witnesses was produced by Ken Mundt, another go-to specialist in product defense formerly with Ramboll Environ and now employed by ChemRisk.[21] In addition to working for the tobacco industry defendants in the case that found the cigarette makers guilty of racketeering,[22] Mundt was the epidemiologist whose work for the chromium industry purported to show that there was a threshold below which hexavalent chromium didn't cause lung cancer, meaning of course there was no need for OSHA to reduce that standard either.[23]

While citing huge costs for any OSHA standard, industries also recognize that such claims probably aren't adequate for swaying the public against regulatory standards. It is necessary, therefore, to also claim enormous job losses, since those affect workers directly, rather than executives and shareholders. New OSHA standards are always predicted to drive firms to cease operations in the United States and move them overseas, where regulation is lax. One of the fiercest opponents of the silica standard was the National Association of Home Builders (NAHB), a politically powerful lobby, with wealthy members in virtually every congressional district willing to donate to politicians who will carry their water. The homebuilders could not make the argument about jobs driven overseas, since their work is right here, so they tried to claim that protecting workers from silica exposure would increase the cost of construction so dramatically ($5 billion a year) that many projects would become too expensive, the industry would slow down, and 50,000 workers would lose their jobs.[24] At OSHA, we knew that this number was coming, as it always does, and that it would be concocted for the homebuilders' group by an economics firm paid to come up with a high estimate. And we were ready with the rebuttal. Prior to the hearing, we asked an economics group at the University of Maryland to look at the question. That academic group's investigation concluded that the proposed silica standard would actually yield a very small positive employment impact.[25]

There is a long history of industry claims that new OSHA health regulations will be job killers. The PR staffs at Washington trade associations, along with "free trade" organizations (often the same ones who defended tobacco and disparage the science around climate breakdown), are trained to label every standard as "job-killing" no matter the number of lives saved, or the fact that many standards end up *increasing* rather than decreasing employment. OSHA standards do increase costs for some firms. Accordingly, many of those firms want the standards killed, no matter how many lives are saved. But for some mysterious reason, even when the standards pass, the sky never does crash down on them. I have never heard of a single firm moving offshore to avoid OSHA. (Rather, they move primarily to take advantage of drastically lower wages.) Instead, companies end up with perfectly affordable ways to save lives, if that happens to be of any interest.

———

The evidence-gathering process around silica was long and exhausting, but very useful. The information obtained through the hearings and subsequent rounds of comments resulted in significant changes and greatly strengthened the proposal. Large teams of experts worked on draft after draft, each reviewed by OSHA's attorneys, back and forth, around and around multiple times until everyone was fine with the product. At least fifty staffers were totally committed to this process. (I thank them in the Acknowledgments.) And by then—late 2015—we were all aware of a new time constraint: if the standard was issued too close to the 2016 presidential election, and if Republicans won the presidency and control of both houses of Congress, the standard might be overturned through a maneuver called the Congressional Review Act.

In December, we sent the White House a 1,700-page draft of the final standard, which, after a few more changes, was published in the *Federal Register* in March 2016: 600 dense, small-print pages. Almost all of that material is preamble, background, and the evidence justifying the decisions we made. The actual "regulatory text"—the part that employers have to follow—is short and straightforward, altogether a few dozen pages.

And then, after the rule was issued, came the inevitable court cases that my tenured OSHA colleagues warned me would come. They came from all sides: lawsuits in which industry claimed that the new exposure limit was unsupported by evidence and that the sky will fall if the rule goes forward, and others in which worker advocates argued that components of OSHA's new standard were not protective enough.

A total of six suits were filed, each in a different federal appeals court. Such venue-shopping is something of a game: potential litigants file their cases in what they hope to be more sympathetic courts. In this instance, industry groups filed in New Orleans, Atlanta, St. Louis and Denver; the labor groups filed in Philadelphia and Washington, DC. (Labor believed the proposal did not go far enough in its requirements around medical surveillance and should include wage protection if a worker had to stop working with silica because they were already getting sick.)

With all the cases filed, a lottery assigned the case to the DC Court of Appeals. Then came the election and President Trump. The Department of Labor filed its briefs supporting the standard before the new president took office, but once Tom Perez stepped down and Alex Acosta became the new administration's Secretary of Labor, all bets were off. Other incoming cabinet secretaries had reversed positions on important legal cases. It is ugly and partisan, but it happens. (A prominent example with the Trump administration is his Justice Department's switching position on whether federal law bans sexual orientation discrimination in hiring and firing.) But Secretary of Labor Acosta respected the rule-making process and permitted the department's attorneys to defend the silica standard.

By now I was out of OSHA and back in my faculty position at George Washington University. As a civilian, I waited for the court case with great apprehension. Shortly before the day of the oral arguments before the three-judge panel, I learned that the panel's chief would be Merrick Garland—suddenly famous as President Obama's Supreme Court appointee whom Senate Majority Leader Mitch McConnell refused to consider for the ten months prior to the 2016 presidential election. He was joined by Judges David Tatel and Karen Henderson. Garland and Tatel had been appointed to the DC bench by Bill Clinton, Henderson by George H. W. Bush. The windows of my old office at

OSHA looked directly at the entrance to the courthouse where the arguments would take place. Walking through the doors I had looked at almost every work day for the seven plus years I was at OSHA, I was greeted by dozens of Department of Labor and OSHA staff who had worked on that silica rule for years or, in a few instances, decades. Sitting at the front of the august courtroom representing the Department of Labor and prepared to defend the standard were three attorneys, all young women who had been deeply involved in writing and reviewing the document. On the other side were a crowd of high-priced corporate lawyers, hired by the Chamber of Commerce, the National Association of Home Builders, much of the construction and foundry industries—men representing employers who did not want to increase protections for their workers.

In the courtroom, each set of lawyers had 30 minutes. The opponents of the rule who brought the litigation went first. Offering their initial argument was William Wehrum, who had been nominated, but not yet confirmed, to the position of assistant EPA administrator for air and radiation. Arguing against the same government he was about to join, Wehrum's job was to convince the court that OSHA's risk assessment was not supported by the evidence. First, he downplayed the risk of silica, asserting it isn't dangerous at all—it is simply dust. "People are designed to deal with dust," he told the court. "People are in dusty apartments all the time and it doesn't kill them." This was pretty unimpressive.

Wehrum went on to claim that OSHA had made mistakes in its estimates of the risk of kidney disease caused by silica. Again, strange. You could throw out the entire discussion about silica exposure and kidney disease risk without having any impact on the evidence supporting the standard. Wehrum's point was secondary at best, irrelevant at worst. After only a few minutes I was perplexed but pleased, even a little relaxed. The three judges seemed to agree with me. They asked if his complaints about OSHA's kidney disease risk assessment were the best he could do. It was. None of Wehrum's mud was sticking. The presentations of the rest of the industry team were just as weak—reiterating the same claims industry had raised in the hearings and OSHA had refuted in the final rule. The three judges made it very clear there was no need to repeat them there.

The industry attorneys were then followed by two attorneys for the labor unions. The judges seemed more sympathetic to their arguments across the board. It is widely understood that appellate judges' questions can mislead anyone trying to gauge their thinking; attempts to read their thinking based on their lines of question or demeanor don't easily foretell outcomes. But as the courtroom emptied, even the industry people acknowledged to me that only a miracle could pull this out. One even suggested they should ask for their money back from these attorneys, who had done such a poor job.

Three months later, the unanimous final decision was a complete and total victory for OSHA. Industry had raised dozens of claims, and the judges rejected every one of them. The years of diligent data collection and analysis, followed by endless writing and editing, had paid off. The opposition could not poke a single hole in our arguments. The judges did, however, rule favorably on one union assertion that OSHA failed to adequately explain why we did not provide medical removal protection, as we had done in previous standards. They sent that portion of the standard back to the agency for additional work, either to add medical removal protection for workers with early signs of lung disease or to better justify the agency's decision not to include medical removal protection.[26]

The new standard went into effect in September 2017. OSHA is now enforcing the new rules and issuing fines when it finds employers out of compliance. Two years into the new silica standard, new inexpensive construction tools with vacuum or wetting devices are flying off the shelves and are now standard equipment on construction sites. Small contractors discovered that meeting the new requirements was far easier and less expensive than they had been told by their scare-mongering trade associations. I have not seen one iota of evidence that these small additional costs have resulted in any layoffs or appreciable rises in housing prices. And in a few years, everyone will have forgotten that the *only* reason power tools on construction sites have vacuum attachments, and silica no longer threatens worker health, was the standard that OSHA issued in 2016.

Coal miners have not been so fortunate. Since 2011, thousands have developed a severe lung disease called progressive massive fibrosis, mostly from drilling in mines where large amounts of quartz rock must be drilled to get coal from poorer and poorer veins. The quartz is silica, and the effects are disastrous. As mentioned earlier, MSHA, OSHA's sister agency, planned to use OSHA's studies and analyses to issue a strengthened silica standard to protect miners. That plan hit a wall in the form of Donald J. Trump. In September 2018, the conflict between science and money at MSHA was laid out for all to see during an appearance at West Virginia University by David Zatezalo, the former coal executive and industry lobbyist appointed by Trump to run MSHA. Speaking to an audience of mining engineering students, agency employees, and industry executives and lobbyists, Zatezalo said, "You hear the phrase in health circles of 'progressive massive fibrosis,' these sorts of things.... I believe those are all clearly silica problems. Silica is something that has to be controlled."

But then immediately after his speech, when reporters approached Zatezalo, the chief could not simply say he was going to do nothing while so many miners were disabled or dying. He needed some way to justify inaction—and, as usual, scientific uncertainty was his choice. "I don't think that the science of the causation is that well-defined," he told the reporter. Asked about the clear affirmation of the link in his speech, he became defensive and replied, "No, I said I suspect silica. I didn't say it was.... I think until such time as you figure out what it is you don't really know."[27]

9

Working the Refs

HOW DO WE know if a substance causes cancer? With some difficulty. Rarely does one single study yield a result so conclusive that there is no debate. In most cases, the task of proving a substance's danger requires interpretation of lots of studies.

Two institutions lead the difficult work of evaluating the scientific literature to identify carcinogens: the International Agency for Research on Cancer (IARC) and the U.S. National Toxicology Program (NTP). Both have rigorous processes to review and evaluate the literature and make the required judgment calls. And it necessarily follows that both have been the target of highly sophisticated doubt and uncertainty attacks from the product defense industry and its corporate sponsors.

IARC is a branch of the World Health Organization and is based in Lyon, France. With a full-time staff of hundreds, it coordinates and conducts research that focuses on identifying the causes of cancer and improving its diagnosis, treatment, and prevention. As part of this work, it regularly convenes groups of expert scientists to review published studies and evaluate whether the weight of the evidence warrants labeling a given substance (or mix of substances, or environmental exposure, or even lifestyle) as a carcinogen. Since 1971, IARC panels have evaluated more than 1,000 agents and labeled more than 400 with one of three designations: carcinogenic, probably carcinogenic, or possibly carcinogenic to humans.

The National Toxicology Program (NTP) is a comparable U.S. program that is housed within the National Institute of Environmental Health Sciences (NIEHS). NTP is unusual in that its executive committee is composed of heads of other federal agencies that rely on NTP's assessments. This means that NTP's board is made up of the heads of the Department of Defense, the Environmental Protection Agency, the Food and Drug Administration (FDA), the National Cancer Institute, the Consumer Product Safety Commission, and the Occupational Safety and Health Administration. (I served as chair of the NTP executive committee for more than five years while I ran OSHA.)

In 1978, while Jimmy Carter was president, Congress passed legislation requiring the NTP to publish the *Report on Carcinogens*, an annual update on substances either "known to be human carcinogens" or "may reasonably be anticipated to be human carcinogens," and to which a significant number of U.S. residents are exposed. Listing in the *Report on Carcinogens* (today issued biennially) is the culmination of a rigorous process with multiple internal and public reviews of the agents nominated for inclusion.

Having government agencies label carcinogens is significant for two reasons. First, it is a vital component of cancer prevention, for the straightforward reason that many consumers will avoid purchasing products that are labeled as causing cancer (which is good). Two, manufacturers of consumer products will respond to the market dictated by consumers and will try to find substitutes for these suspect agents—which may impact their profits.

Corporations do not want their products labeled as cancer-causing, for obvious reasons. Accordingly, the scientific and regulatory process leading to a cancer-causing designation can quickly become contested terrain. The first instinct of many corporate executives is to deny the problem by denying the science; to do so, they engage product defense scientists and PR experts for help. Corporations, especially ones that make or market chemicals, have learned the hard way that a designation from IARC or the NTP is very bad news, so they will make great efforts to prevent it from happening.

Think of this strategy as "working the refs." In basketball, coaches storm up and down the sideline, complaining about the referee's last call with the hope of affecting the next one. The same is true in industry. Working the refs is a necessary and sometimes elaborate component of any corporate campaign to manufacture doubt and uncertainty. And it can be harassing, even suffocating, for the targeted agency.

Talc is a clay mineral that, in powder form, absorbs moisture and reduces friction. It has widespread industrial applications in the manufacture of products including rubber, paints, plastics, paper, ceramics, and
construction materials. Talc is also present in about 2,000 cosmetic
products, including antiperspirants, lipstick, and concealing makeup.
And of course, baby powder.[1]

Talc also has some issues. The presence of asbestos fibers in talc deposits has long been a public health concern. So are the fibers that are
not asbestos but have similar structure to asbestos, often called asbestiform fibers. These are also commonly found in talc deposits, and they
are also worrisome.

Talc made front-page headlines in 2018 after a jury in St. Louis
awarded $4.7 billion (yes, *billion*) to 22 women who claimed that use of
Johnson's Baby Powder contributed to their ovarian cancers. The baby
powder, an iconic American product present in many American homes,
is produced by Johnson & Johnson, headquartered in New Brunswick,
New Jersey. In the case that resulted in the large award, the primary
focus of the case was not the talc itself, but the asbestos contamination.
To many people who use Johnson's Baby Powder and other products
that contain talc, the decision, as well as the revelation of asbestos in
talc, likely came as a surprise. There had been a few previous lawsuits
from women with ovarian cancer, some finding for the women, some
for the manufacturer, but baby powder and other talcum powder products have contained no warning that these products may contain asbestos and could cause cancer.

There was a reason for this missing warning: when talc had been
under consideration for the NTP's *Report on Carcinogens*, the agency's
effort was stopped by a sophisticated product defense campaign fi-
nanced by the talc industry, including both the companies that mine
and produce the mineral and the businesses that use it in their products. The internal documents revealed in that lawsuit provide a comprehensive road map to how their strategy worked.

I had not been closely following the talc/ovarian cancer epidemiology when I received a call in early 2018 from an attorney in Houston
whom I had never met, Mark Lanier, who asked if I would testify as an
expert witness in an upcoming trial in St. Louis involving exposure to
talc. I explained that I was not up to date on the epidemiologic studies

and turned him down. Lanier then explained that it wasn't the epidemiology he wanted me to address; he wanted me to speak as an expert witness to the issue of manufactured uncertainty in general. On this subject I *am* up to date, but I turned him down again. Lanier persisted, asking then if I would object to being subpoenaed as a *fact* witness. (Expert witnesses can offer opinions; fact witnesses cannot, and must base their testimony only on personal knowledge.) Nor would I be compelled to go to St. Louis for the actual trial. Subpoenaed witnesses can't be compelled to travel, so my testimony could be filmed in Washington, DC, where I work.

Having never been a fact witness at a trial, I was intrigued, so I agreed. I had no idea what to expect. And I certainly wasn't expecting a call a few days before my testimony from Johnson & Johnson's attorney, asking what I planned to talk about. I explained what little I knew: Lanier planned to ask me questions about the product defense industry and how corporations use it to manufacture scientific uncertainty.

Arriving at the downtown Washington hotel room, I was greeted by Lanier, a team of attorneys for the defendants (Johnson & Johnson and a company that mines talc), a court reporter, a videographer, and, to my surprise, a judge from St. Louis who would preside over the testimony. After just a few minutes, I understood exactly why Lanier asked me to testify. Several of the leading product defense experts had been brought in to help defend talc, and the documents unearthed during discovery had revealed exactly how they did it. I realized that Lanier intended my testimony to demonstrate how their excellent map for the talc uncertainty campaign carefully followed the template instituted by Big Tobacco and perfected over the years by many industries—all things I had written about previously. Over the course of a few hours, I was shown many documents, including the ones I discuss below, and asked to comment on them. I was told that some of the documents were considered confidential, and I could not discuss them with anyone unless they were later used in court, at which point they would become public.

In the end, my videotaped testimony was never used. Lanier later told me he was saving it for rebuttal, when he would have the opportunity to refute the material presented by the other side. Evidently, he felt his case was strong enough, and the defense's case sufficiently weak, that he didn't need a rebuttal. He was clearly correct: the jurors awarded the plaintiffs $550 million, or $25 million to each of the women or the families of six women who had died, plus $4.14 billion in punitive damages. One juror explained the message they were trying to send to Johnson & Johnson, the only remaining defendant at that point in the trial: "We were just trying to find something they would feel." Johnson & Johnson is, of course, appealing the award.[2]

In that hotel room in Washington, I had been shown only a small fraction of the documents that entered the public record. After the trial, I asked Lanier if I could review the entire corpus that had been admitted into evidence, which he generously shared with me. Examining them was an eye-opening revelation, especially as many of the documents involved the National Toxicology Program. As noted, while running OSHA I served as the chair of the NTP's Executive Committee. After returning to academia, I was appointed by President Trump's Health and Human Services Secretary Alex Azar to NTP Board of Scientific Counselors (BSC), which provides scientific advice to the director and evaluates NTP programs (including the *Report on Carcinogens*). But, needless to say, I had never seen the secret details of a campaign like this.

In the early 1970s—before the NTP was created in 1978—asbestos had become a national concern. Much of the research on the health effects of asbestos was centered in the laboratory of Irving Selikoff at New York's Mt. Sinai Medical Center. Following Selikoff's advice, New York City's Environmental Protection Administration banned spraying asbestos to insulate buildings in 1971, part way through the construction of the World Trade Center. Around the same time, the administrator of that agency reported that Mt. Sinai had tested two brands of commercial talcum powder and found asbestos, naming Johnson's Baby Powder as one of them.[3] One of the mineralogists in Selikoff's laboratory wrote to J&J that he had found a "relatively small" amount of asbestos in its product, although he subsequently told reporters that he detected asbestos in several samples of commercial talcum powder, but not in Johnson's Baby Powder.[4] The public furor around these reports created pressure on the U.S. Food and Drug Administration, which, in addition to foods and drugs, is charged with ensuring that cosmetic products are safe. Johnson & Johnson assured the federal agency that no asbestos was "detected in any sample" of talc tested in the company's laboratories. However, this assurance neglected to mention that at least three tests conducted between 1972 and 1975 by three outside laboratories did find asbestos in talc samples from Johnson & Johnson—including one in which the lab reported the level as "rather high." In addition, Johnson & Johnson's own testing methods were not up to the task of monitoring for asbestos, as they routinely allowed trace contaminants to go undetected. Moreover, the firm tested only a tiny fraction of the talc it used in production. Eventually, the FDA decided not to issue any regulation limiting asbestos in cosmetic talc, essentially deferring the Cosmetic, Toiletry & Fragrance Association's voluntary guidelines that encouraged use of the industry's testing protocols.[5]

In 1979, OSHA's sister agency NIOSH (a research institute situated under the Department of Health and Human Services, like NTP) first nominated talc for review by the newly created NTP. Studies leading up to the NIOSH recommendation had found increased risk of lung cancer and mesothelioma—a cancer caused by asbestos—among talc miners. This was followed in 1982 by a new and very major concern: a study finding increased risk of ovarian cancer among women exposed to talc through perineal applications, or use on sanitary napkins or diaphragms.[6]

This new threat presented a significant foundational problem for Johnson & Johnson. Its Johnson's Baby Powder shapes the public's image of the firm, and it connotes a reassuring image of purity, reminding people of an earlier, less complicated time. (Few people think of Johnson & Johnson as a firm that also manufacturers drugs, including opioids, and medical devices.) The company has long contended that its baby powder is free of asbestos, and the cosmetics and personal care products industry adopted a voluntary asbestos-free standard in 1976. However, special reports published by the *New York Times*, Reuters, and *Bloomberg Businessweek* have revealed a very different story. Investigative reporters examined thousands of documents obtained through Freedom of Information Act requests or civil litigation and spoke with individuals involved in testing talc over several decades. These reports all concluded that Johnson & Johnson recognized as early as 1971 that there had been many indications that the baby powder was in fact contaminated with asbestiform particles (again, not technically asbestos, but with a similar structure). Johnson & Johnson pressured scientists conducting testing programs to report no fibers, while, in the words of the *New York Times* report, "discredit[ing] research suggesting the powder could be contaminated with asbestos."[5]

In 1987, IARC, the international agency, classified talc with asbestiform fibers as carcinogenic to humans. It did not make a designation for pure talc containing no asbestiform, saying there was not adequate evidence to make a determination.[7] (This may be moot given that asbestiform talc seemingly makes its way to market without consumer knowledge.)

That background brings us to the NTP story. In October 2000, the NTP released publicly its initial document titled the "Draft Background Document for Talc Asbestiform and Non-Asbestiform," which reviewed the evidence related to talc and cancer. Its recommendation: designate asbestiform talc as a human carcinogen and non-asbestiform talc as "reasonably anticipated to be a human carcinogen." (Talc with asbestos is of course a carcinogen. This is undisputed.)

How did the NTP scientists reach these conclusions? In most of the numerous studies that found increased risk of lung cancer among talc miners, the talc they were mining included asbestiform fibers. So it wasn't possible to say definitively that talc *alone* contributed to the excess risk. And while there were a few studies of miners working in settings with no reported asbestos that also found increased lung cancer risk, those same settings also exposed the miners to silica, radon, or other carcinogens—so it wasn't possible to attribute the cancer risk to talc alone. (There was animal evidence as well, but it wasn't as powerful. The draft concluded that there were no adequate experimental animal studies involving talc with asbestiform fibers, and there was only one adequate study of rats exposed to non-asbestiform talc. That one study, however, did find increased risk of cancer in the talc-exposed rats.[8])

And then there was the newer evidence of ovarian cancer. By the time of the NTP draft in 2000, more than a dozen studies found women who used talc for perineal dusting and on sanitary napkins and diaphragms were at increased risk of ovarian cancer. On the other hand, one large prospective cohort study was negative on this issue.

Companies involved in talc production and sales interpreted the NTP's draft document as a dangerous shot across the bow. The fear it generated is captured in a presentation made by Steve Jarvis, head of environmental health and safety at Luzenac America, a branch of a French firm that was (and remains) the world's largest miner of talc and a producer of many talc products for industrial and cosmetic use.

> A listing of talc in the [Report on Carcinogens] would have devastating consequences for the talc market worldwide.
>
> First of all...we would see a virtual immediate loss of our sales to the personal care market—around $10 million in sales in the first year.
>
> Secondly...because of the carcinogenic labeling requirements, we would likely suffer a deterioration of sales in all markets...perhaps anywhere from 20% to 50% of all remaining sales by year three.
>
> Additionally, a listing in the U.S. by NTP would likely trigger a carcinogenic status for talc in Europe and the Far East.
>
> And finally...because of our consumer product exposure, civil litigation would likely skyrocket.[9]

The NTP's draft was released in October 2000. Only two months later, in December, the NTP's Board of Scientific Counselors would meet to determine whether talc should be listed for the first time in the annual *Report on Carcinogens*. So time was short—desperately so—for the industry. The Cosmetic, Toiletry & Fragrance Association (CTFA), the leading national trade association, convened a conference call in red-alert fashion to discuss how to proceed. Much of the campaign to stop the NTP designation would be coordinated through this trade association and the talc mining industry. (Of note: CTFA's longtime president, including during the years of interest here, was E. Edward Kavanaugh, father of Supreme Court Justice Brett Kavanaugh. In 2007, two years after Kavanaugh's retirement, the group changed its name to the Personal Care Products Council.)

CTFA had an existing relationship with the Weinberg Group, the product defense firm that did extensive work for the tobacco industry and other industries under duress.[10] By the time of the conference call about the talc emergency, the Weinberg Group had already submitted to CTFA a proposal to manage one component of the campaign:

reviewing the epidemiologic literature to date and finding experts who could testify against the designation at the upcoming NTP hearing.[11]

Of course, Johnson & Johnson had been defending talc, and therefore preparing for this fight, for years. Almost a decade earlier, it had hired Alfred P. Wehner, a toxicologist with experience overseeing animal studies related to talc, to counter the first studies suggesting the link with ovarian cancer.[12] Wehner was a veteran of the regulatory battles concerning second-hand smoke, and had done good work sowing doubt on behalf of American cigarette makers.[13] In 1994, six years prior to the NTP draft, he had dutifully undertaken a literature review focused especially on early talc studies and concluded that the literature "does not provide any convincing evidence that pure cosmetic talc, when used as intended, presents a health risk to the human consumer."[14]

In 2000, Wehner reprised his work for talc interests, trashing the NTP draft on talc as "a seriously flawed, biased document."[15] Any notion that Wehner's critique was a judgment produced independently or without consideration of its sponsors is soundly disproved by the subsequent internal discussions of how it would be used.

Evidence suggests that the industry people didn't like the tone of the rebuke. One quote indicates that "Wehner's critique needs to be toned down." A Luzenac staff person did just that, rewriting and toning down parts of it, then circulated this accompanying email:

> Attached is my first go at the Introduction to the submission. It is intended to be colaborative [sic], to hint at the legal and credibility issues for NTP and to suggest a fall guy, i.e. the consultants....I expessed [sic] some concern about the strident, some might say arrogant, tone of his original essay. That document failed to convince (although we do not know if the style contributed to that) so this time I strongly recommend we turn it round into a collaborative style that puts the consultants who prepared the draft in the firing line, not the NTP and its venerable Counsellors. *The aim should be to create a reasonable doubt in their minds that they may not be acting on the best of advice from their consultants.*[16][emphasis added]

Short on time, CTFA realized it needed more effective arguments than Wehner or the Weinberg Group could supply. Smartly, it hired one of the deans of product defense, Jim Tozzi, head of an organization called the Center for Regulatory Effectiveness, or CRE. CRE's name belies its actual mission, which is to limit regulation on its corporate clients. Tozzi, a former high-level official in the Office of Management and Budget under President Ronald Reagan, had a hand in designing several pieces of legislation that enable business interests to slow regulatory efforts. When he left the government, he established a suite of consulting firms, including CRE, that worked actively with the tobacco industry to oppose the EPA's efforts to limit smoking in public places. Tozzi was instrumental in advancing one of Big Tobacco's signature efforts to tie the EPA's hands, the Data Quality Act, which permits corporations to challenge and re-analyze the data used as the basis for formulating regulations. In the battle around talc, Tozzi brought a wealth of skills and resources to CTFA and the industry's other defenders. Beyond helping them shape their technical argument, he was well connected to the George W. Bush administration, which would take over in January 2001—the month following the meeting of the NFP committee. He knew how to wield the Data Quality Act to pressure agencies to change findings to avoid a fight with the new White House.

Tozzi was a veteran of pressuring the NTP, having campaigned on behalf of the tobacco industry to block the agency from listing second-hand tobacco smoke as a carcinogen. Between that campaign and this one for talc, Tozzi was also tapped by clients who objected to the designation of the infamous chemical dioxin as a known human carcinogen. As part of that job, Tozzi and his organization CRE sued the NTP over its decision-making procedures—a subterfuge for hiding the litigation's actual sponsorship, the ever-unpopular cigarette manufacturers. The lawsuit was mostly unsuccessful (both dioxin and second-hand tobacco smoke were listed as known human carcinogens), but Tozzi did succeed in exposing a vulnerability of NTP's: lawsuits and judicial review, which under-resourced, under-lawyered agencies of its kind generally try to avoid.[17]

At $12,000 per month, Tozzi and his CRE team didn't come cheaply for the talc companies.[18] Some payments went to another of Tozzi's consultancy groups, Multinational Legal Services, rather than CRE, "in order to have the benefit of an attorney/client relationship" that would protect the work product from discovery in civil litigation.[19]

Tozzi and his various firms delivered for Johnson & Johnson, the talc producers, and the trade association CTFA. The consultants first formulated what was later referred to as the "fatal flaw" in the reasoning of the NTP report: In the studies that found increased risk of cancer among humans exposed to talc—either miners or talcum powder users—many of the exposures occurred long enough in the past that it was not possible to state unequivocally that the talc was free of asbestos. At the time, there were no studies that could adequately evaluate cancer risk in people whose exposure to talc only occurred after the industry started policing the presence of asbestiform fibers although there are now positive studies that include women with more recent exposures.[20] However, given the absence of this evidence in 2000, Tozzi's argument was that the NTP could not meet the burden of proof to show that *non-asbestiform* talc caused cancer. Of course, this argument could only be successful if accompanied by the belief that newer cosmetic-grade talc was asbestos-free. The CTFA stressed that it was, and in doing so they had the reputational high ground. After all, the industry had imposed that voluntary asbestos-free standard in 1976. And any evidence cosmetic talc after that date was contaminated, or that the testing was inadequate, had never been made public.

Tozzi's CRE team formulated the argument and then directly communicated it in a strongly worded letter sent to the NTP before the December vote.[21] Under normal circumstances, a trade association might send a letter and argument like this one under its own letterhead. By having CRE send it, the talc trade group conveyed an additional message: we have political muscle here. NTP administrators would recognize they were essentially dealing with a street fighter who had already sued NTP once (in a mostly losing cause, yes, but one nonetheless burdensome for the agency).

Prior to the vote to list talc containing asbestiform fibers as carcinogenic in the *Report on Carcinogens*, that evidence had been reviewed by two federal scientific review groups: the NIEHS Review Committee for the Report on Carcinogens and the NTP Executive Committee Interagency Working Group for the Report on Carcinogens. The seven members of the first group had voted to designate the tainted talc as a known human carcinogen. The second group, composed of scientists from other agencies, disagreed and voted to designate talc containing asbestiform fibers as "reasonably anticipated" to be a human carcinogen. On the question of talc that does *not* contain asbestiform fibers, both groups had voted to designate it as reasonably anticipated to be a human carcinogen.

At the meeting in December 2000, representatives of the talc producers and product manufacturers focused on talc without asbestiform fibers and raised what they claimed was the "fatal flaw": In the human studies to date, it wasn't possible to know which type of talc was present. An NTP staff scientist reported that before 1976, some samples of talcum powder were found to contain up to 30 percent [asbestiform] fibrous materials. The talc produced after 1976, when the voluntary guidelines were put in place, should not contain fibers—but most studies would not have been able to actually determine that.[22] The single animal study came under attack as well: in a study done by the International Life Sciences Institute (which appears in Chapter 14) that suggested that forcing rats to inhale high doses of poorly soluble particles overloads their lungs, and the overload-induced inflammation leads to cancer—cancer they wouldn't have gotten if their lungs were not overloaded. This study has been widely used to dismiss the results of studies that find increased risk of cancer in rats exposed to these sorts of particles, and this was invoked as well.

The presentations left the members of NTP's Board of Scientific Counselors confused and overwhelmed, which was exactly the aim of the product defense strategy. The committee members could not judge which studies involved exposure to talc with asbestiform fibers and which did not. Accordingly, they voted to defer the *Report on Carcinogens* listing until the issues around exposures could be clarified. As Luzenac America executive Rich Zazenski summarized the meeting: "We (the talc industry) dodged a bullet in December based entirely on the confusion over the definition issue."[23] He gave credit where credit was due: "CRE was instrumental in helping divert an almost guaranteed listing for talc into a deferral."[24]

In recounting the factors that led to their success, Steve Jarvis, head of environmental health and safety at Luzenac America (and the same person who warned of "devastating consequences" after reading the draft NTP report), called CRE the industry's "secret weapon." The industry had "decided to be aggressive. This was a fight we simply could not lose. As such, we retained expert legal counsel to ensure we would have a solid foundation for a legal challenge if necessary . . . it was the same firm which assisted CRE in their court battle with NTP . . . and we also became very aggressive in our communication with NTP and other federal agencies. When [sic] didn't let the windows of 'formal comment periods' become restrictive. We sent e-mails, faxes, overnight letters, and even telephones calls to key players in this battle right up until hours before the final Executive Committee meeting." [ellipses in original][25]

The NTP's deferral of its consideration of talc as a carcinogen was not a final decision. Zazenski recognized that the doubt his consultants had generated might not last. He wrote that "given the issue at hand, the Draft report can be amended to remove the 'fatal flaw assumptions' by accounting for the ambiguities surrounding the content of body powders prior to 1976 in a different context. Essentially, if the report were to be rewritten to state that the possibility of asbestos contamination of cosmetic talc prior to 1976 should simply be accounted for as an additional 'confounding' factor in the epidemiology studies, a re-vote for 'talc not containing asbestos fibers' would likely go the other way."[26]

Jim Tozzi agreed. According to Zazenski's account of an in-house meeting held soon after the big NTP meeting, the CRE product defense wizard warned that the talc industry advocates should "not get too confident just yet." He then laid out a set of very specific actions meant to ensure that talc would *not* return to NTP's agenda. He explained that "for the most part, these agency heads do not attend the meeting themselves, but send alternates in their place. Therefore, some lower ranking agency person (who knows nothing about the substances being reviewed) is voting on the recommendation" . . . "Tozzi recommended that over the coming months, we target specific individuals at each of the agencies on the Executive Committee who might likely be the attendees for the talc review. Then we select an issue which we want that particular individual to become familiar with before the committee meeting. For example, we target individuals within the FDA and the CPSC to focus on the weaknesses of the epidemiological studies. Then perhaps we target individuals at OSHA and NIOSH for pointing out the irrelevance of the NTP animal study." Tozzi also said it was time to bring political pressure, recommending the talc industry "enlist the support of senate and congressional representatives from Vermont and Montana [where talc is mined] to lobby the committee members to 'uphold the findings of the BSC Subcommittee and not allow talc to be listed.'"

In a separate and remarkable document, Eric Turner of Luzenac America explained why it was worthwhile to have Tozzi's group play an active role—rather than behind-the-scenes one—in the talc campaign. Some of the highlights:[27]

> I have no doubt that agencies like NIEHS and NTP recognize CRE for what it really is—an industry sponsored "advocate" group whose purpose is to pursue the interests of its clients. CRE is not unlike CTFA in this manner....While CRE is actively promoting the interests of talc and challenging the NTP review process, NTP does not know for sure who is sponsoring the effort....CRE can afford to be aggressive and visible in their efforts without risking credibility....Tolerance of such tactics is usually only extended to 'insiders' or 'powerful lobby groups.' It is how business is conducted in Washington....CRE has been successful because Tozzi and his network of advisors are fairly well "connected." This networking capability does not go un-noticed by political appointees' and ambitious staffers....I would strongly recommend that we continue our association with CRE in some capacity in the event NTP finds cause to list talc as a carcinogen....I believe we want NTP to be 'looking over their shoulder' and seeing CRE is right there watching their every move until this issue is properly resolved.

Over the next few years, Tozzi and CRE kept up the pressure on the NTP, regularly conveying a message that they could inflict pain, and that the pain would disappear if the NTP dropped talc from consideration. Tozzi wrote to NIEHS Director Ken Olden, invoking the Data Quality Act and calling on the director to notify the public that "further review of the evidence has indicated that the listing is not warranted."[28] CRE also wrote to higher-ups in the Department of Health and Human Services, requesting increased scrutiny on the NTP budget: "The scientific community and [*Report on Carcinogens*] stakeholders, including government agencies with related programs, have raised serious and legitimate issues regarding the usefulness of the [*Report on Carcinogens*] program and the manner in which it is administered."[29]

Bringing out the biggest guns, the Data Quality Act challenges raised by Tozzi and CRE prompted John Graham, the head of the White House Office of Information and Regulatory Affairs (this was now the early years of the George W. Bush administration, remember), in early 2005 to send a sternly worded letter to the secretary of the Department of Health and Human Services, predictably raising concerns about NTP's *Report on Carcinogen* deliberations.[30]

At the same time, the industry paid for production and publication of more mercenary studies aimed directly at the NTP's process. In November 2001, toxicologist-for-hire Alfred Wehner submitted yet another article reviewing the talc literature to *Regulatory Toxicology and Pharmacology*, one of the peer-reviewed journals I cited in Chapter 2 as one that provides a venue for publishing some of the product defense industry's most mercenary studies. This version toned down Wehner's over-the-top earlier effort, but covered much of the same material. His title could not make its message more clear: "Cosmetic Talc Should Not Be Listed as a Carcinogen: Comments on NTP's Deliberations to List Talc as a Carcinogen." The paper makes no mention of the CTFA, which sponsored the original report, or any other organization which may have paid for the work. It was published early the following year.[31]

The talc industry's multi-front assault on regulation succeeded. While the memos show the industry recognized many weaknesses in the arguments of its various product defense advocates, the pressure they applied did confuse the NTP's Board of Scientific Counselors, first inducing them to defer their decision, and then convincing the agency to drop the matter altogether. An NTP staffer commented that his colleagues "wished the problem would just go away."[32] In 2005, it did. Talc was withdrawn from the list of substances being considered by the NTP for inclusion in the upcoming *Report on Carcinogens*. Johnson & Johnson credited the success to its collaborative work with Luzenac America and CTFA.[33]

Of course, the problem facing the industry has not disappeared. Epidemiologists around the world have focused on talc and ovarian cancer, with positive and negative studies now appearing with some regularity. The industry has continued to sponsor papers that question the relationship. The most recent meta-analyses performed by independent researchers have concluded that perineal talc use was associated with a 30 to 40 percent increased risk of ovarian cancer—small in epidemiologic terms but of huge public health significance.[34]

Much trouble would have been avoided, and perhaps thousands of cases of ovarian cancer prevented, if the firms that mined talc or used it in their products had shifted to a safer substitute after the first studies showing increased risk of ovarian cancer appeared. Simply put, this was not the finest hour of either the industry or the federal regulators. In reviewing the documents uncovered by Mark Lanier's lawsuit, it is clear that Johnson & Johnson, its trade association, and the mining companies successfully framed what should have been a scientific inquiry as if it were a criminal trial, essentially demanding proof beyond a shadow of a doubt that talc was a carcinogen. That isn't how the NTP process is supposed to work, but that was the industry's stated strategy: "Time to come up with more confusion."[35] They brought in expert strategists to shape the message and conflicted scientists to seed the literature and promote a very one-sided interpretation of the evidence. Their attorneys used attorney-client privilege to protect actions and relationships. They had no qualms about bullying the NTP staff. The regulatory process they disrupted is important to the prevention of cancer. After all, it's the only one we have. But throughout the process, the objective of these firms was not learning the truth—far from it. They wanted to defend their ability to sell a product, and no matter if it increased cancer risk.

In the spirit of equal time, I should note here that many industries try to influence NTP carcinogen designations. Virtually every NTP *Report on Carcinogens* nomination prompts affected companies and their trade associations to hire product defense experts to send in comments and come to public meetings to plead the industry's case. At the same meeting of NTP's Board of Scientific Counselors that considered talc, two trade associations representing tanning salons showed up to assert that ultraviolet radiation is not associated with increased skin cancer risk. This is a ludicrous position that no one takes seriously. And there is a long list of attempts to make similar, questionable claims to NTP. Talc is different and important because we have access to the inside story—how one well-organized industry and its product defense hires were able to bring NTP to its knees.

Recall that NTP isn't the only health agency to receive industry heat for calling out carcinogens. IARC reviews agents for their cancer risk, then publishes findings in a prestigious set of books called the IARC Monographs. The IARC labels carry all the same heft—and all the same contentiousness—as their U.S. equivalents from NTP.

Perhaps in response to ongoing pressure from the private sector, IARC has taken promising steps to insulate itself from outside influence. Previously, IARC panels included scientists who worked for the companies whose products were under review; these scientists, clearly with conflicts, had an equal vote on these issues. In 2005, responding to questions about the integrity of its work, IARC announced that scientists with "'real or apparent conflicts of interests'" would no longer serve on the panels that produce its famous monographs on the causes of cancer. These scientists, now dubbed "invited specialists," would be welcome to share their critical knowledge and experience but would not draft text or vote on the monograph's conclusions.

Progress, definitely, but still not a panacea. The corporations, even stripped of their inside men on the committee, still launch grenades at IARC, often with success.

A prominent example is glyphosate, one of the largest-selling herbicides in the world, marketed by Monsanto as Roundup and by other brand names in parts of the world. Glyphosate works by killing the grasses and leafy plants it comes in contact with—*except* those that have been genetically modified to be resistant to glyphosate. When sprayed on genetically modified crops, this chemical should kill only the weeds. Monsanto, DuPont, and a few other agribusiness firms have developed and now market those glyphosate-resistant seeds, labeled "Roundup Ready" and including soybeans, corn, and cotton. The USDA reports that more than 90 percent of these crops grown in the United States are now of herbicide-resistant variety, with the value of glyphosate sales worldwide estimated to be almost $10 billion in 2020.[36] As a result of this ubiquity, all of us—consumers and especially agricultural workers—have some glyphosate exposure. Clearly, determining the human toxicity of glyphosate is a most pressing question.

In 2014, IARC announced that it planned to convene a panel of experts to review the published evidence to date on the carcinogenicity of a group of pesticides, including glyphosate. That triggered a secret initiative by Monsanto, outlined in a memo titled "IARC Carcinogen Rating of Glyphosate Preparedness and Engagement Plan." This plan included the familiar trappings of product defense: first the rapid production of three new papers on glyphosate "focused on epidemiology and toxicology," supplemented with a strategic communications effort to "amplify existing studies and new papers." Compared to the defiant tone of the internal communications around talc, the tenor of Monsanto's memo is noticeably more practical, even defeatist: there is hope to affect IARC's decision in favor of glyphosate's safety, but only faint. The plan is largely centered on what the company will do *after* IARC labels glyphosate a human carcinogen, including outlining how Monsanto will "Orchestrate Outcry with IARC Decision." It anticipated the need to "provide cover for regulatory agencies to continue making re-registration decisions based on science." It would use sympathetic scientists, front groups, and trade associations to shape public opinion and pressure regulators to "remain focused on the science, not the politically charged decision by IARC." Monsanto focused on devaluing the decision and portraying it as political, not scientific.[37]

Early in 2015, as Monsanto expected, the IARC panel did classify glyphosate as a "probable" human carcinogen, based on "limited" human evidence but "sufficient" evidence from studies of laboratory animals.[38] Monsanto's plan for response was implemented immediately. It has been the subject of in-depth reporting by, among others, Carey Gillam in the United States[39] and Stéphane Horel and Stéphane Foucart in France.[40]

The Monsanto response was also the subject of a 2018 report issued by the minority committee staff (that is, the Democrats) of the U.S. House of Representatives Committee on Science, Space, and Technology. Much of this reporting is based on the thousands of pages of documents disclosed in a series of lawsuits raised by herbicide-exposed people, including agricultural workers, who believe that glyphosate contributed to their cancers.[41]

The House minority report was triggered by an effort from Republican leadership to pressure IARC to revise its designation. Before they were voted out of power in the 2018 midterm elections, Republican leadership wrote several threatening letters to the newly installed IARC director, Elisabete Weiderpass, demanding the agency send a representative to answer questions about the glyphosate decision and the monograph process. These letters raised the possibility of cutting U.S. government funding for the agency and were followed by a legislative effort to actually do so.[42]

These U.S. efforts to pressure IARC backfired in the face of the remarkable findings of the House minority report. It describes the secret efforts by Monsanto and the American Chemistry Council, the industry's trade association, to villify IARC, including ghostwriting scientific papers and articles in business publications, hiring journalists to discredit the agency, establishing front groups that appear to be independent, and aggressively attempting to silence scientists who were involved in the IARC process or who have publicly agreed with the IARC conclusions.

Monsanto's campaign amounted to a full-employment program for product defense scientists, with work going to Ramboll Environ,[43] Exponent,[44] and a host of private consultants. In one instance, Monsanto brought together 16 sympathetic experts, working in four groups, to review the evidence on glyphosate's carcinogenicity. They all concluded, not surprisingly, that "the data do not support IARCs conclusion" and that "glyphosate is unlikely to pose a carcinogenic risk to humans." The paper, titled "An Independent Review of the Carcinogenic Potential of Glyphosate," was published as part of a special group of five studies (31 authors altogether), all of them minimizing risks associated with glyphosate exposure. The journal: *Critical Reviews in Toxicology*, a known haven for science produced by corporate consultants. Many of the authors had done extensive work for Monsanto, but these conflicts of interest were not disclosed. Monsanto paid the authors through a consulting firm, and when this conduit was later acknowledged, the authors claimed "Neither any Monsanto company employees nor any attorneys reviewed any of the Expert Panel[']s manuscripts prior to submission to the journal."[45]

In fact, documents from the litigation later revealed a singular *lack* of independence. Monsanto scientists were deeply involved in organizing, reviewing, and editing drafts.[46] These revelations were evidently embarrassing even for that journal, which then insisted on an extensive correction which noted the many, many ways in which the authors of the various papers are anything but independent from Monsanto.[47]

As of 2019, the data remain equivocal and the IARC designation has not changed, but we will no doubt hear more about Monsanto's never-ending uncertainty campaign. Nor will the lawsuits end anytime soon. In the first of these lawsuits to go to trial, a San Francisco jury awarded $289 million, including $250 million in punitive damages, to a school groundskeeper with non-Hodgkin's lymphoma. This was followed by a case in which the jury awarded $80 million, and then a third in which a glyphosate-exposed married couple were awarded $2 billion. In each of these cases, the judge reduced the punitive component of the award, but the total for the three still approached $200 million. The German chemical giant Bayer, which purchased Monsanto in 2018, now faces thousands of additional suits by people who believe they were sickened by glyphosate. And of course science never sleeps. The jury is still out but the studies keep coming. And while it's unclear where it will end, this is a perfect example of a fundamental principle in public health: the need to make decisions based on the best evidence available, interpreted by truly independent scientists.

10

Volkswagen's Other Bug

THE HEALTH IMPACTS of diesel engine exhaust extend far beyond miners working underground. The same tiny diesel exhaust particulates that burrow into the recesses of the lungs, along with the same collection of nitrogen oxide compounds (NOx—pronounced "knocks"), are billowed into the air wherever there's a diesel engine at work—in a commercial-trade truck, a school bus, or a diesel passenger vehicle. Whatever their source, the particulates in these diesel exhausts are known to cause cancer.

In fact, the most brazen attack on EPA diesel standards was done in the name of one company's interest in diesel passenger cars, an episode that evolved into "the Volkswagen scandal" (aka, inevitably, Dieselgate). This is a story of profound, cinematic dishonesty. While the tricks and practices revealed in the corporate fight against the science about the particulates involved statistical manipulations of existing epidemiological studies, this new story demonstrates how the ethics of testing laboratories *themselves* can be easily compromised when the checks are signed by corporate sponsors.

Dieselgate is a textbook example of the pitfalls inherent in corporate funding of scientific research—and, importantly, ethical issues around animal testing. As we'll see, it's an important litmus test for real, well-intended science versus mercenary, paid-for science: the former is increasingly sensitive to ethical issues, while the latter doesn't give a damn. After all, ethics are, by definition, never its priority.

In Europe, gasoline is taxed heavily and therefore very expensive. Diesel engines put out less carbon dioxide—a greenhouse gas that contributes to climate change—and European automakers convinced the regulatory authorities long ago to encourage the use of diesel fuel by taxing it at a lower level. The result is that diesel vehicles are the more economical choice in Europe. In the United States, where diesel isn't similarly subsidized, gas prices are far lower, and so diesel vehicles have always been less popular.

This brings us to Volkswagen Group, a multinational auto manufacturer whose executives didn't hide their ambition to become the leading auto manufacturer in the world. To do this, they needed to increase market share in the United States, where they had been relatively unsuccessful. VW's managers in Germany recognized that sales growth across the Atlantic would depend on selling reasonably priced cars that got superior mileage and were fun to drive. Rather than take the route of Toyota, which developed the popular Prius hybrid, VW believed they could achieve the same success with diesel, an older technology they understood very well.

There was only one problem: Even in small passenger cars, a big portion of diesel exhaust are the NOx compounds. These nasty molecules irritate the airways, inflame the lining of the lungs, and increase people's susceptibility to respiratory infections. They also trigger asthma attacks, which makes outdoor play dangerous for many kids. When NOx levels rise, emergency room visits and hospitalizations, especially for respiratory conditions, increase. NOx is also a precursor in the formation of smog and ozone. Exposure to these pollutants increases the risk of heart disease, stroke, and chronic obstructive lung disease. There is compelling evidence that exposure levels *below* our current standards are still causing thousands of people to get sick. The impacts are worse among the poor and vulnerable populations.[1] And as the epidemiology improves, we are seeing *new* associations; there is now pretty convincing evidence, for example, that exposure to pollution in utero or early in life is causally related to autism. Nor are the effects limited to humans. The nitrogen gases react to form acid rain, which acidifies lakes, damages trees and other flora, and corrodes outdoor surfaces—like limestone and marble buildings and monuments. And airborne nitrogen deposited in water systems can lead to dangerously polluted drinking water, as well as algae growths that endanger aquatic life.

While manufacturers of the big commercial diesels were making great strides in improving that heavy-duty technology, VW's engineers teamed with the engineers at the German manufacturing firm Bosch to improve its "light-duty" (passenger car) technology. More efficient fuel injection and advanced software produced a smoother, quieter ride, with less vibration and better mileage. Most important for the atmosphere, the smoke issuing from the exhaust pipe became less and less obvious, less and less unhealthy.

But at the same time, the Environmental Protection Agency in the United States was setting increasingly stringent emission limits for NOx. Equally challenging for diesel manufacturers, the California Air Resources Board—presiding over one of the country's largest markets for car-buying—had its own strong standards and significant penalties for breaking its rules. (In Europe, regulatory standards affecting the atmosphere are weaker than in the United States. The European Commission regulators were also strengthening their standards, but they had little teeth and the regulators had no authority at that time to issue fines for noncompliance.)

In 2008, Volkswagen rolled out a new diesel vehicle engine with great fanfare—but failed to meet the stringent new U.S. standards. Faced with pressure to make good on its technological investment, Volkswagen had an imperative to make it work.

One option was a technological fix called the Selective Catalytic Reduction (or SCR), which is essentially a filter that employs a urea-based chemical solution to trap and sequester the NOx. It would add perhaps $500 to the price of each car, and in addition motorists would be inconvenienced—they would be responsible for topping off the urea solution (a compound also found in human urine) on a regular basis.

Another option was to install the NOx trap *in tandem with* a special "defeat device"—software whose sole purpose was to detect and deceive the equipment in the authorized testing stations. When this software sensed that the car was undergoing emissions testing—situated on rollers, and with the steering wheel never turning—it would kick the pollution control system into high gear, injecting more of the urea solution into the NOx trap. Presto: The engine's emissions as measured by the testing machine would be commendably low—*forty times* lower than under normal driving conditions in the real world. Moreover, the "defeat device" program assured that the NOx trap went into action *only* during testing. It would never run down and need to be refilled.

The rest of the time, the car was a flagrant, deceitful polluter; the company was apparently willing to allow for that. (Why not run the NOx trap all-out, all the time to make the car practically pollution free? To keep the cost of the diesel cars competitive with gasoline-powered ones, VW engineers designed the emission control system to last only a few hundred miles, rather than the 120,000 required by U.S. regulation.)

I consider myself something of an expert on corporate wrongdoing, with an excess of great exhibits to choose from. But for clever, almost unbelievably reckless skullduggery, Volkswagen may claim the grand prize. Of course, their recklessness probably didn't seem so at the time. Since the cars were never tested for emissions while actually driving on a real road, the engineers who designed the software understandably thought they had little to worry about. And Volkswagen certainly didn't invent defeat devices: Many of the truck-engine manufacturers worked with similar tricks in the 1990s, varying the timing of the electronic fuel injection while the engine was being tested, thereby improving the emissions numbers. The settlement cost those firms about $1 billion, including some fines, but mostly in commitments to develop cleaner engine technologies. And they promised to never do it again.

Maybe those truck companies didn't do it again—but Volkswagen did. The company's illicit strategy worked for quite a few years. It was able to market its cars as both green and efficient, since they got terrific gas mileage. As such, VW became an exemplary global citizen, touting its commitment to sustainability. The "nonpolluting" claim was particularly important in the United States, where the price differential for diesel fuel was not as great as it was in Europe. Customers needed another reason to choose diesel, and the "green" claims provided it.

Sales boomed. Between 2007 and 2013, diesel-powered passenger vehicle sales in the United States jumped by a factor of six. In 2016, the German automaker that had first come to the world's attention with its cute, oddly shaped little Beetle (initially prized famously by 1960s hippies) surpassed mighty Toyota as the number-one car manufacturer in the world. Life was good.

Too good. Back in Europe, VW, along with other manufacturers of diesel passenger cars, was still lobbying against stronger emission standards in the E.U., an odd way for them to spend their time and money given that their cars were meeting the considerably tougher requirements in the States. A much-respected advocacy group for global clean air, the International Council on Clean Transportation (ICCT), had the smart idea of using the success of the low-pollution European diesel in the United States to leverage tougher standards for Europe. And why not? If the manufacturers had, as they claimed, perfected the technology at reasonable cost, it would be a campaign for an attainable greater good.

In 2014, ICCT hired a group at West Virginia University to find some European-manufactured diesel cars stateside, hook them up to a *portable* testing device (one that registered real-world emissions, not those of a car on rollers) and take them on the road. The researchers—grad students, actually—had to go to California to find some European diesels because none were available in their home state. By luck (the investigators' luck, not Volkswagen's), they happened to select two Volkswagens: a Jetta because it had a lean NOx trap, and the Passat, equipped with an SCR. When they then drove the diesels up and down the length of that state and around Los Angeles, the NOx readings were so high everyone thought the testing devices weren't functioning correctly. The California Air Resources Board (CARB) had a few questions for everyone involved.

This story is pretty wild, with a lot of drama, and it was dramatically laid out by *New York Times* reporter Jack Ewing in his book *Faster, Higher, Farther: The Volkswagen Scandal.*[2] Suffice to say that VW continually lied and gave evasive answers to the CARB staff that was trying to understand how these astronomical NOx emissions under actual driving conditions were so much higher than those measured in the testing stations. The VW officials, led by Oliver Schmidt, who headed its environmental and engineering operations in the United States, repeatedly claimed that the whole study was flawed, the calibrations were off, anything but the real reason—the defeat device. At one point, VW claimed to find some software problems and announced a recall to fix them. Incredibly, technicians then installed new software that actually made the cheating worse. It was an *improved* defeat device, one that better recognized when the engine was undergoing emissions testing.

By the summer of 2015, both the EPA and the California board recognized, because of the ICCT's work, that the emissions testing results didn't reflect real performance. But the agencies still could not completely understand why that was happening. Finally, the EPA pulled out its biggest stick: it threatened to deny certification of the company's 2016 model diesel autos for sale in the United States.

While VW had to reveal the defeat device and admit some culpability, it initially insisted that low-level employees were responsible; ensuing investigations made it increasingly clear that this was not true. Frustrated and increasingly convinced that officials high up the ladder at the esteemed German automaker were lying, the EPA held firm, determined to find out who the individuals were. Now facing the possibility of being unable to sell *any* cars in the United States, Schmidt, who had earlier been transferred back to Germany, returned to California and confessed to his role in the whole dirty business.

Schmidt and other VW executives had reason to believe that by confessing, their personal and corporate penalties wouldn't be too onerous. After all, the largest fine the EPA up to that time had been the $100 million levied against the Korean auto manufacturer Hyundai-Kia, for overstating fuel economy and understating greenhouse emissions. (That amount sounds punitive, but for a big company, it's not much more than a slap on the wrist.) After his confession, Schmidt returned to Germany. Believing he was safe from prosecution, he returned to Florida for a vacation with his wife in January 2007. The U.S. Department of Justice had other ideas, and Schmidt was arrested at the Miami airport on his way home. He was held without bail, eventually pleaded guilty, and in December 2017 received a sentence of seven years in prison. As I type these words, he resides in the low-security federal penitentiary in Milan, Michigan. Five other VW executives have been indicted by the United States but they are unlikely to ever see jail (unless they're dumb enough to vacation in the country where they've committed federal crimes).

When the dust from Dieselgate finally settled, it appeared that VW had installed defeat devices in about 11 million cars worldwide, including 8 million in Europe and about half a million in the United States. We know that when they were on the road, the NOx emissions belched into the air by VW's diesel cars were about 40 times higher than they were when measured with their defeat devices running, and that that extra NOx has killed people; we just don't know exactly who and how many. The best estimates indicate that approximately 1,200 people in

Europe, and 59 people in the United States, died prematurely because of the excess pollution put out by the company's cars.[3],[4] Through 2018, VW has spent more than $32 billion in criminal penalties, civil compensation, and restitution to federal and state authorities as well as consumers, and they are facing lawsuits for another $10 billion.[5] Customers have received thousands of dollars per car in compensation for a variety of losses, including the deception itself and diminished resale value.

VW also agreed to buy back 400,000 cars from U.S. customers, most of which are sitting in 37 parking lots across the country.[6] The company intends to remove the defeat device software from these cars, upgrade the emissions system with new hardware and modified software, and try to resell them over time, slowly, so as to not overwhelm the market. VW also agreed to pay a €1.2 billion fine in Germany.[7] They sold these dirty diesels globally, of course, and are being punished globally as well. VW has agreed to pay up in Canada and was forced to suspend sales in Korea for two years.[8]

VW wasn't the only European automaker that fiddled with their new diesels' software to keep emissions remarkably low during testing. The ICCT has calculated that actual on-the-road NOx emissions of most diesel cars sold in Europe are 6 to 7 times the maximum level permitted under European standards.[9] In January 2017, days before VW's huge plea deal, the EPA accused Fiat Chrysler of illegally manipulating NOx emission on more than 100,000 Jeep Grand Cherokees and Dodge Ram 1,500 diesel vehicles.[10] The French government has also begun prosecution of the automaker Renault[11] (which also manufactures Peugeot and Citroen), alleging the installation of defeat devices on almost two million diesel vehicles,[12] and both BMW and Daimler (Mercedes-Benz) cars have been accused by German authorities of doctoring their diesels.[13]

In each of these cases, the firms have denied breaking any laws. And they may be able to make a case for that, at least in Europe, where defeat devices are prohibited, except when "the need for the device is justified in terms of protecting the engine against damage or accident and for safe operation of the vehicle." There is similar language in U.S. regulations, although the implementation of those requirements differs dramatically between the United States and Europe. The Europeans have little ability to issue fines, so that route was left to the Americans, who were willing to use it—at least until President Donald J. Trump came to power.

———

I don't know of a single significant case of manufactured scientific doubt in any industry that does not also rely on product defense professionals—attorneys, mercenary scientists, and PR strategists hired to run interference, concoct science, provide cover. In the diesel car scandal, the main such facade was called the European Research Group for the Environment and Health in the Transport Sector (EUGT), a collaboration between Volkswagen, BMW, Daimler, and the engine manufacturer Bosch. It was established in 2007, likely not long after VW's engineers realized that their new diesel engines would be unable to feature both high mileage and low emissions and came up with the defeat device. As such, the European automakers' new "sound science" team was charged with "examining the effects of and interaction between emissions, air pollution, and health and to find ways of avoiding possible health consequences."[14] A more accurate description was later offered by the German news magazine *Der Spiegel*, which in its assessment of EUGT's mission called it "a joint lobby organization that was disguised as a research institute."[15]

The names and backgrounds of the group's leadership staff demonstrated that the new outfit was in no way interested in independent research. Its director, Michael Spallek, had previously spent years employed as an occupational medicine physician at Volkswagen. (He retained his VW email address, even after his move to EUGT.)[16] The results of the institute's research were accordingly one-sided. Spallek himself co-authored several of the lobby's attacks on the classification of diesel exhaust particulate as a human carcinogen, along with other pieces that questioned whether breathing diesel exhaust was even so bad for people.

The low-emission zones in cities that place restrictions on driving cars with high emissions? There's no proof they're effective, according to one study Spallek and his coworkers produced.[17] (Establishment of these urban zones is one of the most promising policies to reduce exposure to diesel emissions. Starting in Stockholm in 1996, scores of cities across Europe have designated areas limiting entrance of various vehicles depending on the pollution they cause.[18] Unfortunately, one of the first evaluations of the zones—negative, of course—was the one published in 2014 by EUGT scientists and disseminated by the industry's lobbyists and PR teams.) Nighttime noise pollution from cars? It's no problem, as long as the racket is continuous. Do diesel emissions cause cancer? Can't be proved. Also recall from Chapter 6 that Spallek's EUGT was one of the funders of the mercenary re-analyses meant to demonstrate the uncertainties of the U.S. government's study that found elevated lung cancer risk among diesel-exposed miners.[19] In addition to Spallek, other EUGT scientists also authored papers attacking the classification of diesel particulates as carcinogenic.[20]

There's a famous quote from the American writer Upton Sinclair that says, "It is difficult to convince a man of something if his salary depends on him not believing it." Psychologists label this phenomenon "motivated reasoning." Our motivations influence our reasoning. In humans, it's a hard fact of life. There is no question that being paid by a polluter (in what is probably a lucrative financial relationship) changes the way a scientist looks at the scientific literature. And maybe those scientists working for EUGT truly believed that all the studies completed by academic and government scientists were wrong—that exposure to the soot spewing out of diesel tailpipes containing dozens of carcinogens does not increase risk of cancer. Maybe. But when their research is paired with the flagrant and concurrent scam of installing defeat devices in new diesel engines, it is certainly reasonable to ask what the EUGT leadership knew. After all, it is now clear that *hundreds* of high-level executives and managers at the German automakers were aware of the subterfuge. And we now also know that even after the scandal was front-page news, EUGT scientists were doing their best to pollute the scientific literature with additional rigged studies, ones designed to make the new "clean diesel" engines look safe—even as their dangers were slowly being revealed.

Much about the VW/EUGT episode was flagrant, but one particular episode demonstrates how far at least some of the industry's collaborating scientists were willing to go to ensure that the scientific literature was polluted with phony studies exonerating diesel exhaust. It ended very badly for the company and the industry, scientifically and ethically. It's worthy of a very close look.

In 2012 the World Health Organization's prestigious International Agency for Research on Cancer (IARC) surveyed the rapidly accumulating studies around diesel exhaust and was prepared to officially label the particulates as a known human carcinogen. Several of the industry's consulting scientists (including those paid by EUGT) attended the IARC meeting where the announcement was to be made. Since IARC limits the role of scientists with conflicts of interest, these attendees were present only as nonvoting observers. These consultants had already proclaimed that any evidence linking diesel exhaust to cancer was faulty, and on the very day of the IARC announcement their employers were prepared with press releases that challenged the new rating and offered expert interviews rebutting IARC's claims to interested media. Their primary message was that the diesel engines whose exhaust was carcinogenic were the old dirty ones, not the newer ones made by modern engine manufacturers—a standard industry talking point for years.

But the automakers wanted more than a strenuous rebuttal. They also wanted a *positive* PR message. They wanted to emphasize that the new engines constituted *progress*. The U.S. corporate communications manager of VW subsidiary Audi sent an email up the chain, asking for help internally with "counter messaging."[21] And the best way to do that: a laboratory study where humans would be exposed to exhaust from the new "clean" engines to demonstrate their safety. But there was a major hurdle: The IARC classification concerned lung cancer, which develops over many years. To disprove any cancer link, a study would therefore have to give the human subjects huge doses of particulate-filled diesel exhaust and follow them for decades. The auto manufacturers didn't have time for that.

Instead, VW decided to study something more innocuous: short-term exposure to NOx emissions, which were well controlled in the new technology engines (at least when their defeat devices were operating). The original plan was to find human volunteers, put them in a chamber where they would ride stationary bicycles to increase respiration, then expose them to air mixed with diesel exhaust (with the particulates filtered out) at levels not thought to cause permanent lung damage. This might have been a reasonable study, yielding what should be an obvious and predictable result, if it had been a *true* comparison of the old (dirty) and new (cleaner) technologies.

But that was never the idea. VW executives did everything in their power to rig the results. And in doing so, at least some of their staff demonstrated a complicity with the defeat devices that were then in mass production. While VW assigned the task of commissioning and overseeing the study to the EUGT, the company was intimately involved from the start. It was their attorneys who vetoed the idea of using human volunteers on exercise bicycles, perhaps because research involving putting people in sealed chambers and then pumping in gas might bring back memories that VW, a firm whose history was so closely entwined with the Nazi regime, would prefer to forget.[22]

Plan B was to substitute monkeys for humans. Spallek, the Volkswagen physician turned EUGT's head man, reached out to the Lovelace Respiratory Research Institute, a private nonprofit research lab in New Mexico also featured in Chapter 6. In exchange for $718,572, Lovelace agreed to a study involving 10 male monkeys. The object would be to compare the effects of breathing air containing exhaust emissions from a new-technology diesel to the exhaust from an old-technology diesel. Both emission samples were diluted with filtered air. Some of the monkeys were exposed to the old engine exhaust, some to the new technology, and some to filtered air only. After each exposure, the animal would undergo medical testing, with a particular focus on the presence of any lung inflammation.

The deal between EUGT and Lovelace was signed in August 2013. From the outset, the ground rules were scientifically and ethically dubious. For starters, the contract required Lovelace to provide a final report, but also required strict confidentiality concerning the results.[23] There's precedent for why this is frowned upon: in 2001, following a series of scandals in which drug companies refused to let researchers publish findings the firms didn't want public, the editors of 13 of the world's leading biomedical journals announced they would henceforth publish only studies conducted under contracts in which the investigators are "free of commercial interest." In short, those editors would no longer accept papers presenting findings from studies such as this Lovelace one on diesel exhaust—that is, ones performed under contractual terms that allowed the sponsor to control whether the results could be published. In a joint statement in 2001, the journal editors asserted that such contractual arrangements "not only erode the fabric of intellectual inquiry that has fostered so much high-quality clinical research, but also make medical journals party to potential misrepresentation, since the published manuscript may not reveal the extent to which the authors were powerless to control the conduct of a study that bears their names."[24]

So while EUGT's deal with Lovelace was bound to raise significant ethical concerns about both parties, the eyebrow-raising didn't stop at the terms of the contract. The most impassioned reporting began with the English-language edition of *Der Spiegel* in July 2018, a year after the study wrapped up. Other newspapers followed, and their reporting focused on the problematic study design. First, these were monkeys, raising ethical issues about using nonhuman primates to test toxic exposures. Second, they watched cartoons on TV while they breathed, because the viewing calmed them down. The image of the laboratory monkeys watching TV while breathing engine exhaust makes an unforgettable impression.[25]

What the journalists could not have known is that VW and EUGT rigged the study with the default device. (This was a couple of years before that scam was discovered and revealed.) VW worked closely with Lovelace researchers to ensure that the experiment would give VW leadership exactly the result they wanted, allowing them to point to what looked like a reputable study, falsely assuring us that their engines didn't cause health damage. It did not work out as they planned.

To do this, the Volkswagen-funded EUGT had to provide the researchers with appropriate vehicles that would give the desired results. The Germans insisted that the old-technology diesel chosen as the comparison engine should not be made by a German manufacturer, because they didn't want to be associated with an admittedly dirty vehicle.[26] So they found and bought a 1997 Ford F-250 pickup truck, which by then was 15 years old. For the new engine they went with a VW diesel Beetle. James Liang, a Volkswagen engineer who helped get the Lovelace study off the ground, selected and personally drove a new red diesel Beetle from Los Angeles to the Lovelace lab in New Mexico. To make sure the defeat device was functioning to perfection and delivering the minuscule NOx emissions numbers the company needed, Liang requested that Lovelace install a signal booster to help transmit real-time data from the engine directly to him in his California office.

(This was an added cost, not to mention a wild breakdown in the wall between funder and experimenter, and Lovelace received assurance that EUGT would pay for that equipment.[27])

VW engineers also helped obtain the equipment for the study that mimicked conditions in emissions-testing facilities: wheels moving, but remaining in place, signaling to the Beetle's defeat device to kick on. Stuart Johnson, who worked with Oliver Schmidt in the engineering and environment office of the Volkswagen Group of America, and who would later replace Schmidt when Schmidt was sent back to Germany (before he was arrested at the Miami airport), picked out much of the equipment used in the testing.[28] Liang made sure it was properly installed and shipshape, most especially the defeat device, which would guarantee its NOx emissions would be tiny.[29]

This was not Liang's first experience with these sorts of efforts. He helped design VW's original defeat device software years earlier. After that triumph, he was sent to the firm's testing facility in Southern California to calibrate the defeat device sold in the States so it would recognize the U.S. test's drive cycles. His title at the company: Leader of Diesel Competence. Presumably, the scientists at Lovelace did not know about the defeat device. Presumably, they did not know that this engine's exhaust emissions were guaranteed to be very low.

The 2018 *Der Spiegel* story on the Lovelace study mentions a small-town Virginia attorney, Michael Melkersen, who was one of the many lawyers suing VW on behalf of consumers misled into purchasing cars that were heavy polluters. Before Melkersen had come across a reference to the study in one of the documents he was reviewing for the case and started to issue subpoenas for additional ones. Eventually, he took depositions of several of the actors in the drama.[30] Thanks to the unethical confidentiality clause in the contract, this story might never have seen the light of day if not for the lawsuits and, more specifically, Melkersen's digging through the evidence. The materials Melkersen uncovered document the comedy and tragedy of the ill-fated research.

Setting aside the ethical issues of using monkeys, not to mention the problematic terms of the funding and contract, the actual *design* for the study was reasonably competent. But reading through the memos and the depositions, especially those of Lovelace's lead scientist, Jacob McDonald, one can reasonably conclude that the actual execution of the study was a comedy of errors throughout. Most ridiculous were the results: even though it was carefully rigged to "prove" that the new diesel engines, such as those in the red Beetle, were exponentially cleaner than the old engines, like the one in the Ford truck, the results demonstrated just the opposite: when inhaled by the monkeys, the new Beetle's exhaust caused *more* lung inflammation than the old truck's exhaust, which was 180 times more powerful in terms of NOx exposure. This made no sense whatsoever.

By 2015, when the Volkswagen scandal was breaking and Lovelace had yet to publish anything from their study, the New Mexico researchers learned of the defeat device the same way everyone else did: in the news. As McDonald, Lovelace's lead scientist in the study, said at the time, "I feel like a chump."[29] But inexplicably, rather than just determining that their VW diesel had been tampered with and the study was therefore invalid, the Lovelace researchers *continued* with the project. EUGT made clear that it had paid good money and wanted what it had paid for, even as the walls were closing in on Volkswagen.

I've seen a lot in the product defense arena in my time. Very little compares to what is contained in the memos and drafts that were uncovered via Melkersen's subpoenas. The public likes to think that scientific research is a straightforward exercise, where the scientists accurately report their findings without shading the results. But through these documents we see how wanting to please the sponsor (and get paid) changes how the results are reported. I can imagine a little of how the Lovelace staff felt, because their world had just been turned upside down. They were dealing with two seemingly contradictory facts, *both* of which made them look like chumps. For one, they learned that the VW's NOx emission levels were fraudulently low, and their study was rigged from the start. And at the same time, the results that their execution of the rigged study produced were the opposite of what they expected: the fraudulently low levels of emissions from the new Volkswagen diesel seemed to cause more inflammation than the poison spewing from the old pickup truck.

What could Lovelace do, especially considering that EUGT was withholding $71,000 (10 percent of the contractual amount for the study) until the lab fulfilled the contract's requirements, one of which was to publish the results in a peer-reviewed journal? Well, one thing they could do, and did, was continue analyzing the data and preparing a report and abstracts, reporting with a straight face the rigged study's finding. The Lovelace staff prepared the first draft of an abstract for presentation at the Society of Toxicology's 2016 annual meeting. It ended with the statement, "Sample analysis continues but, contrary to the hypothesis, [new technology diesel] appears to have induced great inflammation by measurement of several key parameters."[31]

Perhaps recognizing this was not what the study's sponsors were looking for, someone at Lovelace suggested removing the word "great" and disguising their observation that the new engine caused more inflammation by "stating that inflammation was observed after both exposures." The final version of the abstract that appeared in the meeting's actual proceedings—the only version seen by the public—more or less gave EUGT what it wanted. The investigators dropped any mention of having even tested the new-technology diesel exhaust, reporting instead that old-technology diesel caused somewhat more inflammation than simply exposing the monkeys to regular filtered air with no exhaust at all.[32] It is hard to believe this could ever be accepted in a scientific journal; the results are painfully predictable and reviewers would correctly ask how Lovelace's Institutional Animal Care and Use Committee, which reviews studies to protect the welfare of laboratory animals, would have let this study be conducted.

The final reports Lovelace prepared for EUGT also went through a series of changes to make it acceptable to their German funders. The first draft acknowledged that the inflammation was worse in the monkeys exposed to the ridiculously low levels of NOx. The researcher who prepared it explained in an email to McDonald, "I was trying to soften the blow from the results of the study without saying it was a bad study."[33]

Nice try. When that version of the final report was shared with EUGT, the response was predictably negative. The trade group responded with a series of questions and comments that they insisted be addressed before Lovelace could be paid in full. (Along with Spallek, the board that issues these demands included several staunch diesel defenders, who individually had written several papers raising doubts about the studies linking diesel particulates with lung cancer. My favorite is entitled "The European 'Year of the Air': Fact, Fate or Vision."[34])

Did EUGT and its chief Michael Spallek know from the beginning that the Lovelace study was conducted with rigged equipment meant to produce convenient results? We don't know and no one from EUGT has been charged with any wrongdoing. But the documents show that, after the widespread rigging of Volkswagen diesels became front page news across the globe, Spallek still pressured the investigators to publish a paper making the new technology engine appear to be safe to human health. Even though the contract said that the final 10 percent would be paid on submission of the final report, McDonald explained to the contracts office at Lovelace, "We submitted this final report several months ago and they have disputed it because it did not meet their expectations in terms of outcome." In other words, EUGT was holding the $71,000 until they received the final report with the results they wanted.[35]

So what went wrong with the Lovelace test? How was it possible for the monkeys with the minuscule NOx exposure to have more lung inflammation than those heavily exposed? It may have been the decision to purchase 10 female monkeys rather than the male monkeys stipulated in the contract. From the Lovelace lab's point of view, there were practical reasons for this substitution—females are less expensive and less aggressive, therefore easier to handle—but there is also more variability in female monkeys' inflammatory lung response, especially during menstruation.[36] Alternatively, the finding may have been the result of poor execution by the investigators. For each monkey, the scientists did a baseline lung lavage—essentially washing out the lung with a saline solution to measure inflammation—the days before they were exposed to the NOx mixture. It is possible that testing after exposure measured not new inflammation caused by NOx, but inflammation triggered by the baseline examination. Whatever it was, the researchers decided the data were, in lead scientist McDonald's succinct assessment, "garbage."[37]

Garbage in, garbage out? The old saying is true and, from Lovelace's perspective, *another* reason to throw this whole thing out. Many scientists would have done just that. But in New Mexico, under pressure to modify the study's findings and prepare a manuscript for publication in order to get that final payment of $71,000, and only two months after McDonald's one-word condemnation, he wrote to EUGT's Spallek that he was modifying the final report with additional "end points where we saw the increase in 'effect' in the old technology. The endpoint a [sic] we observed are consistent with our hypothesis about diesel and lung injury."[38] (Keep in mind, this is a full year after the scandal broke.)

In other words, this was classic product defense manipulation of the raw data. Spallek approved fiddling with the data, of course, but still wanted the Lovelace team to get the results into the scientific literature before he'd cut that final check.[39] McDonald wrote to another Lovelace scientist in an email, "I need to publish a paper and basically I will have to throw out the lavage data[,] then I have three figures... and a bunch of aerosol stuff... so I am trying to see if I can squeeze out something else that may be interesting and says 'old diesel bad, new diesel good' so I can win the nobel prize. [ellipses original]"[37]

I believe we can take McDonald's Nobel Prize reference as deeply sarcastic. The final report from the Lovelace study, sent on June 30, 2017, by McDonald to Stuart Johnson at VW and Michael Spallek at EUGT, provides the opposite conclusion of the first draft. In fact, Lovelace gives VW and EUGT the conclusion they wanted from the start: "Based on the results shown here, the [old technology diesel—the 15-year-old Ford F250] showed an increase in inflammation systematically and in the lung, while [new technology diesel—the new VW Beetle] did not." The email accompanying the report included a commitment from McDonald to submit the data to the journal *Inhalation Toxicology* and requested yet again the final payment of $71,000.[40] But Lovelace was out of luck. Pilloried in the press for sponsoring the monkey study, EUGT could no longer serve a useful role for the German automaker. It was dissolved days before McDonald sent in the final version of the report, the one he thought the German automakers would find to their liking. It has never been published, beyond the misleading abstract published for the 2016 conference.

I shed no tears for Lovelace. They may have gotten a small raw deal in the end, but it also seems apparent that the principals at the lab were willing to try their best to publish misleading results in order to get their final $71,000. They did not succeed, but this episode raises important questions about testing labs in general.

When the tests with the monkeys made world headlines, animal rights groups were furious. Studies had already been done exposing human volunteers to low levels of NOx; there was no scientific need for additional studies with monkeys to learn the same thing. Executives with VW, BMW, and Daimler were shocked, *shocked* that the study even took place. Volkswagen CEO Matthias Muller called the study "unethical and repugnant."

And how about "rigged"? The monkeys had been put through an experiment with software rigged by VW that ensured a fraudulent result, even if Lovelace was kept in the dark about the emissions control deactivation in actual driving conditions. By this point in what had become the long-running VW scandal, it might have been hard to drive the company's reputation further down, but this story did so. VW apologized profusely: "Volkswagen Group explicitly distances itself from all forms of animal cruelty. Animal testing contradicts our own ethical standards." But VW wasn't blaming its executives, of course. "We ask forgiveness for this bad behavior and for the poor judgment of some individuals."[41]

Which individuals did Volkswagen mean to call out? Initially it was some junior employees at VW and Daimler, who were suspended. This maneuver comfortably shifted the blame from upper management, including those who had attended the regular EUGT meetings where the study was discussed. Subsequently, CEO Muller announced that Thomas Steg, VW's head of foreign relations and sustainability, had known about the study since May 2013 and will "assume full responsibility" for the scandal.[42] Steg was suspended from his position but was fully exonerated by a VW internal audit and returned to his post less than six months later. As the U.S. and German investigations proceeded, though, more details have emerged, contradicting VW's claims attributing the misbehavior to lower level employees. According to the U.S. Securities and Exchange Commission (SEC), then–Volkswagen CEO Martin Winterkorn and other VW executives first learned about the defeat device in 2007, before the first device was even installed. The SEC alleges they were warned that selling vehicles with these devices would be problematic for the car manufacturer if their subterfuge was discovered, but those concerns were ignored.[43]

James Liang, the engineer who wrote the original defeat device software and made sure it was working perfectly in New Mexico, was the first VW employee convicted on criminal charges in Dieselgate. In August 2017, he pled guilty for his role in the conspiracy to defraud both U.S. regulators and VW customers. The judge presiding over the case felt the extent of the fraud was so significant that, even though Liang cooperated with prosecutors to help in their case against Volkswagen (which paid $4.3 billion in civil and criminal penalties in the United States alone) and its executives, he sentenced Liang to 40 months in prison and imposed a fine of $200,000.[44] He and Schmidt will be deported to Germany when they finish their prison time.

The biggest indictment in Dieselgate came in May 2018: former CEO Winterkorn, for fraud and conspiracy relating to his role in deceiving U.S. regulators. He remains a free man in Germany.

Dieselgate has had repercussions. Claims raised since by industry scientists are now looked upon with much more skepticism. European cities, eager to rid their air of dangerous chemicals and furious at the subterfuge advanced by the auto manufacturers, are implementing or expanding the Low Emission Zones that three EUGT scientists had somewhat successfully discredited. The German city of Hamburg has now banned older diesel vehicles from much of its downtown. London, which has long had a Low Emission Zone, has announced an "Ultra Low Emission Zone" in certain urban centers.

On the other hand, the scandal did not have a huge impact on Volkswagen's overall sales. Yes, it lost its one-year reign as the world's leading automaker by volume, but it is still solidly second place. I should also note that the year VW did top the list, 2016, was *after* the scandal broke.

VW may return to its old spot as the world's leading automaker, but the sales should be only for gas and hybrid and electric cars. It is time to recognize that diesel-powered passenger cars have little future. New gas-powered engines with catalytic converters put out a small fraction of the NOx coming from even the new-technology diesel engines. The diesels simply can't be both clean and high-mileage, especially in comparison with electric and hybrid vehicles, which are getting better and cheaper. When European authorities stop subsidizing the price of diesel at the pump, there will be no reason left to purchase a diesel-powered automobile. In the United States, there's not one now.

Have I saved the best for last? Maybe. In May 2018, the same month former VW CEO Winterkorn was indicted in the United States, about three years after the dominoes started falling in Dieselgate, VW subsidiary Audi was pulled over by German regulators on suspicion of employing a *new* defeat device in some of its high-end diesel models sold in Europe, and Rupert Stadler, its CEO, was arrested the following month in connection with the earlier Volkswagen scandal. Audi accepted corporate responsibility for the illegal software and paid a fine of €800 million, or about $930 million, in civil penalties. The prosecution of the now former Audi CEO is still under way.[45]

II

The Climate Denial Machine

THE TERM "CLIMATE change denial machine" was coined by journalist
Sharon Begley in 2007, part of a sweeping *Newsweek* cover story that
shined a light on the industry of denial that now surrounds our world's
most existential threat.[1] This denial machine has been wildly successful
in stymying restorative action, even as its case against the science of
climate change becomes more desperate and fatuous by the day.

The success of the climate change denial machine may have something to do with the public vernacular. The term "climate change" has
a nonjudgmental, inoffensive tone, one that minimizes the forces that
are driving fierce wildfires, famine, and changes in ocean levels that will
soon create millions of refugees. "Change" doesn't capture what we are
witnessing; rather, it is an increasingly rapid, catastrophic breakdown of
the climate, with disastrous impacts on people and environments across
the globe.[2]

But "change" has proven a useful term for those with an interest in
suppressing public action in the midst of our climate breakdown. After
all, change isn't necessarily a bad or unnatural thing. Such was the
denial case as offered by Diana Furchtgott-Roth, formerly chief economist at the Department of Labor in the George W. Bush administration, then nominated to head the Department of Transportation's Office
of Research and Technology under President Trump. (I use this example because climate change denial is a *de facto* litmus test for Trump
appointment.) Representing the free-market think tank Manhattan
Institute, Furchtgott-Roth gave a testimony to a congressional hearing
in 2013 in which she opposed all legislative and regulatory efforts to limit
greenhouse gas emissions, including cap-and-trade, a market-based

approach that a free marketeer might actually support, if they believed that it was imperative to reduce greenhouse gas emissions.[3] Furchtgott-Roth is a labor economist with no particular expertise in climate science. But that did not stop her from asserting in 2015 that "the Earth has been warming and cooling for millennia, certainly before the Industrial Revolution. It has been steadily warming since the Little Ice Age of the 1700s. Over the past 15 years, despite increasing greenhouse gas emissions, the warming by some measures has stopped."[4]

Let's unpack this summary, and with it the persisting argument that climate *change* is somehow not cause for alarm:

Yes, the earth's temperature is somewhat cyclical. It undergoes very slow warming and cooling trends that take place over millennia. That is not what we are undergoing at present. What's happening now is a rapid spike of temperatures globally, a trend unlike anything we've seen in human history.

A common talking point for climate deniers is that this warming actually stopped in 1998—a date evidently chosen because of the record high temperatures that year. And by cherry-picking the data, it was at least temporarily a useful argument for them: 1998 saw a strong El Niño, a warm water event in the eastern Pacific Ocean, which made that year the hottest one to that date, and something of an anomaly. The next few years were slightly cooler, which made the talking point about 1998 wildly helpful and popular. But global temperatures in 2005 soon exceeded those in 1998, and global temperatures remain hotter than those of 1998. Since then, for the most part, each year has been hotter than the one before it. The seven warmest years on record have all occurred since 2010.[5] It seems that the 1998 talking point is an old habit that won't die.

Within the scientific community, there is little doubt that climate change is being driven by human caused greenhouse gas accumulation. Multiple, massive reports have been written on the subject. The overwhelming proportion of papers in scientific journals work accept this premise.[6] Most climate deniers don't even publish in scientific journals, often claiming bias against their positions. (Many others, including the labor economist Furchtgott-Roth, are operating outside their areas of expertise by even entering its public discourse.) Many of their arguments require if not torturing, then cherry-picking data. It would be laughable if it weren't so tragic.

Given all this, there is no need to dig deeper into the scientific manipulations of climate change deniers here. The science is settled, and its refutations are silly. My focus here is the other component of the efforts to manufacture and promote scientific uncertainty: the public relations efforts to convince the public that climate change is, in the words of Senator James Inhofe of Oklahoma "the greatest hoax ever perpetrated on the American people."[7]

At many scientific meetings and conferences, some experts who talk about climate breakdown believe that what we need is *more* evidence in order to convince everyone about its urgency. Conversely, I've been to other meetings with PR specialists who believe that if we can just get the *message* right—if we can make clear that climate breakdown is about more than polar bears, or if we just focus on the human health impacts— people will finally understand and embrace action. I appreciate the optimism of both groups. But new scientific and anecdotal evidence comes in all the time, different messages are floated, news stories proliferate, and none of it seems to be having much impact.

For most of the classic controversies around scientific cause and effect, the development of additional evidence *eventually* results in general acceptance of the causal relationship. Even Big Tobacco's most fervent defenders—pretty much only tobacco executives by then—finally conceded (after about half a century) that the lung cancer cases seen in so many smokers were tobacco-related. No such luck with the climate breakdown terrorists so far. "Terrorists" is a loaded term, I realize, but it's a warranted label. At one time, this small group of fringe scientists (mostly with little training in climate science) were labeled *skeptics*. But skepticism doesn't describe their views. We're no longer dealing with science, really. This is a dangerous ideology.

Prior to 1998, although the evidence was clear if you actually looked at it, it was possible for mainstream politicians to get away with dismissing the scientists who predicted that the buildup of greenhouse gases would result in significant changes in the climate. But no longer. As the weight of calamitous events and statistical evidence for global warming approaches "overwhelming" status, denial becomes harder and harder, just as it did with cigarette smoking during the second half of the twentieth century. But when we humans are threatened in our deeply held beliefs, we tend to double down on our commitment. This is what's happening now. The denial machine has successfully turned climate breakdown into a partisan political issue, and the deniers enjoy and take full advantage of the cover and comfort provided by the Republican Party. (I regret having to call out a specific political party so bluntly, but, in any honest discussion, what's the choice? It's a fact, and in my book, there are no alternative facts.)

That climate denial has become a loyalty test for GOP politicians is a relatively recent development. In the 1980s, even into the 1990s, the U.S. government enjoyed a tenuous, bipartisan consensus on the problem posed by the ever-accumulating greenhouse gases. As recently as 2000, both candidates vying for the Republicans' presidential nomination, George W. Bush and John McCain, recognized the imperative to reduce greenhouse gases. For good reason: if there were ever an instance when the precautionary principle makes sense, climate change would seem to be it. But that tentative bipartisan consensus fell apart for a host of reasons—political and cultural—and rather quickly degenerated into a no-holds-barred confrontation between an alliance of libertarian free-market ideologues funded by the fossil fuel industry and those with the temerity to suggest that factors other than that one industry's profits—public health, planetary health—should be prioritized. Opposing efforts to limit greenhouse gas emissions has become an official plank in the Republican Party platform, and dissenters are unceremoniously drummed out of the party. Remarkably, in the words of Hawaii Senator Brian Schatz, "the Republican Party is the only major political party on the planet that is explicitly dedicated to making climate change worse."[8]

In the old days of cigarette smoke and lung cancer, the broad public awareness around the issue was ahead of the game, recognizing the cancer link years before industry's scientists finally threw in the towel and acknowledged the truth. The same is not true of climate breakdown. Today a solid majority of Americans acknowledge the ongoing climate breakdown, but a substantial minority does not. These citizens deny the science behind anthropogenic climate breakdown, and like the rump group of denial experts, this cohort is locked in; while the scientific evidence increases, this cohort isn't getting much smaller.

Belief in the existence of climate change has become tribal. The issue is perceived as preeminently political, not scientific. This is evidenced by the regular invocation of Al Gore's name in conjunction with climate change. And here I'm talking about the climate changing *at all*, irrespective of causes. Thirty-five percent of Republicans believe the climate is not changing, period, compared with 2 percent of Democrats. On the flip side, 90 percent of Democrats think there is solid evidence, compared with 50 percent of Republicans. Almost four in five Democrats agree that humans are at least partially responsible for these changes, compared to only 35 percent of Republicans. These numbers have changed little over the past decade or more.[9]

How did we arrive at this dispiriting, divided state of affairs? It's pretty simple. The pseudo-scientific and political opposition to acknowledgment of climate breakdown is aligned—ideologically, tactically, and now politically—with the same gang that, for almost three-quarters of a century, has specialized in manufacturing uncertainty when it comes to the science of certain economically important issues. It is the same crowd funded by the same money employing the same tactics. They're playing a long game, and their concerted effort, funded by some of the largest corporations, wealthiest families, and most conservative foundations in the United States, has convinced a substantial and politically potent portion of Americans that government regulations of any kind are an attack on the free-market "liberty" of corporations, families, and individuals. These groups have lots of practice in this double-dealing sleight of hand, having perfected the art of manufacturing uncertainty about the *proven* dangers inherent in human exposure to things like cigarette smoke, lead paint, industrial chemicals—the list goes on and on. And now these identical strategies are being employed in what would be the obstructionists' greatest—and quite possibly most dangerous—achievement: denying and undermining the science that documents the atmospheric buildup of greenhouse gases and the impacts of this accumulation on weather and life on this planet.

Climate-breakdown denial began with and is closely linked to Big Tobacco, which in its decades-long fight to deny the link between smoking and lung cancer established both the playbook and the founding organizations for science and public relations against the public interest. The connections here comprise a long and somewhat winding road, but I want to lay out the essential elements as they have played out over the past three-quarters of a century.

The George C. Marshall Institute, named in honor of the titan of the World War II era, was founded in 1984 by three brilliant physicists— Frederick Seitz, Robert Jastrow, and William Nierenberg—all of whom had long and distinguished careers in science. They were also deeply immersed in the ideological conflicts around the Cold War, and they were vehement opponents of Soviet socialism and threats of expansion. Their visceral animosity toward the Soviet Union blended to an instinctive suspicion of anti-nuclear activists and "environmentalists" in the United States, whom the three physicists viewed as deluded do-gooders at best, socialists and Marxists at worst. In fact, the Marshall founders regarded virtually *all* claims of harmful health and environmental effects associated with pollution or toxic chemicals not just as greatly overblown, but as existential threats to free-market capitalism and the future of Western civilization. As conservative George Will described this ideology in a Washington Post column: "Some environmentalism is a 'green tree with red roots.' It is the socialist dream—ascetic lives closely regulated by a vanguard of bossy visionaries—dressed up as compassion for the planet."[10]

The three famous names on the Marshall Institute letterhead endowed any issue they addressed with a valuable patina of credibility, and the institute exploited that advantage in suppressing science they regarded as threatening. Remember acid rain, a major environmental issue in the 1970s and 1980s? Nierenberg collaborated with another physicist, Fred Singer, who was closely associated with the libertarian Independent Institute, to ensure that a presidential review panel underplayed the severity of it. The report exaggerated the uncertainties in the scientific evidence, which in turn provided the rationale to take no action to address the problem. The same thing happened with chlorofluorocarbons (CFCs) and the ozone hole, also a contentious issue of the era. The narrative that CFCs damaged the ozone layer was deemed another threat—not to the environment, but to the free-market system, and Singer was one of the headliners questioning the studies linking the two. Science historians Naomi Oreskes and Erik Conway wrote that Singer's opposition "had three major themes: the science is incomplete and uncertain; replacing CFCs will be difficult, dangerous, and expensive; and the scientific community is corrupt and motivated by self-in-terest and political ideology."[11]

In their obfuscating on acid rain and the ozone hole, the Marshall scientists and their associates contributed to delaying environmental action for only a few years. Their assertions about the uncertainty of the science and the costs of addressing the problem proved to be greatly exaggerated; their distortions of the scientific evidence were soon over-taken by an accumulation of studies and implementation of environ-mental controls that quickly reduced the problem. (Three of the authors of the disputed studies on CFCs disputed would be awarded the Nobel Prize in Chemistry in 1995.) The United States and 195 countries signed a treaty, the Montreal Protocol on Substances that Deplete the Ozone Layer, which has been remarkably effective in reducing CFC releases and protecting the ozone layer although Singer has long maintained his opposition to it.[12] And according to the U.S. State Department (on a 2018 web page that seems to have survived at least the first half of the Trump administration), the treaty is expected to contribute to preven-tion of more than 280 million cases of skin cancer, approximately 1.6 million skin cancer deaths, and more than 45 million cases of cataracts in the United States alone by the end of the century.[13]

The Marshall Institute's prevarications on acid rain and ozone never appeared in the actual scientific literature and were soon forgotten—at least by the outside world. But in the eyes of the tobacco industry, these failed campaigns amounted to dress rehearsals for the arguments and tactics they'd need in opposition to action on secondhand smoke. And the Marshall Institute had shown itself to be a useful actor.

Frederick Seitz, the most prominent of the Marshall founders, was a former president of Rockefeller University and former president of the National Academy of Sciences. He also had a side job: running a grant-making program for R. J. Reynolds Tobacco, the giant manufacturer of cigarettes. The principal goal of this program, according to numerous tobacco industry documents, was to develop "an extensive body of sci-entifically well-grounded data useful in defending the industry against attacks."[11] Seitz engaged in this work long *after* the causal relationship between cigarette and lung cancer was settled science. He would later claim that conflicting scientific points of view had deserved "equal time" in public discourse. (The "equal time" gambit is pure sophistry—but also a go-to strategy of the product defense industry, one that continues in public discourse today.)

By the late 1980s, studies increasingly showed that nonsmoking spouses of smokers were at risk of tobacco-related illnesses, and the Environmental Protection Agency moved to protect these nonsmokers from the cancer risk arising from exposure to tobacco smoke. As the government geared up to increase these public health protections, Big Tobacco mobilized its response: front groups. Front groups were organizations (or *coalitions*, or *centers*—any name that conveyed authority, with bonus points for "common sense" values) that advanced a worldview in which private industry is unfairly hampered by government regulation. It's noteworthy that even though these front groups were funded by tobacco, they never defended tobacco use per se; that train had left the station. Instead, they opposed higher taxes on cigarettes and restrictions on smoking in public areas because those regulations undermined freedom.

This approach probably wasn't going to work on its own. The cigarette manufacturers also needed to disparage the science of secondhand smoke (also discussed in Chapter 2, above), or at least raise enough questions so that the anti-tax, anti-regulatory front groups didn't have to directly defend a product that caused cancer not just among its users (who were voluntarily exposing themselves), but also to nonsmokers who happened to be nearby.

Here, the famed cofounder of the Marshall Institute was invaluable. Seitz provided the same strategic publication relations (I don't want to call it "science") that many product defense firms offer today. For second-hand smoke, it meant writing a report that disputed the EPA's approach and rejecting many of the studies the EPA considered. It didn't matter that Seitz was a physicist with no background in epidemiology; his name gave credibility to the critiques, and tobacco exploited the imprimatur to the fullest. (They also paid. The Marshall Institute did not accept money directly from private corporations, so something had to be done about that. It was Jim Tozzi, former Reagan White House official who has been a product defense consultant to many industries trying to reduce government regulation of their deadly products, who came up with the idea of having tobacco payments to Marshall pass through his own organization.[14] Tozzi's invaluable work for the talc and cosmetics industry is featured in Chapter 9.) Seitz and Fred Singer also served as scientific advisors to the tobacco-funded lobby groups, including Philip Morris's Advancement of Science Coalition and the Science and Environment Policy Project. The latter collaborated with Philip Morris's public relations firm to issue a report, *Junk Science at the EPA.*

In 2015, with all three of its principals deceased, the Marshall Institute closed up shop, but it quickly morphed into a new organization, the CO_2 Coalition.[15] The coalition's motto: "Carbon Dioxide Is Essential for Life."[16] This is true. Fire is also essential for life, but we try to control fire so it doesn't kill us. In all its guises, the denial machine's objective was and is to manufacture doubt and provide some kind of cover for the funders and the politicians. To a large extent, the machine has succeeded.

Looking back on the secondhand smoke science: none of it was junk.

The Marshall Institute's work for Big Tobacco was the blueprint for today's climate terrorists: provide scientific cover for the industry's larger efforts to oppose regulations, including taxes. Of course, calling the publications of the Marshall Institute "science" is wholly inaccurate; the organization issued technical reports filled with charts, graphs, and citations that look impressive, but few would survive peer review in an academic journal of any repute. Marshall, and the hundreds of front groups it inspired, was in the business of undercutting science.

Climate breakdown has witnessed a condensed application of the Marshall approach because oil companies, including ExxonMobil, Shell, and their trade association (the American Petroleum Institute), did much of the earliest research on it.[17] And while some of the oil giants today publicly acknowledge that anthropogenic climate change is real, they have never apologized for launching and bankrolling the deceitful organizations that have been lying about the science—and are still doing so. In many published versions of the story, ExxonMobil has been targeted as the firm most responsible for the campaign to disparage climate breakdown science. Some of that blame is earned; ExxonMobil was, until recently, the largest corporation in the world, and by virtue of being publicly traded, its behavior can be modified by the demands of its stockholders.

But it's Koch Industries, the largest privately held oil company in the world, that appears to be applying the lessons of tobacco to climate breakdown with the greatest zeal and success. Koch Industries is owned by the brothers Charles and David Koch, who, in 1983, following the proverbial "bruising" courtroom and boardroom battle, bought out their other two brothers 16 years after the death of the founding father, Fred Koch. The money that the two active brothers (along with that of the other ultra-wealthy, free-market ideologues they have recruited) have contributed to undermining climate science dwarfs that contributed by ExxonMobil. In the book *Dark Money*, journalist Jane Mayer impressively documents the Kochs' encounters with regulators attempting to protect the public from the companies' more harmful activities (from illegal benzene emissions and dumping mercury to price fixing), as well as their systematic, generously funded attacks on the U.S. system of public protections and regulation.[18]

Firsthand testimony about the Kochs' personal denial machine comes from Jeff Nesbit, who in 1993 was communications director of Citizens for a Sound Economy (CSE), a front group/"wholly owned subsidiary" of Koch Industries. Researchers at University of California–San Francisco, as well as Nesbit in his book *Poison Tea*, have shown that the tobacco industry and the Koch donor network have been the two primary funders of a local and national chain of anti-regulatory, free-market academic centers, think tanks, and "Astroturf" and "Greenwash" groups, all with names that strike similar chords: Freedom Works, Americans for Prosperity, Enough is Enough, the Coalition Against Regressive Taxation, Get Government Off Our Backs Coalition, International Climate Science Coalition, Center for the Study of Carbon Dioxide and Global Change, and countless more (see Figure 11.1). Each purports to be an independent grass roots operation or coalition, but each is in fact an instrument of one very big business—one with an operating goal of a "small government" that allows people (and corporations) to do what they want, unhindered by government regulation.[19]

The chorus of wealthy corporate entities calling for a return to liberty and small government have two goals: lower taxes and regulation for the "makers"; reduce vital safety net programs for the "takers" (to

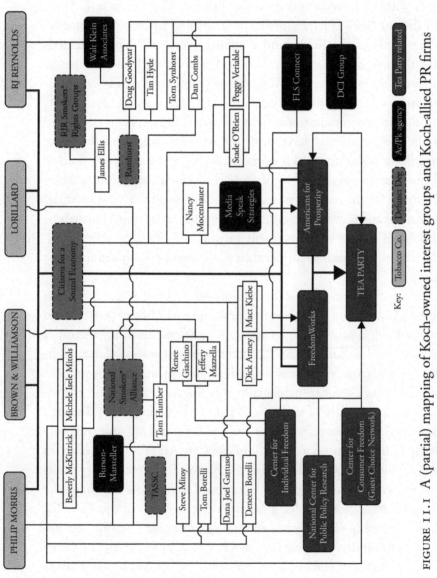

FIGURE 11.1 A (partial) mapping of Koch-owned interest groups and Koch-allied PR firms and political actors. Reproduced from A. Fallin et al., "'To Quarterback Behind the Scenes, Third-Party Efforts': The Tobacco Industry and the Tea Party," *Tobacco Control*, 24: 322-33 [2014] with permission from BMJ Publishing Group Ltd.

employ the language made famous by Mitt Romney in his 2012 presidential campaign). With climate breakdown issues specifically, the fossil fuel industry has led the fight against environmental protections, with both overt and covert campaigns to manufacture doubt and defend "the principles of free markets and limited government" in the words of one Koch-funded advocacy group.[20] Not coincidentally, these free-market principles are consistent with their efforts to maximize their own wealth. Why should these companies be prohibited from operating oil pipelines that leak, or spewing carcinogens into the air of communities around refineries? In fact, firms controlled by the Koch brothers have done all of these, and actually broke some impressive records in the process. Many of the ultra-rich funders of the free market "anti-regulatory" movement are born wealthy but think of themselves as self-made. The wealth of a substantial number of them comes from government contracts and hundreds of millions of dollars in government subsidies.[21] The hypocrisy is blatant. The money spent to further their goals amounts to something more than that.

Thanks to litigation, literally millions of pages of internal tobacco industry documents have given us a new understanding of how tobacco and the Koch family (through Citizens for a Sound Economy and other vehicles) have bankrolled and directed a powerful anti-regulatory campaign in the name of increased freedom and getting the government "off our backs". (Not coincidentally, this litigation also found the tobacco industry guilty of violating federal racketeering laws.) Through these documents, we learned that the Tea Party did *not* spontaneously spring up in opposition to the Affordable Care Act (aka Obamacare) in 2009. Philip Morris first developed the Boston Tea Party analogy for its grass roots operations in 1989 and continued to promote it through the 1990s. In 2002, Citizens for a Sound Economy started the U.S. Tea Party, registering the website www.usteaparty.com. The organization was able to suddenly appear on the scene to oppose President Obama and the Democrats years later because it had been cultivated and developed by the same corporations that had been fighting for lower corporate taxes and against regulation of tobacco and greenhouse gases.[19] All in the name of liberty.

With the repercussions of climate breakdown increasingly visible and palpable and harder to deny, the Kochs' denial machine has had to become more sophisticated. Increasingly we hear from experts, many of whom are economists, who appear to be more reasonable than the "just say no" deniers. Of these accommodationists (also sometimes called "lukewarmers"), the most famous is Danish political scientist Bjørn Lomborg. This class of gadflies doesn't outright dispute the science of climate breakdown, but does argue that the alarmists exaggerate the impacts of this change, which they claim won't be that serious. Often their commentaries focus on a need for "resilience" and emphasize what appear to be clear advantages to warming: ice-free Arctic shipping lanes, longer growing seasons in certain regions offsetting the shorter seasons elsewhere. And their main point: any costs attributed to warming will be insignificant when compared to the economic disruption and bottom-line cost of transitioning from fossil fuel combustion to an all-renewable economy.

This new lukewarmer approach monetizes the value of our planet and its human societies in their infinite wonder and variety—a calculation directly analogous to the cost-benefit analysis free-market ideologues seek to impose on every government regulation. But what are the costs associated with the impending death of the Great Barrier Reef? Is it limited to the lost income for Australia's tourist industry? What is the value of the human life lost in a flood in Boston? In Bermuda? In Bangladesh? Are they the same? As an Oscar Wilde character so famously put it, these accountants know the price of everything but the value of nothing. They are blinded by their dollars. They also generally overstate the costs of renewable energy, which is dropping fast, and would drop even faster with stronger policy incentives. Although the lukewarmers' view sounds more reasonable than the climate terrorists that came before them, it yields essentially the same position: continue our reliance on fossil fuels; better yet, *increase* that reliance. Drill, baby, drill.

Further in from this fringe ideology, some recalcitrant companies like ExxonMobil have changed the tune they sing publicly. At a recent shareholder meeting, CEO Darren Woods announced that he was "committed to being part of the solution on climate change."[22] But as ExxonMobil continues to support right-wing policy groups that deny the existence of climate change, it's fair to say that talk is cheap.[23] Sociologist Robert J. Brulle estimates that industry spent about *$2 billion* (in 2016 dollars) lobbying on climate issues between 2000 and 2016. Peak spending was in the first two years of the Obama administration—2008 to 2010—when it appeared that Congress might pass legislation helping to limit greenhouse gas emissions. That hope died with the off-year elections in 2010 (and the rise of the Tea Party, funded by Koch), so lobbying expenditures decreased accordingly.[24]

But with the rise of Donald Trump, the monster forces launched and nurtured by these industries are going stronger than ever. They have taken control of important components of the federal government. Myron Ebell, a prominent climate change denier who directed the Competitive Enterprise Institute's Center for Energy and Environment (funded by oil and coal companies), was the head of the Trump administration's EPA transition team. He was joined by two of Big Tobacco's leading operatives: Steve Milloy, purveyor of "junk science" stories related to climate breakdown, and Chris Horner, a climate change denier long associated with coal-funded think tanks. Some degree of climate denialism is very nearly a litmus test for a position of authority within the Trump administration.

In the all-out campaign that is under way to roll back the progress that has been made in the face of climate breakdown, the PR talking points are obvious: Climate change is fake news, maybe the original fake news, maybe the mother of all fake news. This argument, floated every day by the climate denialists on the payroll of fossil-fuel companies, is scientifically incoherent, but it doesn't matter. This isn't about the science; eroding trust is much more productive. As Kellyanne Conway, counselor to the president, described President Trump's decision to withdraw from the Paris Accord, "He started with a conclusion, and the evidence brought him to the same conclusion."[25]

Senator Sheldon Whitehouse (D-RI), one of the Senate's most vociferous advocates for programs to limit greenhouse gas emissions, offered a succinct explanation for why the climate breakdown denial machine has established such an iron grip on the political class of the Republican Party: "Campaign contributions," he said. And to be sure, corporate money has a lot of sway in today's politics. But it's also worth noting how the flow of corporate money, in very large amounts, has also

changed the day-to-day lives and responsibilities of politicians, especially Republican politicians. Because a small number of big donors
now in large part finance the campaigns of Republican candidates, the
party's elected representatives no longer have to spend endless hours on
phone calls begging for contributions. This funding network has made
their lives more pleasant (because they hated making the phone calls)
and their campaign treasuries richer. They speak and vote accordingly.
The party had been trending this direction for some time, but the
Supreme Court's *Citizens United* decision made it exponentially worse.
Today there are virtually no limits to a donor who wants to fund campaigns, and, because of certain IRS rulings, they can now do it without
even revealing their identity. Dark money rules. Republican politicians
who expressed concern about climate change have been treated as her-
etics by the base of the party and thrown from office. Republicans who
at one time recognized climate change as a serious problem have aban-
doned that view, at least publicly.[26] The profiles in courage are few; the
new mavericks of the GOP are those who call for civility in conversa-
tions around climate breakdown, then vote to further defund it.
Essentially, many of the same wealthy individuals and financial interests that brought us the climate denial standoff in the first place now
own the Republican Party.

Of course, they have help. The anti-science fervor among the party's
base is not surprising given that the primary sources of information are
Fox News, the Breitbart outlets, the *Wall Street Journal* editorial pages,
and other more fringe platforms, all of which are happy to provide a
platform for scientists whose work isn't good enough to appear in mainstream, peer-reviewed science journals. Why does this matter? Because
this type of unearned visibility has inestimable value, especially when
working synergistically with journalism's (misguided, in my opinion)
"both-siderism" doctrine. The media giants on the right are lockstep in
denying climate breakdown. Steve Bannon, chairman of the Breitbart
News Network before leading Trump's campaign, published pieces
calling environmentalists "greentards" and "totally fucking wrong on
climate change."[27] Rupert Murdoch's media empire, led by Fox News
and the *Wall Street Journal*, delivers the same message, but slightly more
politely. According to an analysis by the website DeSmog, 95 percent
of op-eds about climate change (287 out of 303) published by the

Wall Street Journal between 2012 and 2016 were "full of misleading and debunked denial talking points, conspiracy theories and political attacks."[28]

A stark example: Shortly before the House Science Committee held a hearing on sea level rise in 2018, the *Wall Street Journal* published an op-ed by Fred Singer (among many they've published) entitled "The Sea Is Rising, but Not Because of Climate Change." Singer is a physicist by education, a free-market ideologue, and a professional skeptic. He was vocal in his skepticism about the growing "ozone hole" in the 1970s. He was wrong about that. He was also wrong about acid rain and the effects of tobacco. That's not a good track record, but apparently nothing can thwart his regular appearances in what appear to be respectable publications.

At least Singer's op-ed acknowledged that sea levels *are* rising. This could be news for many Republicans, if not for the millions of residents of Shanghai, Dhaka, Lagos, Miami and other coastal cities where rising waters will soon exact severe consequences. At those 2018 hearings of the House Science Committee, former chair Lamar Smith (R-Oil) denied that sea levels were rising, even while at the same time entering Singer's contradictory op-ed into the record. Perhaps he felt the need to do this to counter the prior testimony of Philip Duffy, president of the Woods Hole Research Center who reported on data showing the rate of global sea-level rise is accelerating. Congressman Mo Brooks (R-AL) then also acknowledged that sea levels are rising—but declared that *rocks falling into the oceans* are a contributing factor. Needless to say, reports from this committee session triggered quite a bit of derision among actual scientists.[29]

———

With the United States pulling out of the Paris Climate Accord and President Trump and his appointees doing their best to roll back any regulation that would slow the accumulation of greenhouse gases, defending scientists and climate breakdown science has never been more important. And in spite of everything, there is reason for hope. There is a global consensus (excluding the U.S. government, of course) that greenhouse gas production must be controlled, and some progress is being made. The cost of renewable energy continues to drop, making

some of the dirtiest and most dangerous fossil fuels financially unattrac-
tive, even with Republicans' desperate efforts to subsidize the industry.
And encouragingly, more and more media outlets have stopped applying the "both sides" approach to presenting climate change stories. The
fringe deniers are quoted less, and when they are, it is common for
them to be labeled as outside the mainstream of science, or confronted
with in-interview fact checks. Reporters are also more often citing climate breakdown as a cause of the extreme weather events that are occurring with increased frequency and intensity.

As we've seen so many times, litigation and the fear of litigation has
had a positive impact on corporate behavior. Aided by research documenting the oil giants' in-house knowledge about the buildup of greenhouse gases, lawsuits demanding compensation for past damage and
financial assistance to mitigate the impact of extreme weather have
sprung up across the country. These suits may not be victorious, but as
a strategy they are powerful. Beyond even the possibility of enormous
monetary awards, these suits have terrified the companies, which quickly
recognize that in defending themselves they will have to disclose many
documents they would far prefer to keep secret. It's a story that has
played out time and again, and a reason for hope moving forward:
damning evidence of wrongdoing brought to light through litigation.
It has brought the oil industry to the negotiating table, and corporations now appear willing to accept a tax on burning carbon fuels
(including oil) in order to cease litigation and avoid further discovery.

Environmental groups are also leading consumer campaigns to pressure firms to stop funding groups that are the worst perpetrators of
climate change denial (including Heartland Institute), and to discon-
nect from the political lobbying organizations like the U.S. Chamber of
Commerce and the American Legislative Exchange Council (ALEC),
the latter a Koch-supported organization. These pressures have produced results: Apple, Levi Strauss and several utility companies have
quit the U.S. Chamber of Commerce because of that organization's
extreme position on climate change. Even ExxonMobil joined Google,
British Petroleum (BP), and Shell in abandoning ALEC over its climate
change policies. Breaking up ALEC is of great value, since it has been
central in advancing some of the most backward public policies on many
fronts, from stand-your-ground gun rights laws to cutting pensions for

public sector workers like teachers and firefighters to slashing benefits for injured workers.

On the other hand, some progress made before the election of Donald Trump has undeniably been wiped away. Many of the corporations that were moving in the right direction have reversed themselves, driven in part by the chance to boost short-term profits in a regulatory vacuum and at the long-term expense of the planet.

It is now a fact of life that destructive weather-driven events will bring tragedy to many and discomfort to countless more. Nevertheless, most climate scientists believe it is *not* too late to head off the most catastrophic effects of climate breakdown if we take immediate, drastic steps to reduce greenhouse gas emissions. But the fossil fuel industry and its closest ally and enabler—the Republican Party—continue to stymie or reverse those efforts. For those of us in the United States, the most important thing we can do is to advocate for public policies that dramatically reduce burning oil and coal. The Republican Party is the party of climate breakdown denial, and it must be routed or completely transformed for the sake of future generations.

12

Sickeningly Sweet

IN DECEMBER 1953, John W. Hill, founder of the public relations firm Hill & Knowlton, shared with his clients in the tobacco industry a brilliant and nefarious strategy to "manufacture uncertainty" about the link between tobacco and lung cancer. To do so, Hill proposed the launch of something called the Tobacco Industry Research Committee (TIRC), to be housed one floor below Hill's office in the Empire State Building, which would promise to conduct rigorous scientific research that would get to the bottom of the health effects of smoking. Less than three weeks later, on January 4, 1954, the industry went public with these plans, buying full-page ads in major American newspapers for what it labeled as a "Frank Statement to Cigarette Smokers." In addition to announcing the formation of TIRC, the industry pledged a commitment to a "research effort into all phases of tobacco use and health," to be directed by "a scientist of unimpeachable integrity and national repute. There was also to be an advisory board of scientists "disinterested in the cigarette industry."[1]

This announcement stirred the interests of one Robert C. Hockett, who had recently retired as the scientific director of the Sugar Research Foundation (SRF), the science arm of the sugar industry. The same morning that the tobacco industry's "frank statement" was announced in every important newspaper in the country, Hockett sent off a letter to the tobacco people (not even knowing the name of the most appropriate recipient). He noted that the tobacco industry had established the TIRC and pitched himself aggressively and perceptively:

> Ten years ago, a very similar industry association, the Sugar Research Foundation, Inc., was formed to investigate charges that refined sugar is a primary cause of diabetes, tooth decay, polio, B vitamin deficiencies, obesity, mid-morning hypoglycemia, and many other conditions. [...]
>
> During a period of nine years, I organized and directed research projects in medical schools, hospitals, universities and colleges which exonerated sugar of most of the charges that had been laid against it. [...]
>
> The challenge of the present situation to the cigarette industry is so similar to that which I helped the sugar industry to meet that I am tempted now to suggest that my experience and background may be useful to the new Tobacco Industry Research Committee.[2]

Hockett's letter must have reached the right department, because his offer was swiftly accepted. His job was to apply the techniques he had employed with sugar, now on behalf of cigarettes. The goal was simple: make the product look safe, or at least question the evidence that it was killing its users.

That the Sugar Research Foundation's former chief could transition so seamlessly to defending cigarettes speaks volumes of the work conducted by the SRF. And indeed, the two industries had similar histories. As documents uncovered and published in 2016 by researchers from the University of California, San Francisco (UCSF) revealed, the sugar industry ran a brilliant, secret disinformation campaign on several fronts starting in the 1950s, if not earlier.

As scientific evidence first began to link sugar with increased risk of heart disease in the 1950s, the Sugar Research Foundation reached out to nutrition scientists as part of their efforts to counter "negative attitudes toward sugar." The industry group provided nutritionists with its own counter-research, which promoted the idea that the primary culprits in heart disease were dietary fats, not sugar. (Conveniently enough, cutting fat intake would also allow everyone to consume more sugar without increasing their caloric consumption.) Although Big Tobacco is now the iconic industry for the dishonest use of science, Big Sugar's subterfuge actually predates that of the more notorious industry. It can now be plausibly argued that rather than merely imitating Big Tobacco's game plan, it was in fact Big Sugar that provided the first full-scale model.[3]

The efforts of Big Sugar also had a profound impact on the American understanding of health across the remainder of the twentieth century.

Until contrary research appeared in the 1990s, the widely accepted scientific conclusion was that fats were the primary dietary contributor to cardiovascular disease. In fact, both fat *and* sugar are culpable, but Big Sugar has spent a fortune going full bore focusing on just one of the two dietary factors. The industry has assured the public that, yes, the sugar in our diet may deliver "empty calories," but the calories are otherwise benign. Other falsehoods: Sugar doesn't cause disease; although diabetics need to cut back on sugar, sugar didn't *cause* their diabetes. Sugar certainly doesn't contribute to heart disease. And while sugar's calories do contribute to weight gain, all you need to do is exercise to burn off those calories. (None of this is true.)

The documents unearthed by Cristin Kearns and a group of UCSF researchers included the text of a speech by Sugar Research Foundation president Henry Hass before the American Society of Sugar Beet Technologists. With the title "What's New in Sugar Research," the speech announced the launch of a new public relations campaign, one spurred by the industry's stance that "(f)ear of obesity is undoubtedly the greatest single deterrent to sugar consumption." He laid out the forthcoming rebuttal clearly and identified a strategic opportunity for the industry: increase sugar's market share by getting Americans to understand that fat, not sugar, is their chief dietary enemy:

> I am unhappy about advertising which implies that sugar is in some unique sense the cause of obesity. [...]
>
> On September 21 [1953] the members of Sugar Association voted unanimously to spend $600,000 [more than $5,500,000 in 2019 dollars] per year for at least three years to tell the story of sugar in the diet....We hope that Leo Burnett [one of the leading advertising firms in the country, who later that year would be awarded the Marlboro account by Philip Morris and would go on to develop the Marlboro Man campaign] can do for sugar what has been done for meat. There will be no bunkum and no ballyhoo, only a process of presenting the facts about sugar in an interesting way. [...]
>
> You have seen our first advertisement. Factual, scientifically correct, simple and easy to comprehend, it is the prototype of many more to follow. At last people who never had a course in biochemistry are going to learn that sugar is what keeps every human being alive and with energy to face our daily problems.[4]

More than a dozen years later, in 1967, the fat-blaming initiative achieved its greatest success with a two-part review of the causes of coronary heart disease, published in the prestigious *New England Journal of Medicine*. Authored by scientists at Harvard School of Public Health, it attributed far more significance to fats than sugars in terms of increasing the risk for heart disease. In the article's fine print, funding for the study from some industry interests groups (including the Special Dairy Industry Board) was acknowledged, as was funding from some non-industry sources. The Sugar Research Foundation was absent from the list.[5] (In that not-so-distant era, conflict of interest disclosures were not required by journal editors.) Later, the financial link between the authors and the sugar industry was confirmed by the discovery of the sugar papers by UCSF researchers.[3]

These claims about the sugar industry's hidden role in cardiovascular disease research—fingering fats, exonerating sugar—and the parallels with Big Tobacco's strategy of manufacturing uncertainty made national headlines. There is some debate within the academic community whether it's fair to ascribe nefarious motives to the scientists involved, especially the high-profile Harvard team. It certainly appears, in the words of one leading nutritional expert, that the "intent of the industry-funded review was to reach a foregone conclusion. The investigators knew what the funder expected, and produced it."[6] Or, alternatively, is any accusation against the scientists an overextension of "the analogy of the tobacco industry playbook" and a failure "to assess historical actors by the norms and standards of their times"?[7]

These two views are not mutually exclusive. Big Sugar used some of the same tools as Big Tobacco. However, that does not necessarily mean that the Harvard scientists changed any of their opinions or shaded their findings to appease their sponsor. It may be that sugar's efforts played only a supporting role in attributing blame for heart disease on dietary fats. But there is little question that this is exactly what the industry tried to do. Big sugar did what tobacco did—funded a secret campaign combining mercenary science and a public relations campaign to raise doubts about the link between sugar and disease. We don't know all the details, and we don't know how much sugar learned from tobacco and vice versa. Much of our knowledge about the strategies and actions of the cigarette industry come from the literally millions of pages of documents disclosed in the giant tobacco lawsuits, and we don't (yet) have those for sugar. But there is little question that the parallels are there.

———

In addition to its misinformation about fats, Big Sugar has long proffered an idea that all calories are equal, no matter their source in the diet. In other words, as it concerns their impact on one's weight, 1,000 calories from a bucket of soda has the same impact as 1,000 calories from a meal featuring, say, fish, salad, broccoli, and fresh fruit. That's the argument. A corollary of this argument holds that increased caloric intake can be balanced by increased caloric *expenditures*, primarily through increased exercise. So, you can consume as many calories as you want, just as long as you exercise and burn away more calories than you eat.

This "energy balance" theory certainly *sounds* convincing, which is why Coca-Cola, needing something—anything—to counter the growing concern among public health experts and the public about the obesity and related epidemics, seized on it as the answer to all its PR problems. According to emails and other documents uncovered by the *New York Times* and US Right to Know (themselves a food industry research group, but funded by the organic food industry), Coca-Cola launched, funded, and provided logistical support to a nonprofit called the Global Energy Balance Network, or GEBN, which operated under the slogan "Healthier living through the science of energy balance." The uncovered documents show how an industry-sponsored nonprofit tried at great expense to shift the public's focus from the link between diet and deleterious health outcomes (obesity, diabetes) to increased exercise as the best way to address these diet-related health problems.[8]

Clearly, Coca-Cola recognized that enlisting scientists to front its ideas would be far more credible than dispensing the same claims through its PR department. To this end, Rhona Appelbaum, who in 2014 was Coca-Cola's chief health and science officer, sent a proposal to a small group of academic scientists describing how GEBN envisioned a concerted campaign to take on "the most extreme public health experts" who advocate "stronger regulation on specific foods." No doubt referring to her employer, she decried the academics who cast "particular food companies as the villain, even likening them to tobacco companies."

Appelbaum's solution: throw money at this problem. GEBN's $20 million endowment would promote new research supporting the hypothesis that reducing caloric input was not necessary to tackle obesity. The campaign's "consistent message" would emphasize that "an energy balance framework is the only framework that makes sense in addressing obesity."[9]

To get this slippery ball rolling, Coca-Cola pulled together what appeared to be an impressive group of university professors, but one primarily grounded in the field of exercise science. The front group's vice president, Steven Blair (then an exercise scientist at the University of South Carolina) said, "Most of the focus on the press is, 'Oh they're eating too much, eating too much, eating too much'—blaming fast food, blaming sugary drinks and so on....and there is virtually no compelling evidence that this is the case." Additional comments in the GEBN press release blamed the media for proliferating stories that focused on nutrition, then described Blair's approach as "an alternative, data-based theory."[10]

These assertions so lacked in subtlety that they triggered multiple inquiries into the organization's funding sources. The first questions came from Yoni Freedhoff, an obesity specialist at the University of Ottawa. And indeed, Coca-Cola's fingerprints were everywhere. Although GEBN's website, Facebook page, and Twitter feed made no mention of Coca-Cola, the group's website was registered to the soda manufacturer, which was also listed as the site's administrator. The *New York Times* reported that two of GEBN's founding members, Blair and Gregory Hand (the latter being the dean at West Virginia University School of Public Health) had received $4 million from Coca-Cola since 2008. This included $500,000 to Hand to help launch GEBN, plus another $1 million to the University of Colorado School of Medicine, employer of GEBN's President James Hill, to fund GEBN activities.[11]

The universities who employed the GEBN executives didn't appreciate being identified in one of the country's largest newspaper as complicit flacks for Coca-Cola. At West Virginia, Hand was demoted from his position as dean. Colorado returned its million dollars. With its cover blown and credibility forfeited, GEBN served little purpose to Coca-Cola. Funding presumably dried up from there, and within a few months its academic beneficiaries folded their tent and announced they were going out of business "due to resource limitations."[12]

Secretly shoveling money to scientists to claim that drinking gallons of Coke posed no threat to anyone's long-term health? It looked bad. The GEBN scandal caused significant damage to the iconic brand's reputation, and Coke committed to greater transparency in future funding. It even released a list of its recent donations, including $3 million to the American Academy of Pediatrics, $3.1 million to the American College of Cardiology, $3.5 million to the American Academy of Family Physicians, $2 million to the American Cancer Society, and $1.7 million to the Academy of Nutrition and Dietetics, the nation's largest organization of dietitians. The grand total of its giving was $120 million over six years; of that, $29 million was designated to support academic research. According the *New York Times*, this "won the company allies in anti-soda initiatives, wielded influence over health recommendations about soft drinks, and shifted scientific focus away from soda as a factor in the causes of obesity."[13]

But was Coke's itemization complete? Researchers at the University of Oxford and the London School of Hygiene and Tropical Medicine suggested that the company was only acknowledging its funding of do-good organizations, while hiding its stacking of the scientific literature with papers promoting their mercenary "energy balance" theory. The team discovered 151 journal articles, published by 468 authors across approximately 100 different journals, that identified the Coca-Cola Company or the Coca-Cola Foundation as a funder of their research, none of whom were included in the company's list of donation recipients. Not surprisingly, many of these papers promoted the "energy balance" message, equating the obesity epidemic with lack of physical exercise.[14]

From a critical perspective, the evidence supporting the "energy balance" theory is equivocal at best. A letter signed by 36 leading nutrition scientists criticized Coca-Cola and the Global Energy Balance Network for spreading "scientific nonsense."[15] Certainly there are cross-sectional studies that show thinner people exercise more than fat ones, but you can't tell from these types of studies which way the causation runs. Does the exercise make people thin or do thin people choose to exercise more? Studies conducted over longer periods of time that attempt to control for this question find little evidence that people who are more physically active gain less excess weight than those who are less active.[16]

On the other hand, there is little question that diet change is a powerful mechanism for losing weight or maintaining a healthy weight. The studies proving this point number in the hundreds, at a minimum.

Just as Big Tobacco lost its battle with the truth about cigarettes, Big Sugar is going to lose its battle with the truth about empty, but nevertheless harmful, calories. On this matter, time will most certainly tell.

———

In recent years, public health experts have focused their overall concerns about dietary sugar on the increase in consumption of the sugar-sweetened beverages (SSBs, as they're generally labeled). With little uncertainty, the science that shows that the amounts of sugar currently consumed by many Americans and people all over the world is harmful to the point of being dangerous. It is widely accepted that obesity and diabetes, not to mention tooth decay, will be prevented if sugar intake is reduced. And while sugar-sweetened solid, processed foods at least play a useful role in curbing hunger, SSBs have little if any redeeming nutritional value. Yes, they quench thirst, but that goal is accomplished better, or at least as well, by water. In short, SSBs are nothing but sugar-delivery systems—not as addictive as nicotine, but certainly playing to humans' built-in sweet tooth.

Given the global scale of the obesity epidemic, the importance of understanding the true health impacts of sugar and SSBs cannot be overstated. For its part, the scientific community has launched large numbers of independent studies. And for their part, the manufacturers of these beverages have gone to great lengths to slow the momentum of scientific understanding. Leading this charge is the American Beverage Association, the trade group representing Coca-Cola, PepsiCo, Dr Pepper, and other SSB producers, which has taken what Big Tobacco did for lung cancer and applied the strategy to obesity.

In 2012, the *New England Journal of Medicine* published three randomized control studies focusing on sugar intake, accompanied by an editorial concluding that the results provide a strong impetus "to limit consumption of sugar-sweetened beverages, especially those served at low cost and in excessive portions, to attempt to reverse the increase in childhood obesity."[17]

In response, the ABA issued long statement, raising criticisms of each the studies—and adding a bold assertion of its own:

Obesity is a serious and complex public health issue facing our nation and the rest of the world, and we all must work together to solve it. We know, and science supports, that obesity is not uniquely caused by any single food or beverage. Thus, studies and opinion pieces that focus solely on sugar-sweetened beverages, or any other single source of calories, *do nothing meaningful to help address this serious issue.* [emphasis added]...The fact remains: sugar-sweetened beverages are not driving obesity. By every measure, sugar-sweetened beverages play a small and declining role in the American diet.[18]

While lacerating the credibility of independent scientific studies, soda manufacturers also sponsored their own studies, ones that offered countervailing science (what we might today call "alternative facts"). A scientific review of these studies prompts the question of whether they were designed by scientists or by public relations firms; they are not good. The methods are weak, and the results are, by definition, highly questionable.

But is anyone else besides scientists looking closely? The results of flawed, industry-backed studies are blasted to the media in glossy, pandering ways, and it works. Outrageous or counterintuitive stories about scientific studies, especially ones that sell an easy path to weight loss, get attention and not all journalists are equipped to assess their rigor. One journalist who is equipped, the Associated Press's Candace Choi, identified, critiqued, and published a few embarrassing claims by the industry that were guaranteed to grab the attention of dieters and would-be dieters: "Study: Diet Beverages Better for Losing Weight Than Water." The headline accompanied a story reporting research funded by, of course, the American Beverage Association. "Hot Oatmeal Breakfast Keeps You Fuller for Longer," described a study paid for by Quaker Oats.[19]

Academic journals are filled with sugar studies. Some are funded by the National Institutes of Health or other independent sources; some are funded by the producers of sugary drinks. The types of studies vary greatly, and the devil is in the details. No single study would, by itself, be sufficient to understand the effects of drinking soda or other sweet-ened beverages. So researchers (and their funders) set out to review and synthesize the accumulated data, often by evaluating the findings and the quality of multiple individual studies. Predictably, studies paid for by SSB producers, or those performed by scientists with links to the industry, reported very different findings from those conducted by nonconflicted scientists. In one analysis of 60 sugar studies, 25 of 26 negative studies (i.e., studies that found no correlation between SSBs and obesity) were industry-funded; only one of the 34 studies that re-ported a positive relationship between SSB consumption and ill health was paid for by an SSB manufacturer.[20] This "funding effect"—finding the result your funder wants—has been true of studies on SSBs, but also for the large-scale reviews of the accumulated studies.

There are now several reviews of the reviews. And what do they show? The first of them was sponsored by a foundation, not the indus-try, and published in 2007. It found that the reviews funded by indus-try were seven times more likely to have a favorable conclusion than those with no industry funding.[21] Over time, the numbers have gotten starker. A more recent analysis of 133 SSB studies published between 2001 and 2013 reported that industry-related papers were 57 times more likely to conclude that the drinks had a weak or no detrimental health effect than did studies by independent scientists.[22] Virtually all industry-funded reviews of the reviews found the evidence linking SSBs to ill health was weak and unconvincing.[23]

In an effort to write its own narrative, Coca-Cola engaged epidemi-ologist Douglas Weed to review the reviews that linked SSBs to negative health outcomes. Weed was an excellent choice: a respected scientist who, before launching his own consulting firm, held a high-level post at the National Cancer Institute. After leaving NCI, he has lent his scientific credibility to the defense of corporations accused of making people sick by exposing them to DuPont's Teflon chemical PFOA[24] and the controversial pesticide glyphosate made by Monsanto.[25] On behalf of the American Chemistry Council, he produced a review critical of a Consumer Products Safety Commission advisory panel's report on the effects of phthalates (chemicals used to make plastics softer and more flexible, common in toys and care items) on children's health.[26] These are but a few of his projects. In short, Weed has transitioned to a career as a product defense scientist. And in that role, it is little surprise that his and two colleagues' review of the SSB reviews concluded that, overall, the quality of earlier reviews was low.[27] If you follow the logic in Weed's analysis, we really can't be sure that SSBs contribute to the risk of obesity, heart disease, or diabetes. And in the absence of certainty, the beverage industry would be quick to remind us, no action can or should be taken.

But Coca-Cola couldn't catch a break. When Weed's paper appeared in the *American Journal of Clinical Nutrition*, it was accompanied by a scalding editorial by Vasanti Malik and Frank Hu, both of the Harvard School of Public Health. They wrote, "[R]ather than shedding more light on this pressing public health issue, [Weed's review] obscured important relations between SSB consumption and harmful health consequences." In short, Malik and Hu said exactly what Coke did not want to hear. The two public health professors argued that the policies the beverage industry is trying to stop, like taxing SSBs, are working and should continue:

Despite attempts from the beverage industry to obfuscate the issue by funding biased analyses and reviews, and by providing misleading information to consumers, many regulatory strategies to reduce intake of SSBs are already in place. Some states are considering taxation as a means of reducing SSB intake and as a method of offsetting some of the high health care costs attributed to regular consumption of these beverages. These measures have a great potential to reduce SSB consumption and their adverse health consequences."[28]

In 2016, when the U.S. government's Dietary Guidelines Advisory Committee recommended a limit or target for "added sugars" of no more than 10 percent of total calories, the sugar industry answered with a long list of challenges. As the tobacco industry did for decades, they focused on the uncertainty of the scientific evidence and the absence of randomized clinical trials—a multi-year study in which some volunteers are assigned to consume large amounts of sugar and others are allowed little or none. Until any such sweeping (very expensive) study is conducted, it is likely that America's sugary beverage manufacturers will continue to do what they're doing: publish their own reviews, then complain that the government didn't pay enough attention to them.[29]

The pushback on sugar is not restricted to the beverage producers. Producers of many other processed foods—dairy products, eggs, breakfast cereals, pork, beef, soy products, dietary supplements, juices, cranberries, nuts, and chocolate—have gone to great lengths to defend their products in the face of threatened regulation or market contraction. New York University's Marion Nestle is perhaps the leading academic expert on nutrition and the corporate marketing of food products. (I should note that she is not a renegade member of the Swiss food juggernaut's founding family, Nestlé; Marion Nestle is American, and her name rhymes with "wrestle.") Nestle was one of the first to bring attention to the food and beverage industry's manipulation of data and promotion of questionable science, including the link between industry funding and favorable results.

One notable, often repeated bit of industry treachery relates to chocolate, and it originated in a study funded by Mars Inc. (now known as Mars Wrigley Confectionary), the maker of chocolate candies, including the ubiquitous M&Ms. The subject of the study was the possible benefits of cocoa flavanols on arterial function and blood pressure. As the researchers concluded, plant metabolites "have the potential to maintain cardiovascular health even in low-risk subjects." This was great news for the people at Mars, who broadcast the findings in a full-page advertisement in the *New York Times* on September 27, 2015. But as Nestle pointed out, "[n]either the press release nor advertisement explained that cocoa flavanols are largely destroyed during all but the most careful processing of chocolate, nor did they mention chocolate at all. They didn't have to. Uncritical readers are likely to interpret the statements as evidence that chocolate is good for them and that its sugar and calories can be ignored."[30]

Vox's Julia Belluz identified 100 studies funded or supported by Mars over the past twenty years, all looking at the health effects of cocoa. Is it surprising that nearly every one of them provided findings favorable to this key ingredient in chocolate? And if these were the only studies you read, you might, as Belluz points out, mistakenly believe that "[r]egularly eating cocoa flavanols could boost mood and cognitive performance, dark chocolate improves blood flow, cocoa might be useful for treating immune disorders, and both cocoa powder and dark chocolate can have a 'favorable effect' on cardiovascular disease risk."[31]

Mars walks a line of legality here. For all the liberties taken by food companies in co-opting research, making claims up without having some semblance of scientific support might induce charges of deceptive advertising by the Federal Trade Commission (FTC). That's exactly what happened to the POM Wonderful company, which asserted in advertisements that its product—pomegranate juice—could cure a host of dreaded diseases, including heart disease, prostate cancer, and erectile dysfunction. In official charges against the juice company in 2010, the FTC asserted that such claims must be supported by at least one clinical trial. Without that justification, the manufacturer must drop its claims. The company disagreed and replied, "We stand behind the vast body of scientific research documenting the healthy properties of Wonderful variety pomegranate. Our research is unprecedented among food and beverage companies, and we take pride in having initiated a program of modern scientific research to investigate the health benefits of this ancient and revered fruit."[32] POM Wonderful took the FTC all the way to the Court of Appeals, losing the legal argument at every level.[33]

Food manufacturers are creative. If the sugar in a product is a problem, they change the subject. A product that's bad for you can suddenly be healthful when viewed in a very specific, narrow way. General Mills, for example, aggressively markets its high-sugar cereals like Lucky Charms and Cinnamon Toast Crunch as "made with whole grains."[34] Yes, whole grains are better than plain white flour. But that matters appreciably less when your toddler is getting walloped with sugar in every serving.

So, should sugar researchers accept funding support from Big Sugar? The question is too narrow. A more important question is, should *any* food and nutrition researchers accept funding support from industry? There is no question that more (and better) science is needed to improve the diet and nutrition of people across the world. For the most part, the studies from which we learn the most are large, long-term, and expensive. Academic scientists can't do this work without support, and with government funding decreasing, at least in the United States, these sorts of sweeping studies aren't coming anytime soon. It would be fair to argue that the food industry firms should pay for the research, because they are the ones who benefit from research that finds new, improved products. Providing data that show a product is safe is the reasonable cost of doing business if they want to exploit it in a free-market economy.

But industry funding brings with it the inherent conflicts of interest. There are too many ways studies can be kneaded and shaped to fit the needs of the sponsors, and there are not enough people with the expertise and platform to officiate such matters. Firms certainly won't hire scientists whose studies have a track record of finding that food products are unsafe or not particularly nutritious. Industry *will* commission studies that answer the questions the industry *wants* answered. More often than not, these questions are posed in ways that produce results more suited to marketing materials than nutritional goals. Scientists who receive industry money are likely, consciously or not, to produce the results their sponsors expect. Research funding is hard to come by, and they want to keep the financial support flowing.

The answer in all this, I believe, is not simply to *allow* industry to fund nutrition research; food manufacturers should be *required* to do so. Our system for scientific inquiry needs to move past the current ethical controls, which are applied inconsistently at best and which allow independent researchers to design studies, apply for funding, and publish the results no matter what the outcome of the work. In this model, the industry gets to set the research agenda and select who does the study, with little public disclosure, all but guaranteeing that the firms will get the results they want.

An alternative system could require all components of the food industry to contribute money to a research institute, one with pooled funding and a board of experts stewarding the research agenda and deciding which independent scientists will be funded to conduct the studies. In terms of model, the precedent of requiring producers to contribute to a fund for the collective good of the food industry is already well established. Congress has authorized 22 industry-funded research and promotion (R&P) boards that collect mandatory contributions or fees in a range of industries—beef and pork, dairy and eggs, all sorts of fruits and vegetables—even the firms that produce the paper and packaging for food products have an R&P Board to which they all contribute.[35]

These R&P boards work, in that they promote the sales of crops and products. The new board or boards would have to be independent of the funders, directed by scientists with no financial conflict of interest. Controversial? Yes. But impossible? No.

In the most remote, poorest village in Latin America or Asia or Africa, you can buy a Coke. It will cost more than pennies, but not much more. Sugary drinks (along with other processed foods, but especially SSBs) are present almost everywhere, which in itself explains why the obesity epidemic is also global.

The price paid in terms of medical and disability costs and lowered workforce productivity is much more than pennies. In considering the toll of sugar-laden products on human health, and especially the ensuing costs saddled on municipalities, states, and national governments, it is important to consider how healthier diets can be encouraged more actively—in other words, how barriers to unhealthy habits can be constructed. The most straightforward is an excise tax in order to raise the price of the product for which decreased consumption is deemed a public good. The reasoning is straightforward: demand is elastic; higher prices mean less consumption. With cigarettes—the most obvious example—the problem is that once addicted, it's difficult to stop, and smokers end up paying a sizable portion of their income to satisfy their nicotine fix. A key strategy with cigarettes, therefore, is to discourage that first puff, or at least that first pack by raising the price. It has worked. According to the U.S. Centers for Disease Control and Prevention, "increasing the price of tobacco products is the single most effective way to reduce consumption."[36]

Today, the most prominent experiment with an excise tax on a food product is the "soda tax" on sugar-sweetened beverages. It's designed to discourage SSB consumption while generating revenues for public health programs often aimed at the diseases and conditions associated with sugar consumption. Among processed food products that are logical targets of market intervention, the sugar drinks are the low-hanging fruit. They provide little or no nutritional value, and the tax is easy to levy.[37] School districts, goaded by PTAs and nutritionists, are going even further, limiting or banning these products from school cafeterias and snack machines. Make it harder to tank up on sugar.[38]

The opposition has been fierce, predictably, with millions of dollars spent to convince the public and legislators that the science behind the soda taxes is doubtful, that the causation between sugar and obesity has never been proved, that taxes will be woefully ineffective in fighting obesity, and that thousands of jobs will be forfeited in a (failed) experiment in social engineering. Nor, critics argue, does the government have any right to interfere with the workings of the free market. This last salvo can be an effective argument, but it's a real howler in its hypocrisy. Most consumers probably do not know that many, *many* food products, with sugar products high on the list, enjoy subsidies and market protections of one sort or another. The producers know this very well, of course. Sugar producers benefit from one of the commodity support programs common across the food industry, *and* from tariffs on competing exporters (in effect in the United States since 1789, in fact). They are subsidized by the government and protected from their competitors. Now that is a sweet deal.

The tobacco and liquor industries don't pay the costs of the diseases their products cause; they have shifted much of this cost to the public, especially through safety net programs like Medicaid. The same is true for manufacturers of the sugar drinks and other sugar-added products. They want it both ways: Privatizing profits, socializing risks. This should be stopped. (Only the mammoth lawsuits against Big Tobacco forced the cigarette manufacturers to repay states for a small portion of the money laid out by Medicaid systems for millions of cases of lung cancer, heart disease and a host of other illnesses caused by tobacco. Is this in the future for Big Sugar?)

Despite the unflagging opposition, momentum for these soda taxes is growing. They have been enacted in countries around the globe, including Barbados, Belgium, Chile, Dominica, France, Great Britain, Hungary, Kiribati, Mauritius, Mexico, Portugal, and Tonga. Several U.S. jurisdictions, including a growing number of cities, states, and tribes, have done the same. The World Health Organization has recommended that all governments enact taxes to raise the retail price of SSBs at least 20 percent.[39] And the taxes appear to work. After Mexico implemented its one peso per liter tax on SSBs, sales decreased 5 percent the first year and almost 10 percent the second year, with the largest decreases seen where the price increases probably have the biggest impact: low-income neighborhoods.[40] Decreases in consumption also occurred after soda taxes went into effect in Berkeley (the first American city to embrace this approach)[41] and Philadelphia.[42] The success in low-income neighborhoods is used to support the argument that soda tax disproportionately impacts the poor. Well, yes. The rich are never going mind paying a few extra cents for every gulp, but the poor may. The two most notorious excise taxes—tobacco and liquor— also impact the poor disproportionately. However, this is only part of the complicated calculus. Lower disease rates associated with healthier diets will benefit these consumers in the long run, both physically and monetarily, and less illness will mean less societal spending on medical costs associated with sugar-related diseases.

Governments are getting smarter in their implementation of the tax. The first ones simply raised the price of all sugary beverages. Newer ones use a sliding scale to reflect the relative amount of sugar in a given product.[43] When Great Britain began consideration of a soda tax, industry's response was predictable. The British Soft Drink Association commissioned a report by a consulting group affiliated with Oxford University that forecast the new tax would have little positive impact (decreasing daily consumption by a mere five calories per person, on average) but would kill 4,000 jobs.[44] These conclusions were widely promoted, with many in the media mistaking this public relations effort for actual, impartial analysis.[45] Recognizing the need to maintain their market share, Britain's leading soft drink manufacturers, including Coca-Cola and Pepsi, reformulated their soda, dramatically decreasing their sugar content. Just the threat of the law had a major impact on sugar consumption.

People who oppose sugar taxes are quick to label the legislation paternalistic. "The government shouldn't tell people what they should and shouldn't eat," cry the soda manufacturers. "Let them choose for themselves!" This sounds good, but the producers' argument is blatantly hypocritical. The argument is valid only if the associated risks are widely available and publicized—and they aren't, because Big Sugar spends tremendous sums manufacturing uncertainty about the health impacts of its products. It's the same old story: sow doubt and confusion in order to slow down or eliminate requirements to provide the better information they claim they want.

———————

I will conclude here with a modest suggestion relating to the U.S. Department of Agriculture, which holds the mandate to protect the nation's food supply and promote healthy diets. Enforcing that mandate is tricky, however, because the agency is also in the business of promoting the agriculture industry. The USDA is thus tasked with serving two masters, the industry and the public. The resulting danger is "industry capture," which is an abiding risk within any regulatory structure. The political power and financial influence of a given industry are too powerful, and they overshadow concern for the public good within the oversight agency. The industry ends up in *de facto* control. In the past, when it has become clear that an agency couldn't serve both masters, Congress has subdivided the agency into one serving the industry and a second one, presumably independent, whose primary mission is safety. Where this doesn't happen, the public gets the short shrift as the government goes to great pains to accommodate corporations. In 2010, for example, the Deepwater Horizon explosion and subsequent monumental oil leak illuminated the conflicted mission of the Interior Department's Minerals Management Service (MMS), whose job was to both promote and regulate offshore drilling. The predictable result was lax oversight of the offshore wells. Less than one month after the explosion, Interior Secretary Ken Salazar split the MMS into three independent agencies. But imposed independence isn't guaranteed. Soon after taking office, the Trump administration rolled back many restrictions on the deep wells, clearly at the behest of the drillers.

Given that tens of thousands of Americans are killed annually by the diseases related to obesity and eating unhealthy foods, and given that the USDA is given the impossible task of serving Big Sugar and the other Big Food producers *while also* promoting standards for healthy diets that might not serve the interest of the producers, the imperative is evident: break up the USDA. Create an agency that's independent of the producers and promotes *only* healthy eating.

13

The Party Line

DONALD TRUMP HAS been portrayed by some as "hijacking" the Republican Party. This argument casts the forty-fifth president of the United States as a radical populist whose views and methods belie the history and ideological roots of the Grand Old Party.

On matters related to science and regulation, this claim is patently false. The Trump administration's policies reflect a half-century of Republican hostility toward any scientific evidence that does not align with the needs of the party's financial benefactors. The coalescence under Trump amounts to nothing more than a rebranding.

Disdain for science isn't new in American society; it has been a long-running thread in its social fabric throughout modern history. Here I am not talking about the populist anti-intellectualism described by historian Richard Hofstadter in his Pulitzer Prize–winning book *Anti-Intellectualism in American Life*. This is a different strain of anti-intellectualism, first identified by neoconservative Irving Kristol, through which leaders of corporate capitalism defend their power by stirring opposition to another elite that he labeled "the new class"—intellectuals, journalists, scientists and others who attempt to change the society in ways that adversely impact the corporate class.[1] What is notable today is that this strain of anti-intellectualism, intertwined with white nationalism, is now a core component of the platform of what used to be the party of Lincoln.

I had a first-hand encounter with the Republican ideology when I testified on OSHA's policies and performance before the House of Representative's Education and the Workforce Committee (since renamed the Committee on Education and Labor). This was in 2018, after I had returned to academia after heading OSHA for more than seven years. I was the sole Democratic witness on the panel that day. I was joined by the three Republican witnesses, one representing the Chamber of Commerce and the other two industry trade associations. At one point, Representative Glenn Grothman (R-WI) walked into the hearing room after missing much of the testimony, looked at the panel, and noted with a loud sigh that the Democrats had done it again: they had invited a professor, a word he enunciated with some derision. His attitude was clear: the business representatives were expert, knowledgeable, and worth listening to, while I was but yet another pointy-headed intellectual who couldn't really know much about OSHA, seven years at the helm of that agency notwithstanding. Grothman, unsurprisingly, is a soldier in the Republican campaign to defend the tobacco industry. He opposed legislation for increasing spending on anti-smoking campaigns from $10 million, a pittance, to $30 million, a larger pittance. His reasoning: "Everybody knows you're not supposed to smoke!"[2] Grothman was one of a handful of Republicans who opposed 2009 legislation that outlawed smoking in bars and restaurants in Wisconsin.[3]

Grothman's anti-intellectualism and defense of tobacco are linked. Antipathy to science for the sake of corporate (and political) profit was honed and perfected by Big Tobacco and the fossil fuel industry in the second half of the twentieth century. This has become the ideology of the Republican Party. And in the latter days of the tobacco industry's peak lobby efforts, it had no greater ally in government than Trump's vice president, Mike Pence. Pence was a favorite of the industry and its aligned network of exceedingly wealthy individuals and families, led by the Koch Brothers.

Before assuming the vice presidency, Pence was a congressman from Indiana, a chair of the House Republican Conference, and then the state's governor. His benefactors showered him with financial support, and his political positions returned the love. As a congressman in 1997, he parroted the industry line and opposed efforts by state governments (including that of Indiana) to force the tobacco industry to pay the costs of smoker's diseases paid by Medicaid—litigation that eventually delivered billions of dollars to state treasuries. In an op-ed in the *Indianapolis Star*, he equated the health effects of smoking to those of eating candy, contending, "Our government was not established for the purpose of eradicating bad personal habits."[4]

Pence showed no sympathy for victims of secondhand tobacco smoke, whose only "bad personal habit" would have been breathing in the presence of smokers. In a position piece published on his personal website in 2000, he wrote:

> Time for a quick reality check. Despite the hysteria from the political class and the media, smoking doesn't kill. In fact, two out of every three smokers do not die from a smoking-related illness and nine out of ten smokers do not contract lung cancer. This is not to say that smoking is good for you...news flash: smoking is not good for you. If you are reading this article through the blue haze of cigarette smoke you should quit. The relevant question is, what is more harmful to the nation, second-hand smoke or back-handed big government disguised in do-gooder healthcare rhetoric?[5]

In 2009, Pence and 89 of his Republican colleagues in the House— about half of the Republican caucus at the time—voted against the Family Smoking Prevention and Tobacco Control Act, the landmark legislation that gave the FDA authority to regulate tobacco products.

Make no mistake: the Trump administration's policy agenda on science is fundamentally the same as the Republican Party's policy agenda. For evidence, look no further than what happened after the president pulled out of the Paris Agreement on climate change in 2017: the controversial, ecologically devastating move was met with widespread cheering—and nary a few whispers of dissent—from Republican elected officials. The party has long been the political vehicle of choice for industries whose profit margins increase when they're left unregulated by environmental and public health agencies. These corporations, typically polluters and manufacturers of dangerous products, have long relied on GOP efforts to defang such public health and regulatory agencies. Republicans' primary objective, cloaked in phony rhetoric about "liberty" and "personal responsibility" and "free-market enterprise," is to lower corporate taxes and reduce regulatory "burdens," thereby enabling manufacturers to market dangerous chemicals and polluters to dump the waste haphazardly with little fear of regulation or litigation. This stratagem shifts the burden of protection from the government to the individual—who, in the very hollow American lore, is encouraged to think of regulation as an attack on individual liberty.

But can everyday consumers decide what food additives are safe? Or prescription drugs? Perhaps a few can, with some help. By and large, however, the core problems of public health and the environment cannot be solved by individuals. In fact, we are mostly powerless in protecting ourselves and our children. Air pollution, clean water, climate change, safe food, and so many other issues are problems "of the public good," as economists put it. These issues must be addressed by the government, in all of our names. To pretend otherwise is sheer sophistry.

But the genius and deviance of the GOP is that they don't often engage directly with ugly, specific issues. Rather, they police the public discourse *around* these issues, framing proposals for regulation as the encroachments of a reactive nanny state. In other words, you won't see any Republicans defending unfettered smoking *directly*; that would be utter stupidity. No, if you want to make the argument that people should be free to smoke wherever they want, you disparage the evidence showing that secondhand smoke kills innocent nonsmokers. When you are defending an industry under attack for killing people or harming the planet, science is your adversary. So Republicans take steps to neutralize it by litigating scientific consensus and scientific expertise. And even though it might seem ludicrous to prop up the dying coal industry, since it is clear to everyone, most of all the residents of the coal-producing states, that many of its practices are destructive to the environment and human lives, the GOP is up to the task. Be bold—be best! (Note here: The Department of Interior under Ryan Zinke, former Republican congressman from Montana appointed by Trump, and who later stepped down amid concerns around alleged ethics violations, killed a half-completed study on the impacts on humans of the most extreme form of strip mining, which removes the tops of mountains, undertaken by the National Academies of Science, Engineering, and Medicine.)

It helps that Republicans can back up their attacks on science with hundreds of millions of dollars, perhaps more. With total lack of transparency, the Koch network, Big Tobacco, the U.S. Chamber of

Commerce, and their allies have funded nonprofit groups to elect politicians sympathetic to their positions and then ride these issues unrelentingly. This largesse has launched lawsuits to stop government action on tobacco and climate change. More importantly, it has funded the phenomenally successful movement to pack the federal courts with judges hand-picked to back the corporate position in almost every case. And these donors' magnum opus is the creation of a Supreme Court majority that is hostile to regulatory action on behalf of human health and the environment.

My personal experience with Brett Kavanaugh, President Trump's second Supreme Court appointee, suggests that he will very likely uphold his part in this dreadful progression. In the winter of 2010, a few months after I began work at OSHA, we were notified about a tragic death at SeaWorld in Orlando. In front of a live audience, the 12,000-pound killer whale (or orca) named Tilikum violently dragged trainer Dawn Brancheau underwater and killed her. Orcas have had their informal name for a long time: Pliny the Elder, the great Roman military commander and naturalist, so described them after witnessing these fierce creatures attack mother whales and their calves near the Straits of Gibraltar.[6] We now know that in captivity, the appellation is also all too accurate: in closed settings, there have been multiple killer whale attacks.

Given that only a tiny number of U.S. facilities house captive killer whales, OSHA did not have a specific standard requiring employers to protect their workers from these animals. So government inspectors issued two citations under the agency's general-duty clause, which requires employers to maintain workplaces free of "recognized, serious hazards." SeaWorld's lawyers challenged the citations, claiming that the company didn't recognize that working closely with a killer whale was hazardous. The case was eventually argued before the three-judge District of Columbia Court of Appeals, where Judge Merrick Garland (President Obama's ill-fated nominee to fill Justice Scalia's seat on the Supreme Court) and Judge Judith Rogers strongly affirmed the validity of OSHA's citations (and the measly $14,000 fine).

Dissenting, though, was Judge Kavanaugh, who, as he almost always does, found for the corporation over the regulatory agency trying to protect the public. He claimed that Sea World trainers could and had willingly accepted the risk of violent death as part of their job. This was not only a clear misreading of federal law, but also an example of the valuing of corporations' rights over human rights in his judicial decision-making.

———————

In Donald J. Trump, the United States electoral system produced a president who questions the benefits of childhood vaccines. (Indisputably, the benefits *greatly* outweigh any risks.) Peter Navarro, Trump's top trade advisor, described his role as an advisor in these terms: "My function, really, as an economist is to try to provide the underlying analytics that confirm his intuition. And his intuition is always right in these matters." In this era, this is dismal science indeed, but in this administration, economics is in good company. The sciences are mostly unappreciated, and if Trump's budget proposals were enacted, they would be disastrously underfunded. Unwelcome science is dismissed as "shoddy" and "politicized,"[7] challenged at every turn by "alternative facts."

Researchers at the Rand Corporation have termed this phenomenon "truth decay," and it has spread across government with Trump at the helm.[8] Purveyors of "alternative scientific thinking" were placed in countless important government positions, often endangering the basic work of the agencies they direct. As R. Alta Charo, Professor of Law and Bioethics at the University of Wisconsin–Madison, has noted, the allegiance to "alternative science" has been particularly endemic in the area of human reproduction. Teresa Manning, former lobbyist for the National Right to Life Committee, "insists that contraception is ineffective, despite evidence that hormonal methods are 91% effective and long-acting reversible contraceptives such as intrauterine devices (IUDs) are 99% effective at preventing pregnancy." Under Trump, Manning played a central role in shaping federal family-planning programs. Similarly, Charmaine Yoest, assistant secretary for public affairs at the Department of Health and Human Services, "asserts that condoms (which can reduce the risk of HIV transmission by at least 70 percent) do not protect against HIV or other sexually transmitted infections." According to Charo, Yoest also claims contraception does not reduce the number of abortions and that abortion causes breast cancer, despite the overwhelming evidence to the contrary.[9]

Manning and Yoest are two examples of lobbyists who were allowed to play scientist in Republican government. They're not alone in this path. Sam Clovis, a former right-wing talk show host who had been national co-chair of Trump's campaign, was nominated as chief scientist at the Department of Agriculture. (He was forced to withdraw his name not because he is utterly lacking in scientific expertise, but because he was the direct supervisor of campaign aide George Papadopoulos, whom he reportedly encouraged to arrange a meeting of campaign staff with Russian officials.[10] Papadopoulos later pled guilty and served prison time for lying to federal agents about his contacts with the Russian government during the campaign, and Clovis would have had to answer questions about those matters under oath had he continued with his nomination.) Another memorable nominee was Kathleen Hartnett-White, selected to chair the Council on Environmental Quality and serve as the president's principal environmental policy adviser. Previously, she directed the Texas Public Policy Foundation's "Fueling Freedom Project," whose goal was to "end the regulation of CO_2 as a pollutant" and "explain the forgotten moral case for fossil fuels."[11] "Fossil fuels dissolved the economic justification for slavery," Hartnett-White has opined with absolutely no evidence. "The productivity made possible by fossil fuels led to the institutionalization of compassion and respect for the inalienable rights of each human individual."[12] This nomination did make it to a Senate confirmation hearing—but disastrously. Hartnett-White suggested that the evidence of the human contribution to climate change was "very uncertain," then could not answer a series of basic scientific questions that a science advisor would certainly be expected to know: she could not say, for example, whether ocean water expands as it warms. She withdrew her name from consideration shortly after the hearing, and the post remained unfilled for almost a year thereafter.

The list of Trump's appointments of totally unqualified individuals to important government science or science-related positions posts is a long one. While many were lobbyists, many more were corporate scientists or attorneys with expertise in product defense. Their pronouncements are couched in traditional scientific terms that seem reasonable to lay listeners; in reality, they are flawed window-dressing science, carefully constructed for the purpose of creating a space that protects the sales of a product or defends it against costly litigation.

Pushing through the nominations of hacks and charlatans to run federal science agencies is damaging enough. What happens to scientific advisory panels within these agencies adds profound insult to injury. Until recently, most of the scientists on these panels were in academia. Their voluntary service represents a serious commitment, and they are not paid for this time-consuming work. Nevertheless, in *most* past administrations, the federal government had been able to call on these scientists to ensure that the government had access to the latest and best nonconflicted scientific advice. (I emphasize "most" because there have been exceptions. The George W. Bush administration was a notable one.[13]) You will not be surprised to learn that the Trump administration is, for the most part, dismissive of the entire *idea* of a federal advisory system. As an illustration: during my time as OSHA administrator, I relied on four safety and health advisory committees, plus another one focused on whistleblower protection, each of which was required to meet at least twice per year. In the first two years of the Trump administration, one of them held a brief telephone conference; and the other four had no meetings at all.

Then again, no advice is sometimes better than bad advice. The EPA has traditionally relied heavily on its Science Advisory Board (SAB). During Scott Pruitt's tenure as President Trump's EPA administrator, Pruitt turned conflict-of-interest rules on their heads by announcing that scientists whose research was funded by the EPA (presumably because they were doing studies of most value to the agency—and because they were good scientists) would be barred from serving on the SAB. Several of the members Pruitt inherited were thus pushed out and replaced by industry scientists with conflicts of interest so significant they would not have been seated in previous administrations, even that of George W. Bush. Others named to SAB held views so far outside the scientific mainstream as to make their advice questionable, if not dangerous. Consider Michael Honeycutt, Texas's chief toxicologist and Pruitt's choice to chair the board. Honeycutt has a long history of advocating for the loosening of EPA regulations on many known hazards, including mercury and arsenic. He believes the EPA's rules on ozone are unnecessary because "most people spend more than 90 percent of their time indoors."[14]

The Trump administration's choice to chair the Clean Air Scientific Advisory committee was Louis Anthony (Tony) Cox, a long-time industry consultant who clings to uncommon opinions, like lowering ozone and the belief that $PM_{2.5}$ exposures would not improve public health.[15] Cox was well-known at the Labor Department for his testimony on behalf of the National Mining Association, predictably claiming that the government's risk assessment on respirable coal dust was flawed.[16] Not just his science, but Cox's integrity was called into question by the FDA following his efforts on behalf of Bayer to defend the use of an antibiotic in poultry production that the FDA believed would increase the development and spread of antibiotic-resistant campylobacter infections in humans. Taking an action that almost never occurs, in 2005, President George W. Bush's FDA commissioner actually excluded Cox's testimony from the proceedings; the agency found that he "intentionally misquoted published articles," and "Dr. Cox's credibility was such that his testimony was so unreliable that it was inadmissible."[17] (He's also the same person who argued against OSHA's new standard for silica in Chapter 8. This issue ended up in federal appeals court, where his position was rejected unanimously. But it's worth noting that these same mercenary scientists have a way of popping up in front of almost every regulatory agency.)

Amid preposterous appointments and the stacking of advisory committees, including the firing of some of the nation's leading scientists, congressional Republicans haven't complained. That's not to say that the regulatory rollbacks that followed weren't taken to court; all of them were. And in most of the initial cases, usually involving the EPA or other agencies simply ignoring the law, the judges have ruled against the rollback and ordered the agencies to follow the law as written by Congress. In the long run, however, given President Trump's appointments of arch-partisan federal judges who almost invariably prefer the arguments of corporations over those of the regulatory agencies, the outlook is grim.

On June 9, 2017, President Trump appeared at an event at the Department of Transportation that was organized as part of an ongoing campaign for infrastructure investment—specifically, infrastructure investment executed with reduced regulatory oversight and at lower cost. At one point during his remarks, Trump flipped through, then dramatically dropped to the floor, a thick binder containing something called an *Environmental Impact Statement*—a federal agency's documentation of how they've examined possible ecological and social impacts on the surrounding area before embarking on any large construction initiative. "Nonsense," he announced. "These binders on the stage could be replaced by just a few simple pages."

I have long felt that the most important little-known environmental law is the National Environmental Policy Act (NEPA), which requires federal agencies planning major construction projects to conduct a public process to consider the ecological and social impacts of the proposed activities, along with possible alternatives. The product of this process is an Environmental Impact Statement (EIS). The legislation does not require the agency to select the option least harmful to the environment, only to at least *consider* the impact of different options in planning the project. A pretty reasonable position, we might think—but according to Republican ideology, we would be wrong.

Trump's stagecraft was unquestionably effective in the service of deregulation. But one of the most dangerous long-term impacts of the administration's policies has been its unrelenting attempt to change the processes through which agencies evaluate scientific evidence, then use it to minimize the potential impact on human health and the environment. The long-term changes driven by these reports often do not get much public attention. The reports themselves are sometimes obscure and their details hard to follow. But one also saved the country from what might have been one of the worst environmental disasters in our history. And that particular environmental impact statement was overseen by the office I directed while working at the Department of Energy in the late 1990s, during the final years of the Clinton administration. The Los Alamos National Laboratory in northern New Mexico was founded in secret in 1943 to lead the development work on the atomic bomb. Half a century later, the facility was still an important part of the nation's ongoing nuclear weapons program, and as a result it had produced a vast amount of plutonium-contaminated waste material over the course of more than half a century. This waste was stored in thousands of standard-issue metal barrels sitting on wooden pallets in the government-owned forest nearby, where they were exposed to all the elements. In the late 1990s, the laboratory was planning some construction projects, and the parent Department of Energy conducted the mandated process to develop an environmental impact statement for the entire site. As part of the NEPA process, the plans were opened for public input. At one of the hearings that followed, local residents asked troubling questions about the potential impact of wildfire on all the toxic waste stored out in the open. (After all, wildfires were then, as they are even more today, endemic throughout the forested American West.) Had Los Alamos not asked this question of itself? Amazingly, perhaps, it had not. But now it did, and the final environmental impact statement for the Los Alamos construction was issued in December 1999. (With more than 900 pages, it filled a set of large binders similar to the ones President Trump would deride almost twenty years later.)[18]

With this process, the fire threat at Los Alamos was brought to the official attention of the DOE for the first time. And within months, appropriate actions were taken. The wooden pallets were replaced with aluminum pallets, and trees and brush cleared to make the storage area more open and safe. Not long after all this work was accomplished, the western United States suffered through what at the time was an unusually dry and severe wildfire season. Almost 7 million acres burned during that summer of 2000. One of those infernos, the Cerro Grande Fire, started as a controlled burn at the Bandelier National Monument in New Mexico, less than 10 miles south of the lab and the stored nuclear waste. On May 4, high winds drove this blaze out of control. The massive fire swept through Los Alamos, burning 50,000 acres of forest and residential land, including 30 percent of the laboratory's land. The conflagration destroyed many of the historic buildings where the atomic bomb was invented and tested, along with more than 200 homes. The smoke plume reached the Oklahoma panhandle, several hundred miles away. The fire's damage was estimated at $1 billion.

But with the brush cleared and the wooden pallets replaced, the huge fire could not reach the newly protected nuclear waste. If it had, the consequences would have been truly disastrous. That smoke plume would have transported plutonium particles across a large swath of the Southwest, contaminating everything and exposing millions of people to increased risk of cancer. Instead, the precautions developed through the NEPA review were successful. No radiation was released.[19]

Less than 1 percent of public works projects—only very large ones—actually require these environmental impact statements. And for those few, there is little question that the process can be made more efficient and less time-consuming. But the requirement that government agencies consider the environmental impacts of their major projects and involve the public in those discussions is valuable. Discarding this process would be reckless and costly—but Republicans in power are going to try.

The Republican marketing of deregulation as a return to individual rights has been highly successful. One of their new, more cynical efforts to ensure that federal agencies get off the backs of polluters and manufacturers of dangerous products is an EPA proposal speciously entitled "Strengthening Transparency in Regulatory Science."

A word here about transparency. As a scientist who has been deeply involved in promulgating regulations that protect the public's safety, health, and environment, I recognize the importance of open science and providing access to the best available research findings. That's not what this new proposal is about. In fact, the new EPA regulation would do the opposite of what its title suggests: it would make it more difficult for EPA to use the findings of scientific investigations to protect public health. It is part of a larger tack utilized across the political right, one that can only be characterized as *weaponized* transparency: making the data underlying scientific conclusions publicly available, then hiring mercenary scientists to re-analyze it in faulty, specious ways.

The broad strategy was hatched by—who else?—the tobacco industry, then embraced by polluters of all types. The history is highly revealing. By the mid-1990s, there could no longer be any doubt that secondhand cigarette smoke was causing cancer among nonsmokers. The industry was still claiming it wasn't true (heck, they were still claiming that nicotine was not addictive!), but they understood this was a rear-guard action; they were destined to lose eventually if it was their only defense. In other words, Big Tobacco needed new ways to stop the government from applying the science to disease prevention, including in this case the EPA, which was focused on environmental exposure to second-hand smoke. Chris Horner, the tobacco attorney who would later apply his disinformation skills to the climate change debate, came up with a nefarious solution. In a memo to his client R. J. Reynolds,

Horner proposed a legislative effort to "construct explicit procedural hurdles the agency must follow in issuing scientific reports." The idea was to require the EPA to provide access to all the raw data in all the studies used to protect the public so that corporations could hire their own scientists to re-analyze the results and make the ones they didn't like disappear. Horner recognized that this plan would never work if it were seen as an effort to defend tobacco smoke, so "our approach is one of addressing process as opposed to scientific substance, and global applicability to industry rather than focusing on any single industrial sector."[20]

Horner understood this strategy would appeal to other industries facing regulatory challenges. Sure enough, it was immediately picked up by the most polluting energy companies—fossil fuel producers and the coal-burning utilities—in their efforts to slow the EPA's regulation of the particulates that cause thousands of premature deaths every year. And these companies found a new champion in Congressman Lamar Smith (R-TX), who assumed the chairmanship of the House Science Committee in 2013 and introduced legislation forbidding EPA from using any study unless the authors submitted all the raw data, computer programs and analysis tools for the EPA to post on the Internet. He called it the Secret Science Reform Act.

Smith promoted his bill by claiming that sound science requires transparency and replication—and since the polluting companies couldn't access the raw data of the studies on which EPA relied, how could we trust that the findings were accurate? But this justification is a caricature of how science really works. While in theory most studies *could* be reproduced, they rarely are, because it is a waste of resources. Instead, scientists try to approach the same topic from *different* angles, using different methodologies, to determine if the results acquired support each other. As Bernard Goldstein, associate administrator of the EPA under President Reagan explained, reanalyzing the same study over and over is about as useful as checking on a surprising newspaper article by buying additional copies of the same paper to see if they all say the same thing.

Polluting corporations that conduct their own research, if pressed to defend their products and emissions, would no doubt be able to provide whatever data and materials that this new legislation might require.

But for independent researchers, this bill's requirements would place demands that would render much of environmental science, particularly epidemiologic studies, outside the evidence base available to the EPA. In other words, they would become irrelevant to efforts by the agency to protect the public and the environment. Why? Because most studies involving humans provide the subjects with assurances of confidentiality, with the investigators agreeing in advance to keep raw, identifiable data secret; EPA promises to redact the information before posting would not be sufficient to meet the scientists' obligations to the subjects. Moreover, it is unlikely that Canadian or European scientists would turn over their raw data to a U.S. agency for "independent validation," especially with that agency increasingly known for anything but independent evaluation. And because important studies on disasters like Deepwater Horizon or Chernobyl are, fortunately, not reproducible—well, sorry. Great work on that once-in-a-lifetime disaster, but not good enough for the EPA.

When Smith introduced his proposed legislation in 2015, a slew of the nation's leading science organizations came out in strong opposition, as did President Obama's EPA. But with the Republican majority at the time, it still passed the House of Representatives with only a single Republican voting no. It then died in the Senate, thanks to the standing threat of a filibuster by Democrats. And even if it had passed the Senate, President Obama would have vetoed it.

But that was then. As of January 20, 2017, we no longer had that confidence. Lamar Smith lost no time reintroducing the legislation, but with a new title: "Honest and Open New EPA Science Treatment Act," aka the HONEST Act. Hoping to mobilize the scientific community, Tom Burke, who served as EPA science advisor under President Obama, and I prepared to write an editorial opposing the legislation at the request of the editors of *Science*, the leading U.S. science journal.[21] In researching the new version of Smith's legislation, it became clear how the Trump administration planned to use the bill, and it was exactly what all of us had feared. The EPA would use only studies *provided by industry* that met the new requirements, and not even that many of them. When Smith's first version was under review, the EPA provided the Congressional Budget Office (CBO) its estimation for the cost of gathering, redacting and posting the data on a public website: $250 million annually.[22] The Trump administration's estimate of the implementation cost for the second version dropped to $1 million annually. How could this be? Here's the candid, shocking explanation from the CBO:

> EPA officials have explained to CBO that the agency would implement the legislation with minimal funding and generally would not disseminate information for the scientific studies that it uses to support covered actions. That approach to implementing the legislation *would significantly reduce the number of studies that the agency relies on* when issuing or proposing covered actions for the first few years following enactment of the legislation [emphasis added].[23]

This was no doubt music to the ears of the House Republicans, and they passed the HONEST Act in a hurry, although the opposition did manage to convince seven out of the 232 Republicans to vote no. But again the Senate stood in the way, so the Trump administration decided to do an end-run around Congress and implement this drastic change through regulation. This effort has generated even more controversy. The same science organizations weighed in against the bill, of course, but now the Pentagon broke the informal rule against publicizing interagency conflicts and also openly opposed it.[24] (Different departments generally don't oppose each other's proposals—it's not good form—but try to resolve their differences through the White House.) Lawsuits are inevitable in this case, and there is a chance this administration's end-run around Congress will not be upheld by the courts.

These truly are perilous times. The direct impacts of the Trump administration's actions—and more broadly, those of Republicans across the preceding decades—on health and life on this planet will be measurable only with the benefit of time. For now, the rejection of science in order to enable industries to operate unchecked has already delayed action to slow the buildup of greenhouse gases for years beyond what would have been optimal. We are already paying the price in rising sea levels, more fierce and frequent wildfires, new patterns of vector-borne illness, and extreme weather events in virtually every part of the globe. If Trump's efforts to roll back EPA clean air rules prove successful, increased air pollution will result in tens of thousands of premature deaths and hundreds of thousands of cases of respiratory disease in children across the country.[25]

Beyond these obvious health and environmental impacts, the Republican efforts to dismiss science and ravage federal science agencies will make future repair of a damaged regulatory system that much more difficult. The exodus of the country's best and brightest from many federal agencies will, in the best scenario, take time to build back. Senior scientists and high-level managers, men and women with decades of expertise and willing to make the sacrifices required by a career in public service, are being forced out. Many others are leaving of their own accord, often in frustration or disheartened by the policy changes dictated from the top of the agencies. If and when American government becomes the mostly level playing field it was in past administrations, rebuilding the science-based agencies with talented, qualified people will still be difficult.

And what of the even more fundamental damage done by President Trump and the Republicans to the scientific enterprise itself? There are no "alternative facts" in science. Well-meaning observers can interpret the same data differently, but that isn't what is going on now. We need the best science and the best scientists to solve the problems facing the world. To be successful, the climate change and evolution deniers, the defenders of secondhand smoke, and the product defense industry as a whole, must disparage science and scientists. Just as Trump's attacks on fact-based journalism increase disbelief (if not animosity) toward the news media, attacks on science feed dangerous myths and misunderstanding about vaccines, abortion, climate change, and a host of other pressing issues. The result is cynicism about science and rejection of science-based policy. The costs to people, the environment, and our future are enormous.

14

Science for Sale

SCIENCE, IN ITS pure form at least, is about asking questions, designing experiments, and scrutinizing the evidence to find an answer. This book has mostly focused on product defense scientists, whose full-time and lucrative employment involves manufacturing uncertainty. But only a small portion of the studies examining harm from exposure to products or pollutants are done by product defense scientists. Many are produced by academics with government, corporate, or foundation funding, or no outside funding at all. Many other studies are undertaken by scientists in the laboratories of government agencies or corporations.

Not surprisingly, no matter who performs the study, those paid for by a private sponsor tend to deliver the results the sponsor wants. This was seen in the tobacco literature, when the tobacco industry was still holding firm to the idea that secondhand smoke did not increase lung cancer risk.[1] Within the field it's called the "funding effect," or, maybe more cynically, the Golden Rule: those who have the gold make the rules. In broadest terms, it's the main subject of this book. There have been so many studies documenting the funding effect in evaluating risk associated with tobacco, food products, chemicals, and pollutants that it is almost surprising when manufacturers of a product sponsor a study that does not find the results they desire.

We know the impact of the funding effect because, for many studies, the authors acknowledge who paid for their work. This is more common now that journals are insisting on it, but there are still, as discussed below, plenty of studies with incomplete or misleading disclosures.

Disclosure of conflicts of interest are important, but are they as important as the conflict itself? No way. The disclosure figures into the assessment of the scientific research as published, but it is the actual conflict that shapes the course of the research itself. It's a huge difference, and one that's easily forgotten.

I have been asked why we should care about financial conflicts of interest. Doesn't the work stand or fall on its own, and shouldn't it be evaluated on its own, without regard to who paid for it? Well, no. Some scientists will say pretty much whatever someone pays them to say. But the broader "conflict" issue is much more nuanced than that. Theoretically, a scientist conducting an experiment and following certain accepted methods will find the same results as anyone else who does the same experiment the same way. That's the theory. In most laboratory experiments, however, even more so in field studies involving humans, the investigator must make many decisions along the way that can shape the outcome. And we look at the world through our own prior beliefs (a perhaps kinder way of saying prejudices), theories, and experiences, and these can impact all of our decisions while conducting the research. A relatively new label for this dynamic is "motivated reasoning." And, to get to the point of this book, the funding source for any research—who's footing the bill—is a powerful motivator of anyone's reasoning. Any of us would look at the same data differently than someone with a different set of financial relationships.

But why is it that scientists produce the results their sponsors want? In some cases, the studies are designed, essentially rigged, to find certain results.[2] But in other cases, scientists look at the same data and see different things. The impact of motivated reasoning on the interpretation of data has been powerfully demonstrated in an experiment involving very respected scientists, some with financial conflicts and others without, who provided differing interpretations of a data set before the truth was known. At the center of this experiment was Vioxx (the brand name for rofecoxib), the non-steroidal anti-inflammatory drug (NSAID) that was introduced to the market by Merck & Co., Inc. in 1999. NSAIDs are pain killers, especially important for alleviating osteoarthritis pain because many of these sufferers can't take other NSAIDs (aspirin, for example) because they cause gastrointestinal problems. Merck marketed Vioxx as an effective, safe alternative: a painkiller that doesn't cause GI problems. That story follows, in extreme brief.

Most pharmaceutical companies don't want to test a proposed new drug head-to-head against an existing one. The new drug, even if it's effective in its own right, might still be found *less* effective than the old one. Not good, because it loses the possibility of touting that "our drug is better than theirs." Trials against placebos are better for pharmaceutical companies, but in a market with already proven performers, including aspirin, the FDA requires a head-to-head test against at least one of the competitors. The choice of the opposition in such trials is complicated and, clearly, very important. In the case of Vioxx, one obvious factor was aspirin's widely known cardiovascular benefits; Vioxx would be unlikely to beat it in that regard. Many other factors were also considered, and in the end, Merck chose naproxen (sold over the counter as Aleve) as the competition. The drug company set up a large randomized trial comprising 8,000 participants.

The early Vioxx results available in 2000 were not clear-cut; conflicting interpretations were possible. From one perspective, test subjects taking Vioxx had 2.4 times the risk of a cardiovascular event compared with those taking Aleve. This was the interpretation of three scientists not associated with Merck who published a review of the Vioxx trial in the August 2001 *Journal of the American Medical Association*.[3] The stunning conclusion was not welcome in Merck's headquarters and laboratories.

But wait a minute. Couldn't that interpretation of the data be challenged? Merck could and did argue that the trial demonstrated not that Vioxx was *bad* for hearts relative to Aleve, but that Aleve was extraordinarily *good* for hearts—on par even with the famously heart-friendly aspirin. Merck-affiliated scientists wrote, "Differences observed between [Vioxx] and [Aleve] are likely the result of the antiplatelet effects of the latter agent."[4] In effect, Merck and its consulting scientists chose the interpretation that improbably credited the comparison drug with preventing disease over the interpretation that much more plausibly indicted its own drug for increasing the risk of cardiac problems. The Merck scientists (the lead author was actually an academic physician consulting for Merck) wrote, "We believe that the analysis of [the independent scientists] provides no substantive support for their conclusions."[5]

The truth dramatically and tragically appeared not long afterward. There was and is reason to believe that Vioxx also prevents colon polyps, which are precursors to colon cancer. A new clinical trial was initiated, and since no agent is known to prevent these polyps, this trial used placebos as the comparator. Even before the trial was scheduled to end, the experimenters halted it. Halfway through the trial, participants who took Vioxx for more than eighteen months had suffered twice as many heart attacks and strokes as those who took a placebo—seven excess heart attacks per thousand users per year. The correct interpretation of the original study was now beyond question: Vioxx causes heart attacks. These results were front-page news around the world. The drug was removed from the market, but too late. FDA scientists estimated that Vioxx caused between 88,000 and 139,000 heart attacks, probably 30 to 40 percent of them fatal, in the four years the drug was on the market.[6]

Indisputably, Merck did play fast and loose with the data to make its drug look far safer than it was. If its scientists had truly believed that Aleve reduced the risk of heart attack by 60 percent (there were numerous reasons to be suspicious of that finding, and it did turn out to be groundless), Merck should have lobbied the government to pour the drug directly into the water supply. Instead, they launched a concerted attack on the independent scientists who first identified the problem with Vioxx, while manipulating the data to obscure the risks when it published flawed and incomplete results of the trials. It turned out that Merck ghostwrote papers published under the names of academic scientists and several of the studies contained such serious mistakes that two respected journals were forced to issue corrections.[7] The *New England Journal of Medicine* issued two "expressions of concern" in which the editor criticized Merck because it "did not accurately represent the safety data available to the authors when the article was being reviewed for publication."[8] Merck pled guilty to criminal charges over marketing and sales of Vioxx and paid a $950 million fine. It also paid almost $5 billion to settle lawsuits by people taking the drug or family members.

All that said, it is not unreasonable to give the benefit of the doubt to the humanity of the academic scientists who were consultants to Merck. I think, or would like to think, they would never have kept pushing a drug that they knew doubled the risk of heart attacks. They did not consciously lie (I hope). They *did* convince themselves the drug was safe. They looked at what is in retrospect powerfully clear data and simply didn't see the obvious.

I don't mind giving product defense scientists the same benefit of the doubt. They may not be intentionally misinterpreting the data or issuing misleading conclusions. And in some cases, maybe their interpretations will someday turn out to be accurate. But, as the philosopher Cyndi Lauper explained, "Money changes everything." Given what we know about how conflict of interest shapes how one looks at data, and given who is paying their generally substantial fees, the conclusions of these scientists about the toxicity of a product produced by their client simply cannot and should not be treated as valid.

———

But sometimes, I believe, scientists do intentionally misinterpret data or issue misleading conclusions. It is not an exaggeration to say that in the product defense model, the investigator starts with an answer, then figures out the best way to support it. As often as not, the product defense investigator starts with *someone else's* answer, then reviews the evidence or subjects an important study to a post-hoc "re-analysis" that magically produces the sponsor's preferred conclusions—that the risk is not that high, the harm not that bad, and/or the data fatally flawed. These are the studies that are flogged to regulatory agencies or in litigation.

What follows here is a modest overview of some of these firms' specific methods (and the conventional identifiers of those methods) for repackaging science as something more malleable. While this is unquestionably some "inside baseball," my hope here is to provide a field guide to the behaviors of mercenary scientists and product defense firms in the wild. Recognizing these behaviors can be tremendously valuable in trying to frame public discourse in today's toxic political environment. It can also be kind of fun.

What follows is the product defense disinformation playbook.

The Weight of the Evidence

One popular tactic—maybe the most popular—is some version of "reviewing the literature." The basic idea is valid; we *do* need to consider the scientific studies to date to attempt to answer important questions. The questions that come up in regulation and litigation are complex; they go way beyond simply asking, "Does this chemical cause cancer or lower sperm count or cause developmental damage?" With public health issues, the important and tricky part is determining at what level an exposure can contribute to the undesired effect, and after how much time and exposure. Is there a safe level of exposure, below which a chemical cannot cause disease (or has not, in the case of litigation)? No single study answers such questions, so reviews are warranted. Sometimes these literature reviews are labeled "weight-of-the-evidence" analyses, with the authors deciding how much importance to give each study. But if your business model—your whole enterprise—is based on being paid by the manufacturers of the product in question for those reviews, your judgment is suspect by definition. More specifically, if a review was undertaken by conflicted scientists in business to provide conclusions needed by a commercial sponsor to delay regulation or defeat litigation, the findings are tainted and should be discarded. How can we know if the weight they've assigned different studies, intentionally or unconsciously, is impacted by the fact that their sponsors want a certain result?

I have seen product defense firms use "weight of the evidence" analyses to create uncertainty about virtually every common toxic exposure, no matter how strong the evidence. Take, for example, ozone, the invisible atmospheric gas. Ozone can inflame and damage airways and aggravate existing lung diseases like asthma, emphysema, and chronic bronchitis. Countless studies have confirmed that emergency room visits and hospitalizations for asthma spike with increases in ozone level in the atmosphere. But the leaders of the Texas Commission on Environmental Quality (TCEQ), a government agency that acts as if it is a wholly owned subsidiary of the oil and gas industry (and perhaps, as a branch of the Texas state government, it is), have long held that the dangers from ozone, as well as other pollutants from fuel combustion, are greatly exaggerated. The commission's top toxicologist, Michael Honeycutt, who was later appointed by President Trump to chair the EPA's Science Advisory Board, is on record saying that lowering ozone levels will *increase* the risk of lung disease.[9] This is exactly the opposite of what accepted wisdom, and the evidence at hand in Texas and elsewhere, has to say.

In need of scientific backup to give oil and gas companies relief, the TCEQ hired the product defense firm Gradient to question this otherwise widely accepted relationship between ozone concentrations and asthma severity. But even Gradient (which received more than $2.2 million from the TCEQ[10]) couldn't make this evidence completely disappear. The best they could do, in light of overwhelming evidence, was to take the tobacco road and stress the uncertainty: the evidence was "not sufficient to conclude that a causal relationship exists. The substantial uncertainty in the body of evidence should be taken into consideration when this evidence is used for policymaking."[11]

Gradient seems to have a particular expertise in weighing the evidence on air pollutants and concluding the studies that find harm are light and filled with flaws and uncertainty. Working on behalf of the trade association representing electrical power companies (they burn fossil fuels and contribute to ozone exposure), Gradient scientists published a study titled "Critical Review of Long-Term Ozone Exposure and Asthma Development." The conclusion: the studies are inconsistent and more research is needed to address "key uncertainties."[12]

Of course, the true purpose of these literature reviews is to help stop government agencies from strengthening public health protections, so corporations that produce and burn fossil fuels will not be forced to change their economic model. Gradient scientists are confident that "available evidence does not indicate that proposed lower ozone standards would be more health protective than the current one[s]"[13] and they weigh in with the EPA on behalf of the American Petroleum Institute and the TCEQ each time the EPA considers a strengthened ozone standard.[14]

Gradient has also long worked for corporations that pollute the environment with lead, an exposure that can impact children's neurological development even at low levels. The Gradient clients with a financial interest in showing that lead exposure is not as dangerous as most research concludes include the Battery Council International (consisting of firms that manufacture, sell, or recycle lead batteries),[15] and smelters which have been cited for environmental lead pollution.[16] When EPA was tightening its environmental lead standard during the Clinton administration, Gradient experts went to the White House on behalf of the Association of Battery Recyclers. Its presentation highlighted "unresolved potential math errors" and the uncertainties in the scientific literature used by EPA to justify the stronger standard.[17]

Some studies have also suggested that lead exposure is associated with autism spectrum disorder (ASD);[18] Gradient's team has developed a different viewpoint. In a presentation at a scientific meeting entitled "A Weight-of-Evidence Evaluation of the Association Between Lead Exposure and Autism Spectrum Disorders," the conclusion said: "Lead exposure is not associated with the development or severity of ASD." (The client for the study was not identified. Instead of that disclosure we have this: "The underlying work for this poster was supported by a private client, but the opinions presented here are solely those of the authors. Dr. [Barbara] Beck was named as an expert witness in a matter for which she relied, in part, on results from this analysis."[19]) It could very well be true that lead plays no role in the development of autism but, given the provenance of Gradient's work, and their history of minimizing the neurotoxic effects of the neurotoxic metal on behalf of the lead industry, how can anyone accept this literature evaluation as unbiased?

The Risk Assessment

Weight-of-the-evidence reviews generally include both human and animal studies, and the attribution of weight to any given study is generally a subjective, qualitative decision. A more quantitative approach to reviewing the literature entails risk assessment, which in its earnest form attempts to provide estimates of the likelihood of effects at different exposure levels. Importantly, risk assessments attempt to estimate the levels below which exposure to a given substance will cause no harm. But as William Ruckelshaus, the first head of the EPA, famously said, "A risk assessment is like a captured spy: Torture it enough and it will tell you anything."

This much is true: there is tremendous variation in the results of many risk assessments. There are also individual scientists and firms who can be counted on to produce risk assessments that, conveniently for their sponsors, find significant risk only at levels far above the levels where most exposures are occurring. And if these risk assessments are accepted by regulatory agencies or jurors, the sponsors will be required to spend far less money cleaning up their pollution or compensating victims.

One purveyor of mercenary literature reviews and risk assessments who merits discussion is Michael Dourson, toxicologist and founder and principal at the nonprofit Toxicology Excellence for Risk Assessment (TERA). Dourson has made a career of manufacturing doubt to defend toxic chemicals. Over and over again, chemical manufacturers have paid him and TERA to help make the case for weak, inadequately protective public health standards.

Dourson's *modus operandi* is ingenious. With funding in hand from a firm or an industry producing a product under scrutiny, his TERA team reviews the studies and produces a risk assessment that almost without exception minimizes the risk, pinpointing a level for "safe" exposure that is almost without exception many times higher than the risk assessment level determined by academic or government scientists. Sometimes TERA's risk assessment is provided by a panel of "independent" experts, many of whom are not actually independent. The work is presented as legitimate science and often published in one of the industry-controlled journals discussed in Chapter 2.

An example: Dourson and his colleagues published a paper about "managing risks of noncancer endpoints at hazardous waste sites" focused on the widespread and very dangerous solvent trichloroethylene. In the paper, he proposed a range of safety standards up to 15 times weaker than EPA's for the same exposure. Cleaning hazardous waste sites to meet these weaker standards would be advantageous to the members of the American Chemistry Council. How was the paper funded? By "a gift from the American Chemistry Council."[20]

TERA provided risk assessments that determined a safe level that would be less protective, often hundreds of times less protective, than the risk assessments done by public health agencies for numerous toxic chemicals. The firm has provided this service for Dow AgroSciences (for the pesticide Chlorpyrifos that EPA staff had recommended banning until they were over-ruled by both of President Trump's EPA Administrators); Koch Industries (petroleum coke); ACC's North American Flame Retardant Alliance (the flame retardant tetrabromobisphenol A); Cargill, Coca-Cola, ConAgra Foods, Frito-Lay North America, General Mills, J. M. Smucker Co., Land O'Lakes, Procter &

Gamble, and Unilever) (diacetyl, which causes bronchiolitis obliterans, or popcorn lung, in exposed workers), and, of course, DuPont (for the PFAS used in manufacturing Teflon) that I discuss in Chapter 3. The list goes on and on.[21]

Dourson became industry's go-to hired gun for this kind of product defense "science," always ready to minimize the risks of exposure to their toxic chemicals and to weaken standards that should be protecting the health and safety of Americans. Having provided so much help to the chemical industry, Dourson was a logical selection to be President Trump's nominee for the EPA's assistant administrator for chemical safety and pollution prevention. Following his nomination, activists around the country organized against his nomination, bringing to Washington people who had been hurt by the same chemicals whose risks he minimized. This was too much for even some Republican lawmakers, and, as discussed in the following chapter, his nomination failed.

The Reanalysis

By its nature, epidemiology is a sitting duck for the product defense industry's uncertainty campaigns. Epidemiology's studies are complicated and require complex statistical analyses. Judgment is called for all along the way, so good intentions are paramount. Both epidemiologic principles and ethics require that the methods of analysis be selected before the data are actually analyzed. One tactic used by some of the product defense firms is the re-analysis, where the raw data from a completed study are looked at again, changing the way the data are analyzed, often in the most mercenary of ways. The joke about "lies, damned lies, and statistics" pertains.

The battle for the integrity of science is rooted in these sorts of issues around methodology. If a scientist with a certain skill set knows the original outcome and how the data are distributed within the study, it's easy enough to design an alternative analysis that will make positive results disappear. This is especially true with findings that link a toxic exposure to disease later on—which also happen to be among the most important results for public health agencies. In contrast, if there is no effect from exposure, post hoc analysis to turn a negative study positive is generally difficult and often not possible, since the effect of interest is equally distributed across all parts of the study population.

As with most things about product defense, the re-analysis strategy dates back to tobacco, whose strategists recognized that they needed a means to counter early findings related to smoking's dangers, in order to shirk responsibility and regulation for lung cancer risk among non-smoking spouses of smokers. From a public health perspective, a 25 percent increase in cancer risk is a big deal. To industry, making it disappear would be a huge deal, and that's why they brought in the re-analysts. The tobacco strategists also realized that they couldn't mount their own studies, which would take years and millions of dollars, so they figured they could get the raw data from the incriminating studies, change some of the basic assumptions, change the parameters, tinker with this and that, and make the results go away. Tobacco's approach is now commonplace; "re-analysis" is its own cottage industry within product defense.

An early, non-tobacco example came following a 1987 study by NIOSH's Robert Rinsky and colleagues, published in the *New England Journal of Medicine*. This report showed that OSHA's workplace benzene-exposure standard, then 10 parts per million (ppm), was inadequate and estimated that benzene exposure increased risk of leukemia even at lifetime exposures below 1 ppm. OSHA then leveraged this study in setting a new standard of 1 ppm, which posed massive financial implications for the oil industry. Since then the petroleum producers have spent millions of dollars and hired several of the leading product defense firms to re-analyze these results in order to convince regulators and courts that low levels of exposure to benzene simply aren't so dangerous. The American Petroleum Institute (here they are again) or another branch of the oil industry have commissioned the same product defense firms that appear in virtually every chapter in this book, including Exponent, ChemRisk, Ramboll, and Gradient, to pull apart Rinsky's study. They have produced at least nine papers in the scientific literature as part of this campaign to make Rinsky's results go away.[22] But they are all *post hoc* analyses and none of them are very convincing. Since the scientific community (outside of the oil industry and their consultants) recognize the causal link between low levels of benzene exposure and leukemia, there is little additional epidemiologic research under way in this area. Actual studies of benzene-exposed workers (rather than these mercenary re-analyses) published subsequently by researchers *not* paid by the oil industry continue to find benzene effects at very low levels of exposure.[23] Based on these studies, the European Union has announced plans to cut the allowable maximum workplace exposure level by 95 percent, to 0.05 ppm.[24]

The Back-in-Time Simulation

In many mercenary re-analyses of epidemiologic studies that find increased risk of disease associated with low levels of exposure to a given chemical, the product defense scientists decide that the actual exposures in the study were in fact far higher than those estimated by the scientists who did the original study. This is farcical, of course, but highly useful: a retrospective adjustment to the exposure level is guaranteed to change the results of the study, making the exposure look safer because now only those higher levels cause disease. And, of course, the conflicted scientists doing the reanalysis know very well this is exactly what will happen if they juice up the exposure estimates.

But when there is no longer debate whether exposure to a substance causes disease at a given level, a firm whose product is under attack may want to show that historical exposures in the past were lower, not higher. These types of studies, usually conducted by attempting to re-create historical exposure levels in a laboratory, are generally done only for high-stakes court cases, since there is little if any scientific interest in revisiting settled science around old exposure levels. The basic model sometimes involves finding the original product—often that is no longer manufactured or in use—and then simulating the exposure that a plaintiff in a court case would have experienced decades earlier. Pretty much the only reason these studies get published in a scientific journal is so the expert can testify that their study was peer-reviewed.

As a rule, litigation-generated studies like these receive little response in the scientific literature and have no significance in setting regulations. Critics of these efforts, like Brown University physician David Egilman, have shown how the studies can be manipulated to underestimate exposure and thus produce the outcomes desired by whomever is paying the bill. Egilman demonstrated this in a study of asbestos exposures associated with working with Bakelite, a synthetic plastic made by Union Carbide. The exposure was simulated by the product defense firms Exponent and ChemRisk.[25] Egilman documented that the experimenters had access to but ignored actual asbestos measures taken in the 1970s in order to claim that the exposure levels found in their simulation were low and therefore presumably safe. Union Carbide paid about a million dollars for this paper, but it was worth it. In fact, Dennis Paustenbach, a leading purveyor of these exposure recreations and co-author of the Bakelite paper, boasted that as long as a recreation indicated that historical exposures were minimal, "I'm not aware of a single case that has been lost in litigation in the U.S. when a high-quality simulation study was done."[26]

The "Independence" Gambit

Many papers produced by the product defense firms contain the disclosure that individual scientists may be testifying for the corporations being sued, but that the research itself was done *independently* of the corporations. This sleight-of-hand provides a fiction of independence that might provide a fiction of objectivity. But the research was almost certainly paid for by the product defense firm out of the fees it was paid by the corporation. It's a charade, but also standard practice.

An example is tucked within a letter written to a Ford Motor Company attorney by ChemRisk's Paustenbach. As part of his request for more money for his firm, Paustenbach cites the value of producing these sorts of studies, which are of great value to their clients. In Paustenbach's words: "Over the past 5 years, I have personally spent (in hard or soft dollars) a little more than $3M in profits (which would have been distributed to me or my staff) in asbestos-related research which has been enormously illuminating to the courts and juries. I did this because I believe that the courts deserve to have all the scientific information that can be brought to the table when reaching conclusions. In my view, these papers have changed the scientific playing field in the courtroom. You know better than anyone as you have seen the number of plaintiff verdicts decrease and the cost of settlement go down." He then goes on to discuss a paper which had been used in 30 or so cases in the 90 days after it was published, and that cost ChemRisk $300,000 in effort.[27]

Similarly, manufacturer Georgia-Pacific (GP) launched a secretive $6 million program to produce papers that would increase its ability to win suits in connection with asbestos exposure from a joint compound it marketed in the 1960s and 1970s. Using Exponent, ENVIRON (now Ramboll), and other consultants, the manufacturer developed a comprehensive research agenda to conduct a suite of 13 studies, all aimed at showing that the risk from their product was low.[28] ENVIRON was tasked to attempt to recreate the levels of exposure that workers might have had when they were working with the joint compound. David Bernstein, a toxicologist hired to study the effects on lab animals, was lead author on several papers published in the *Journal of Inhalation Toxicology* for which the disclosure statement read in its entirety: "This work was supported by a grant from Georgia-Pacific, LLC." A coauthor on these papers was Stewart E. Holm, who headed this research initiative for GP, but didn't exactly make a scientific contribution. In documents that later came out, it turns out his work was "directed solely by GP's in-house counsel." Eventually, Holm sent a correction to the journal acknowledging he worked for GP (although not saying he was part of the legal team), which then published an apology for not including the relevant information.[29]

The truth about Holm's role and the fact that all the studies were commissioned as part of a legal effort came out in a legal dispute in New York, where Georgia-Pacific tried to claim that many of the documents underlying the studies were subject to the attorney-work-product privilege. This is one of the older tricks in the playbook, again perfected by the tobacco industry: hiding suspect scientific work by claiming attorney-client privilege. The New York court did not see it that way:

> GP should not be allowed to use its experts' conclusions as a sword by seeding the scientific literature with GP-funded studies, while at the same time using the privilege as a shield by withholding the underlying raw data that might be prone to scrutiny by the opposing party and that may affect the veracity of its experts' conclusions.[30]

Occasionally authors of industry studies leave off the conflict-of-interest disclosure entirely. One stunning episode was a paper written by two well-known Italian epidemiologists who have been deeply involved in product defense, Carlo La Vecchia and Paolo Boffetta. Boffetta (now associated with Cardno ChemRisk), has published literature reviews paid for by firms or trade groups eager to dispute independent studies that found cancer risk from exposure to, among other toxic chemicals, beryllium,[31] diesel exhaust,[32] formaldehyde,[33] styrene,[34] and the non-stick PFAS chemicals used to make Teflon and Scotchgard.[35]

In one instance, the two epidemiologists analyzed the patterns of death in several populations of asbestos-exposed workers in Italy, concluding that "for workers exposed in the distant past, the risk of mesothelioma is not appreciably modified by subsequent exposures, and that stopping exposure does not materially modify the subsequent risk of mesothelioma."[36] In short: once you're exposed to asbestos, might as well be exposed a bunch more later on; it's all the same. Putting aside the public health implications of such an argument, this paper was conspicuously useful to corporations (and corporate executives) responsible for exposing workers to asbestos in the last few decades: the cancers among these workers could be attributed to earlier exposures, before the period covered by statutes of limitations.

In La Vecchia and Boffetta's conflict-of-interest disclosure, they stated, "There are no conflicts of interest." The authors did note that the "work was conducted with the contribution of the Italian Association for Cancer Research (AIRC), project No. 10068." This sounds high-minded enough, but both authors had also been witnesses for the defense in a high-profile trial of an asbestos company executive in Italy, so their work defending an asbestos producer facing criminal charges was no secret within the scientific community. The study itself came under extensive criticism by Benedetto Terracini and other prominent Italian epidemiologists,[37] and, in addition, the unacknowledged conflict of interest resulted in much censure of the authors and the journal, which (two years later) published an extensive correction. The correction acknowledged the testimony on criminal defense work done by the authors and withdrew the statement that AIRC had funded the study, since it had not.[38]

Front Groups

A different kind of conflict of interest, and a different kind of disclosure trickery, is the use of front groups by many industries to advance their interests while hiding their involvement. These fronts are generally incorporated as not-for-profits, with academic scientists in leadership, and innocuous-sounding names, but they are bought and paid for by their various corporate sponsors, many of them sponsoring "research" to be used in regulatory proceedings or the court. In addition, there are the all-corporate-purpose think tanks devoted to "free enterprise" and "free markets" and "deregulation." Dozens of them work on behalf of just about every significant industry in this country. Each year these entities collect millions of dollars from regulated companies to promote campaigns that weaken public health and environmental protections.

Always, the idea is to portray front groups as serious, independent purveyors of scientific research. And some *do* produce legitimate science, while at the same time producing purely questionable science that its sponsoring organizations rely on to promote their unhealthy products. It's a delicate balancing act. Perhaps the most successful of these mixed-purpose outfits is the International Life Sciences Institute, "a nonprofit, worldwide organization whose mission is to provide science that improves human health and well-being and safeguards the environment." ILSI was founded in 1978 by Alex Malaspina, Coca-Cola's senior vice-president, and it long has had significant funding from the beverage giant.[39] It is also notably open about its funding sources and sponsors, which include hundreds of food and pesticide producers, including ConAgra, Kellogg, Kraft, McDonald's, Nestlé, PepsiCo, and Unilever, along with the pesticide and seed companies Bayer (which purchased Monsanto in 2018), Syngenta, and Dow.[40] CropLife International, the global trade association of pesticide manufacturers, is a major contributor.[41] ILSI's membership confirms that the organization has met Malaspina's objective "to unite the food industry" by doing work that no single manufacturer, not even Coke, could have accomplished on its own.

With support from these and other corporations and associations, ILSI funds genuine academic research. It also convenes conferences and brings together experts to produce research and reports. There is no question; some of the studies have value. But under this guise of addressing important scientific issues, they also promote positions that greatly benefit their sponsors. True to its roots, ILSI has always been a faithful advocate for the sugar industry, but it doesn't fund scientists to defend something outrageous, like the proposition that unlimited sugar consumption is safe. Instead, it comes at the issue indirectly, surreptitiously, by questioning the quality of the science underlying the dietary guidelines that recommend limiting sugar intake.[42] That particular ISLI literature review was paid for by its technical committee on dietary carbohydrates. Sitting at that table are Coca-Cola, Dr. Pepper, PepsiCo, Archer Daniels Midland, Campbell Soup Company, General Mills, Hershey, Kellogg Company—in combination, a major source of carbohydrates in the diets of most Americans.[43] This is one more example of the funding effect. The organization's critics have succinctly captured what is actually occurring here: ILSI's claims that there is inadequate evidence to justify placing limits to junk food is based on junk science.[44]

15

Future in Doubt

HISTORICALLY, HUMAN HEALTH has taken a backseat to economic growth and product sales. Whether the product is tobacco or cosmetics, baby formula or a pesticide, we have allowed firms to use, produce, and emit potentially harmful products, then ask questions later if things go wrong. This system, capitalism, has the capacity to produce extreme wealth and economic development, but at a severe cost to human health and the environment.

Today many widely used consumer products (and the chemicals used in the production of those products) are safe only when encountered at low levels of exposure. At higher levels, they are harmful. For some of the toxins I've written about in this book, like asbestos or PFAS compounds, there is compelling evidence they cause harm to humans at absurdly low exposure levels. Most people alive today have already been exposed, many more will be, and the health of a significant number of people will be affected over time.

And that's just the old stuff. New chemicals and new hazards enter the market every day. With each of them, we won't know—and to some extent, we cannot know—their harmful effects until long after they are on the market. By then, perhaps millions or even billions of people will have been exposed.

One could argue that we could maintain economic growth and our modern lifestyle with much lower industrial use of some of these chemicals. Defenders of the status quo, while perhaps acknowledging the social costs of these products, argue that the consumer and economic benefits greatly outweigh the harms. Such cold cost-benefit analyses are loaded with unstated values and assumptions, and the calculations are typically conducted imperfectly and indirectly, through litigation and government mandated programs (e.g., the "polluter pays" approach to cleaning up of Superfund sites where toxic waste has been left to foul the surrounding environment).

The premise of this book is that corporations, when faced with the reality that their products are doing damage to customers, employees, or the environment, too often respond with denials and defenses that are disingenuous at best, reckless at worst. Corporations can't do this alone. They enlist hired guns—scientists along with attorneys, public relations specialists and others—to help undermine evidence, shape public opinion, delay protective regulation, and defeat litigation from people alleging current or past harm.

None of this is to say that corporations are inherently bad, or that corporate leaders are bad people. Most problematic corporate behavior happens through a series of small decisions made over a long period of time by many individuals. One challenge for publicly traded companies and corporations, and consequently the rest of us, is the pressure they face to deliver consistent, growing profits on a short-term basis. The free market economist Milton Friedman argued that a publicly held corporation's primary objective is to maximize shareholder value. In fact, Friedman viewed it as a fiduciary responsibility, one limited only by the boundaries of law and regulation—in essence, *do whatever it takes that isn't illegal.* In this sort of corporate ecosystem, there are consequences for companies that don't perform to expectations. They can face insurrection from shareholders or, increasingly, predatory actions from hedge funds or corporate raiders that have been known to leverage shareholder disquiet into changes in ownership or leadership.

Where short-term profit is valued above all else, it is too easy to make decisions that result in harm to others in order to live another day. This philosophy has driven the executives across countless industries to do everything in their power (except breaking the law, at least theoretically) to produce products that harm humans. For fossil fuel industry executives, this includes marketing products that will have disastrous consequences for the future of life on earth.

Is it always this way? Are there companies that respond to early warning signs around the safety of their business, conduct a truly unbiased independent investigation of the facts and, if appropriate, pull a profitable product on the basis of reasonable (but perhaps not yet compelling) evidence regarding likely harmful impacts? Yes, a few. The outdoor clothing company Patagonia, which describes itself as an activist company "in business to save our home planet," is transparent about potential harms associated with its products. For example, as it has become increasingly clear that microplastics and tiny fibers from synthetic textiles are a significant source of ocean pollution, Patagonia has highlighted the problem and the company's efforts to address it.[1] Similarly, Seventh Generation, maker of ecologically minded household and personal care products, advertises its removal of potentially toxic contaminants from its products. The efforts of both these companies are laudable, if not easily transferrable: both cater to markets willing to pay more for environmentally friendly products - individuals who are also likely to be drawn to companies that champion social responsibility. (Also worth noting that Patagonia is privately owned; Seventh Generation was purchased by Unilever in 2016.)

Interestingly, some of the firms that have been most commendable in ensuring the safety of their workers have *not* appeared to make the best choices when it comes to producing and selling toxic chemicals. The 3M Corporation, for example, has a world-class worker safety program: I asked them and they generously shared some of their strategies and approaches with representatives of Chinese manufacturers under the auspices of a 2015 bilateral initiative in which OSHA collaborated with our Chinese counterpart, the State Administration of Workplace Safety. This bears stark contrast to the company's continued production of PFAS compounds until 2002, long after it was aware of the hazards and much too late to allay the harm already perpetrated. As laid out in Chapter 3, 3M has retained several of the more notorious product defense firms in order to minimize the dangers posed by the firm's PFAS water contamination; it has settled the lawsuit brought by the state of Minnesota for more than $800 million, but faces many others in all parts of the country.

The same dissonance could be cited in the behavior of Johnson & Johnson, which for decades has maintained an exemplary safety program for its workers. (During my tenure at OSHA, I appointed Joseph Van Houten, former head of Johnson & Johnson's environment, safety, and health office, to the federal agency's national advisory committee, where he helped shape regulatory activities.) But Johnson & Johnson was also one of the companies that funded the over-the-top promotion of opioids (Chapter 7), and was central to the manufacture of uncertainty around the cancer-causing potential of talc (Chapter 9).

There is a small movement under way in which some corporations seek to separate themselves from the myopic motivations that have been known to define them and toward acknowledgment that corporations may and should have other objectives beyond increasing shareholder value. Many firms at least give lip service to the goals of the sustainability movement: to meet the needs of the present without compromising the ability of future generations to meet their own needs. Corporate social responsibility has become a common talking point— if not full-fledged behavior—for larger companies, and it is too often part of a trend in which acknowledgment of sustainability's importance is a passable substitute for actually pursuing sustainability in earnest. Every major corporation now issues an annual sustainability report, which in theory at least encourages them to take positive steps— reducing their carbon footprint or water use or signing union contracts— because these behaviors are publicly disclosed.

These are positive developments, but *major* changes in this realm are not going to happen soon, at least not soon enough, or on a sufficiently large scale. What do we do in the meantime? The answer to that question has to begin with the laws and regulations that govern corporate behavior, because they're the primary levers of power that free-market theory acknowledges as viable. These laws not only need to protect health and the environment, but must also apply penalties high enough to discourage future lawbreakers. If the penalty is the loss of whatever profits accrued due to the illegal activity (and the penalty is often not even close to that amount), there is little disincentive for the illegal action, since in many cases the offending corporation will never be caught. To have any impact, the penalties have to be far *greater* than the earnings that were enabled by the transgression.

Of course, the writing of these laws and regulations is mightily influenced by the firms that are subject to them. This catch-22 is for another day—and another book. My subject here is the use and abuse of science in the public health realm. In order to have a system that protects people and the environment from harm, we must ensure the production and application of the best science possible, produced by independent, un-conflicted scientists. So how do we accomplish that?

Build the Evidence Base

In the simplest system, manufacturers would be responsible for estab-lishing what exposure to a product or substance is safe—with "safe" being established by an independent evaluation, not someone they oversee. Just as "polluter pays" is the governing principle in cleaning up contaminated land, producers should pay for toxicity studies and risk determinations. Make it "producer pays" and require manufacturing and importing firms to establish the safety of their products before they are allowed to capitalize on their sale.

The tests used to investigate the effects of chemicals on humans—generally involving nonhuman animals or cells, or even using computer models to estimate an effect or mechanism—are largely standardized and typically conducted in laboratories. Even though the interpretation of laboratory data can be influenced by financial relationships, it may be acceptable for manufacturers to conduct these standardized toxico-logical tests—as long as there are severe penalties for lying about the results, hiding studies or cooking the books. To be most effective, top corporate executives would have to sign off on the test results just as they must affirm the accuracy of their financial accounting, under the threat of criminal sanctions for wrongdoing

Selecting and designing studies beyond the standardized core re-quires decisions that can unquestionably impact the outcome; scientists control these experiments. Their choices include deciding the test methods and subjects, the types and levels of exposure, the length of exposure, the time frame for the study itself, and the health effects or physiological changes of interest, among other variables. And the choices scientists select make a big difference: short studies may provide certain information but offer little information about a chemical's abil-ity to cause cancer, for example.

So that's what we need: a system in which producers pay for the studies but do not control the scientists who do them. Because, if this book has demonstrated anything, I hope it is that the impact of financial conflict is present any time a scientist has a financial tie to an organization that would benefit from a particular outcome. There are several ways to address this issue. One is to have research overseen by parties with no financial interest in the results, as was the case in the lawsuit against DuPont that was detailed in Chapter 3. These studies were paid for by DuPont but performed by three epidemiologists chosen jointly by DuPont and the attorney suing the company on behalf of residents of West Virginia and Ohio, whose water was fouled by DuPont's chemicals.

In the early 1990s, I was involved with a similar effort related to DuPont, this time at the company's Chambers Works plant in New Jersey, where the workers manufactured organic lead. This was long before my tenure at OSHA, but I was brought in when the federal agency found unacceptably high levels of organic lead exposure among workers. (Decades earlier, the plant was labeled the "House of Butterflies" because of the hallucinations common among lead-exposed employees.[2]) DuPont agreed to commission a series of studies on the health effects of the exposure, to be overseen jointly by the company and the union. I was paid (modestly) by DuPont, but because I was selected by the union, DuPont could not fire me. I worked closely with my counterpart, DuPont epidemiologist Elizabeth Karns, overseeing the data collection for a series of important studies conducted by faculty at the Johns Hopkins School of Public Health, who themselves were able to decide on the method without direction from DuPont or the union.[3] There were many hands involved, each with limitations on what they were allowed to influence.

A more ambitious approach would be building independent institutions to commission and oversee studies prior to product release. In the United States, the best known of these is the Health Effects Institute (HEI), a research group originally established in 1980 by the EPA and the automobile industry to study the health effects of motor vehicle emissions, with each party contributing half the budget. HEI has since expanded to collaborate with more firms and industries, and it continues to produce research of great importance. Institutes like HEI are not a perfect solution. The corporations involved still wield undue influence, in that they can withdraw from HEI if they don't approve of a research project or its findings—a fact that must shape the thinking of HEI's leaders.

Could government scientists conduct the research, with industry paying for it? In the United States, it's probably not realistic. Even the U.S. National Institutes of Health, the country's most powerful health-research entity, struggles with ensuring that the integrity of its studies is not compromised by private funding. It has been burned at least twice—by the National Football League (Chapter 4) and the alcoholic beverage industry (Chapter 5)—and is currently re-evaluating whether it should continue to accept donations for funding these sorts of studies.

In the short and medium term, we will have to accept the fact that scientists, and especially those working for product defense consulting firms, will do studies for corporations that have a deep stake in finding a specific outcome (generally, that their product is perfectly safe, or at least the evidence showing risk is weak). For as long as this is the case, we need rules governing how industry-funded studies are performed. Let me suggest two:

First: No studies should be paid for by or through attorneys on behalf of a client. The only reason for money between a corporation and a scientist to flow through a law firm is to ensure that important information, including possibly unfavorable results, can be withheld from the public, regulatory agencies, and court cases. If only the favorable results are allowed to see the light of day, the science of record is potentially incomplete or misleading.

Second: Put an end to rigged data re-analyses. As we have seen time and again, product defense epidemiologists, provided with the raw data, will re-analyze the results of a government-funded study to produce results an industry needs in order to counter the original, damaging results. (As a legal matter, the government must provide these data when asked, thanks to tobacco industry prevarications discussed in Chapter 6.) The only objective of these re-analyses is to force regulators or jurors to doubt studies that provide unfavorable conclusions. Within the epidemiology community, it is widely understood that data analyses that use methods and comparisons selected *post hoc*—after studying the distribution of the data—are suspect and are not afforded the same credibility as those that test prior hypotheses. Some regulators understand this, too, but industry sponsors don't need to convince everyone in order to meet their ends; their audiences also include federal judges reviewing regulatory actions, or juries considering whether a chemical caused an illness. Moreover, once a re-analysis is done, that's usually where the issue ends. Federal support for occupational and environmental epidemiology is limited and shrinking as we speak. The government agencies and institutes that fund scientific research are generally unwilling to spend more public money to conduct additional studies to clarify the confusion and uncertainty caused by the re-analyses.

It should be noted that re-analyses are not *all* corrupt; there are circumstances justifying such studies. When honest scientists conduct them in an objective and transparent manner, they can make a useful contribution to the scientific literature However, for re-analyses to be recognized as valid, the sponsors and investigators must afford honest and deliberate consideration of the complex issues involved. There are ways to re-analyze a study's raw data in ethical ways, as opposed to "data dredging" to find a preferred result—easy alchemy for the experienced if unethical epidemiologist.[4]

Have Unconflicted Scientists Decide What the Evidence Means

Decisions around causation and then the appropriate protections require reviewing and synthesizing the scientific literature. One study is rarely adequate and there are inevitably inconsistencies and gaps in the overall picture. The financial success of product defense firms requires producing "strategic literature reviews" that exonerate chemical exposures. They may not all be corrupt, but they are unquestionably under pressure to produce a certain result, which in a fee-for-service setting makes the conclusions questionable. I don't believe corporations hire Gradient, Exponent, ChemRisk, or any of the other product defense operations to give them an honest, unbiased appraisal of the literature; they choose these firms knowing the firms' experts will almost never conclude the product in question causes illness, or at least causes illness at levels at which people have been exposed. I am not saying that these scientists are being paid to lie. Let's give them the benefit of the doubt and say they were selected because their firms are known to produce results favorable to their clients, and they likely believe the results of their own analyses. As Upton Sinclair famously said, "It is difficult to get a man to understand something, when his salary depends upon his not understanding it."

The system of regulatory science needs to account for financial relationships in a clear-eyed manner, one that allows for the best scientists to opine while also providing a check on any conflicts they might have. In the example of the World Health Organization's cancer agency IARC, conflicted scientists are allowed to participate in discussions to provide expertise and input to the expert panels, but not to write the reports or vote in the panels' conclusions. To a large extent, this is the case in the processes through which agencies like the EPA, OSHA, and the FDA evaluate exposures and issue regulations. These agencies follow procedures in which federal staff and contractors, all of whom, at least theoretically, are free of financial conflicts as they review the scientific evidence and draw conclusions about levels of risk. But all of these agencies are under-resourced and can't provide nearly the number and range of analyses needed to help ensure that our air, water, food, and workplaces are safe.

Other approaches to evaluating the evidence of risk are problematic as well. In addition to its role in commissioning studies, the Health Effects Institute (HEI) is often brought in to examine and evaluate particularly important studies—especially when industry doesn't like what a study has found. HEI is theoretically more trustworthy to industry because industry has a seat at the table. Polluting industries embrace HEI's analyses when they like the results. When they don't like the results, what happens is fairly boilerplate: they reject the new analysis then hire more product defense specialists to go back on the attack. This obstruction took place in both the Six Cities study of the effects of atmospheric pollution and the Diesel Exhaust Miners Study (Chapter 6) Such behavior isn't enough to warrant discarding the HEI model, but it is certainly more evidence that polluting industries have an incentive to subvert the truth, and in these cases they will manufacture as much scientific uncertainty as needed to avoid regulation.

Complete Disclosure of Funding and Control

Every scientific and medical journal requires disclosures of who paid for studies and whether the authors have financial conflicts of interest (or competing interests, as they are sometimes called). This convention is no longer controversial or even debatable; every published study should be accompanied by a statement by the authors of sources of their funding and their financial ties that might be perceived as posing a conflict of interest. Disclosure does not cleanse a study; the fundamental concern is the conflict, not the failure to disclose. But it at least allows readers to recognize issues that need to be further examined.

It is common to see a statement that a product defense firm is involved or consulting in consumer litigation on a certain topic, but that it paid for a study out of its own funds—a suggestion that no conflict exists. It is important and laudable that these firms acknowledge their consultation around related litigation, but again, the disclosure does not eliminate the conflict. It mainly reminds readers that the firm is doing work that helps it obtain or maintain funding from corporations whose product needs defense. That funding most certainly informs the portfolio of studies that they undertake, and the results they provide.

While science journals require authors to disclose financial conflicts, the U.S. federal government does not require any such disclosure when accepting public comments on proposed regulations. This policy should be changed, requiring disclosure of financial conflict of interest for comments sent into government agencies.

In proposing OSHA's silica regulation during the Obama administration, I issued a request that all public comment submissions be accompanied by a disclosure of financial conflicts. We recognized that we could not *require* submitters to include information on who paid for their work, because under the terms of the Administrative Procedures Act we were obliged to consider every comment. But nothing prevented us from *requesting* information on the funding sources behind individual comments, and nothing prevented us from giving weight to the information provided (or not provided). Knowledge of the funding sources helps evaluate the validity of the comments; any submission that did not provide sponsorship information might plausibly merit a red flag and a much more intensive examination of the claims it made.

To industries trying to manufacture uncertainty and slow regulation, challenging their secrecy represents an existential threat that they fight tooth and nail. Shortly after the proposed new rule for silica, including the request for disclosure of conflicts, was announced, I received a letter signed by 16 Republican senators, complaining that "disclosing the funding sources of commenters who submit scientific or technical research raises questions about whether OSHA will use that information to prejudge the substance of those comments and could result in dissuading stakeholders from even submitting comments," and summoning me to a meeting to explain myself. I was fortunate to have the strong support of the Obama White House, as well as the backing of the scientific community. *Nature* soon after issued an editorial titled "Full Disclosure: Regulatory agencies must demand conflict-of-interest statements for the research they use."[5] I didn't back down and the provision stayed in the rule. Most of the submissions included the information we requested. (We were also able to include the same provisions in the proposed beryllium standard we issued in August 2015.)

Authors of news articles, op-eds, and other commentaries shouldn't be exempt from disclosure, either. There are endless examples of corporations and product defense firms who hire experts, ostensibly independent, to write such documents, or to put their name on ghostwritten documents without acknowledging the funding source. Of course, any hypothetical disclosure means a lot less in the age of dark money, which flows more secretly as public awareness increases. Big Tobacco, Koch Industries and other fossil fuel firms, chemical manufacturers, food and beverage makers, and other industries that produce dangerous products—all have secretly funded groups that advocate for their positions. Front groups like the American Council on Science and Health resist revealing their funders, but when they are revealed, they inevitably show that the firms being defended and those writing the checks are the same.

In some cases, the scientists—and perhaps even the front groups—may not even know their funders' actual identities. At the time the United States was competing for the right to host soccer's World Cup in 2022, Dennis Coates, an academic economist associated with both the University of Maryland and the Mercatus Center (a think tank infamous for producing studies that benefit its corporate funders), was paid to write a report and at least two op-eds casting doubt on the financial projections made by the U.S. bid's backers. His message: "U.S. taxpayers are better off saying no to an expensive and secretive World Cup bid." A later investigation by the *Times* (London) found that the government of Qatar was behind the campaign. Coates was paid through a New York PR firm and claimed not to have known who put up the money, but the fact that he didn't even name the PR firm in his report or op-eds is symptomatic of the problem.[6] Disclosure has to go deeper than simply the source who, as in Coates' case, hands you the check. Scientists must inquire and reveal the sources of their funding, and in cases where the money has flowed through several hands, what the true source of the money is.

Protect the Public from Entire Classes of Chemicals, Not Just Individual Ones

In America, individuals are innocent until proven guilty. Products, especially chemicals, have no such rights, but it's not for lack of effort from the chemical industry. Chemical companies and their powerful trade groups manufacture doubt in order to cloak the industry with the same presumption of innocence afforded to people. While in our system of criminal justice, people are innocent until proven guilty, chemicals are not people and they have no inalienable rights. Why should that presumption of innocence apply to chemicals and other products that might be reasonably predicted to be harmful? Waiting for proof of harm before taking action will too often permit harm to occur.

There are currently tens of thousands of chemicals in commerce. OSHA maintains workplace standards on only a tiny fraction of these chemicals, and under the current rules it takes years and tremendous resources to issue a new standard for any single chemical. But while we have inadequate toxicity information on most chemicals, we know a tremendous amount about others—and those facts don't encourage optimism about what their unregulated relatives are doing to human health. We know, for example, that some PFAS compounds hurt children's immune systems and increase exposed adults' risk of several types of cancers, among other effects. But what of the other 4500 or so similar PFAS compounds? For most, there is little direct evidence they are hazardous, but there is *no* evidence they are safe—since they have never been tested.[7]

The answer to this contradiction is to move away from regulating individual chemicals and to regulate classes of chemicals as a whole. In terms of worker protection, this is known as "control banding," or developing protection requirements for classes of similar chemicals together, even though specific hazardous properties for some of them may be unknown.

Of course, regulating classes of chemicals generates the predictable opposition from chemical manufacturers, who demand proof over precaution. In September 2017, the U.S. Consumer Product Safety Commission (CPSC) held a hearing to consider banning all organo-halogen fire retardant chemicals—a class of chemicals consistently found to be toxic, but which manufacturers have altered chemically in increments in order to return the testing process to square one. In the hearing CPSC Commissioner Robert Adler asked an American Chemistry Council representative whether the ACC could provide a list of organo-halogen chemicals believed to be safe.[8] As of 2019, Commissioner Adler is still waiting for that list.[9]

Recognize the Role of Litigation in Protecting Public Health

The U.S. regulatory system is a vitally important lever for encouraging corporations to take proactive responsibility for the products they man-ufacture or discharge into our water or air. But this system works only in one of three ways: slowly, very slowly, or not at all. Regulation is not nimble. And when government regulators do catch up with companies that have hidden science, the penalty is rarely much more than a slap on the wrist. When DuPont was caught hiding a trove of studies on the health effects of C8/PFOA in West Virginia, the EPA fined that giant corporation all of $16.5 million, a tiny percentage of the profits gener-ated by Teflon. In some cases, there is no penalty at all; after colleagues and I discovered that product defense scientists working for the nation's leading producer of Chromium 6 had taken a study that found in-creased lung cancer risk at low exposure levels and played with the data to make the most important finding disappear,[10] the EPA's chief ad-ministrative law judge fined the chromium manufacturer $2.5 million for failing to report the study. The fine was later overturned on appeal, essentially because the carcinogenic effects of chromium had already been documented, just not at the low exposure levels found in the study.[11] Meanwhile, the environment was despoiled, people were harmed, and some people died.

For workers who become sick and discover that studies have associated their disease with chemicals to which they have been exposed, the workers' compensation system provides inadequate benefits, and most workers with occupational illnesses never receive compensation at all. And under that system, they are barred from suing their employer.

This leaves one other force to discourage corporations from their most antisocial behaviors: fear of litigation. Workers cannot sue their employers for making them work with inadequately regulated chemicals, but they *can* sue the manufacturer of the product that made them sick, especially if that manufacturer knew that the product was harmful but failed to issue warnings. Community residents and consumers can launch these types of suits as well. If the ill effects of corporations' toxic products shift the real costs of these products onto individuals and communities, then litigation is a means to return those costs to their source.

These "toxic tort" lawsuits suits begin with a discovery process in which the defendant firms must provide relevant documents as requested by the attorney for the people alleging damage or harm. These discovery documents are the reason we know so much about the efforts by Big Tobacco and other industries to launch and maintain, often for years, campaigns to hide data and convince regulators that their product is safe. These documents are vital in court cases because they hit home. Finding that a person's illness was caused by the toxic exposure results in compensatory damages for losses and direct costs incurred. Such compensation is vital for the plaintiffs, but it's usually not enough money to seriously influence a corporation's future behaviors. But if the court determines that the defendant acted irresponsibly (again, an understanding generally rooted in the discovery documents), the jury can award punitive damages in order to, in the vernacular, *send that company a message* about its bad behavior. These awards are often several times higher than the compensatory damages, and they do send a message—sometimes so large that the company's share price drops precipitously. This is what happened to both Johnson & Johnson and Bayer, who were on the receiving end of large punitive damage awards in the talc and glyphosate lawsuits detailed in Chapter 9. Likewise, it was lawsuits, including large ones filed by state governments for medical costs borne by taxpayers, that first brought the tobacco industry to the table and is now forcing those firms to shift their focus to creating and marketing alternative nicotine delivery devices.

All this is sometimes called "regulation by litigation," and it is despised by the corporate world. I do not claim that it is perfectly fair in meting out justice. Most cases of environmentally caused disease are clinically identical to ones that would have occurred had there been no exposure, so it often not possible to say with absolute certainty that a chemical exposure was responsible for a particular case. The best we can do is a probability statement. There are also huge "frictional" costs with litigation, for better or worse: the attorneys for the plaintiffs receive large amounts of money if their clients win, nothing if they lose. The attorneys for the defendant corporations are paid very generously as well, win or lose. These lawsuits are also the revenue motor behind much of the product defense industry; corporations hire certain scientists and firms to help them win in court. (We know this, of course, from all the documents revealed in the cases themselves.)

There is no question that we would all be better off if we had a system that discouraged bad corporate behavior and provided fair compensation without having to resort to litigation. But we don't. Our regulatory agencies are weak and under siege, especially from corporations whose behavior is threatened by regulation, and the courts can be a faster and more effective regulator. OSHA provides a powerful example. In 2000, public health officials discovered that diacetyl, the artificial flavor used to make microwave popcorn taste like it is buttered, was causing among workers exposed to the chemical *bronchiolitis obliterans*, a lung disease as terrible as its name implies. OSHA started moving slowly—very slowly—toward issuing a regulation limiting workplace exposure. Simultaneously, dozens of workers whose lungs had been destroyed sued the manufacturers of the product and diacetyl makers hired product defense firms Exponent and ChemRisk to attempt to exonerate the chemical.[12] Those efforts may eventually help limit their costs, but after $100 million in settlements and awards, the flavor industry virtually stopped selling the product.

By the time I took over leadership at OSHA, it was not worth our while to continue pouring resources into a new standard for a chemical no longer widely used. The industry had switched to a substitute, 2,3-pentanedione. We know very little about the toxic effects of this new additive chemical, so OSHA couldn't even consider issuing a regulation, and still can't. But the industry, chastened by the lawsuits around diacetyl, is likely looking more carefully at this substitute, and doing much more to help limit worker exposures.

I am proud to have contributed to setting up a compensation system that did not rely on attorneys or the courts. When I was Assistant Secretary of Energy for Environment, Safety, and Health under President Clinton, I developed a proposal to compensate workers and the families of deceased workers who became sick after exposure to radiation, beryllium, silica, or other hazards when they were working to produce the nuclear weapons that helped the United States win World War II and the Cold War. I shepherded it through Congress, which passed it almost unanimously in 2000, and helped launch it at the Labor Department. This program, in which the claimants don't need and generally don't use an attorney, has provided more than $16 billion to sick workers or their families in compensation and payments for medical expenditures.

Alas, this experience has been the exception, not the rule, at the intersection of individual well-being and federal regulation. Until the United States adopts a regulatory system strong and reliable enough to discourage corporations from hiding evidence and running campaigns to manufacture uncertainty about their products, litigation must play a central role in protecting us from harmful exposures. Lawsuits do provide monetary compensation to individuals sickened by a product, correctly shifting the costs to the source of the problem. Equally or perhaps more importantly, they serve an important public health purpose: discouraging companies from knowingly selling or discharging a toxic product and hiding what they know about it.

Organize

Much of the work of researching toxic exposures, and the resulting advocacy for clean air and water and safe food and workplaces, is done by scientists employed at universities or nongovernmental organizations (NGOs). Their efforts are invaluable and irreplaceable in the larger societal efforts to prevent illnesses, injuries, and premature deaths. They testify at hearings, send comments into regulatory dockets, write op-eds for local newspapers, and assist environment, community, and work organizations trying to reduce dangerous exposures. These scientists are heroes. They speak truth to power, taking on huge corporations whose manipulations and machinations of scientific evidence slow efforts to protect the public's health.

But it isn't individual scientists' job, let alone that of individual citizens or unions or NGOs, to make sure our environment is clean and that food and workplaces are safe. The solutions to problems like these must be societal, and the government must take the lead in strengthening our public health and environmental protections.

The challenge today is to push legislators and government agencies to require corporations to stop producing and marketing hazardous products, and to clean up the dangerous mess they've already made. And good, strong science is necessary but not sufficient to drive change; change requires organizing. The voices of unconflicted scientists are best amplified by the organizations focused on environmental, public health, and community concerns, the same ones that have been the driving force behind stronger public health protections in the past. Historically, the strongest advocates for safe workplaces have been labor unions, although their strength has substantially lessened in recent decades. Where scientists join forces with unions, public health—and society—benefit.

Activist citizens with or without scientific credentials play an essential role in exposing the exposures (and the lies about those exposures). Joining together, working with and in NGOs, they can have a significant effect on government policy and corporate actions. Two notable examples:

Jerry Ensminger is a former marine who was stationed at Camp Lejeune, North Carolina, when his six-year-old daughter Janey developed leukemia in 1983. Janey died in 1985. When Jerry Ensminger later learned that the drinking water on the base had been contaminated with several solvents, including the degreaser trichloroethylene (TCE) used on the base, he started a campaign to press the Marine Corps to investigate the exposures and their effects. Ensminger's persistent public advocacy helped launch the scientific studies that later confirmed elevated cancer rates among the camp's residents, and led to Congress passing the Janey Ensminger Act, which provides benefits for Camp Lejeune marines and their families who may have become sick because of exposure to chemicals in the contaminated water system. Predictably, the American Chemistry Council hired an ace product defense team—Michael Dourson and his firm TERA—to estimate risk from TCE exposure. Dourson's study predictably found that the exposures in the range of the ones at Camp Lejeune were safe.[13] Years later, when Jerry Ensminger heard that Dourson had been nominated by President Trump to run EPA's chemical safety office, Ensminger traveled to Washington to lobby North Carolina's senators against the nomination. Not long after his visit, Republican Senators Richard Burr and Thom Tillis announced they were voting against Dourson's nomination, essentially killing it.

Beginning in 2017, residents of Willowbrook, Illinois, learned that the air levels of ethylene oxide (EtO), a carcinogen, were far higher than allowed under EPA standards. The source of the pollution was a plant in which medical equipment was sterilized. Sterigenics, the owner of the plant, along with other EtO users and their trade association (the American Chemistry Council), employed Exponent and Ramboll to argue that the studies showing high risk from EO were wrong, and the exposure levels were safe.[14] Led by Gabriela Tejeda-Rios, Neringa Zymancius, and other Willowbrook residents whose children and neighbors had health problems they attributed to the exposure, the residents organized into a powerful force, rejected these claims and were able to convince the governor of Illinois to close the facility. Once the plant was closed, EtO levels in the town's air dropped rapidly, also refuting Sterigenic's claim that the plant was not the primary source of EtO pollution. Unfortunately, the residents' fears appear to have been well founded: the Illinois Department of Public Health issued a report finding higher rates of cancer among women and girls living around the plant.[15]

Confronted with product defense scientists attesting to the low risks associated with a given exposure, how can affected individuals know whether these experts are acting in good faith or in defense of corporate interests? Several websites have become depositories of documents uncovered in lawsuits, and their cumulative power is staggering. The first and most famous is the Truth Tobacco Industry Documents (formerly the Legacy Tobacco Documents Library), housed by the University of California, San Francisco (UCSF). Whistleblowers working for cigarette companies sent the earliest smoking guns—damning documents revealed in states' lawsuits, plus the famous suit brought by the Department of Justice in which the tobacco firms were found guilty of racketeering. That initial anonymous contribution seeded a repository that now includes 90 million pages and has been the basis for important studies revealing corporate behavior on a range of issues, from marketing sugar-sweetened beverages to children, to the tobacco industry's efforts to manipulate and exploit the Americans with Disabilities Act.[16] Recognizing the value of making documents revealed through litigation public, UCSF has expanded its collection to include thousands more documents related to the subterfuges of chemical, pharmaceutical, and food corporations. Among their holdings are papers documenting product defense campaigns waged by DuPont for its PFAS compounds, Monsanto for the pesticide glyphosate, Shell Oil for benzene, and Coca-Cola for sugar-sweetened beverages.

A newer and rapidly growing source of documents is Toxic Docs, launched by historians David Rosner and Merlin Chowkwanyun of Columbia University's Mailman School of Public Health and Gerald Markowitz of the City University of New York. It includes extensive material on industry's defense of lead, asbestos, silica, talc, vinyl chloride, polychlorinated biphenyls (PCBs), pesticides, and a host of other dangerous products. (Toxicdocs.org is also the host of the unpublished primary documents that I reference in this book.)

When I want to know more about a particular scientist, I first search for their publications and hope they include honest conflict-of-interest disclosures. I then run their names through both these archives, since it is rare for product defense specialists to work solely for one product or firm. Since their expertise is defending products, these individuals will typically work for a range of industries, reliably finding that the evidence is uncertain and that there is no reason to take any action to protect or compensate people exposed.

To better understand an individual scientist or firm, one question I always ask: have they worked with or for the tobacco industry? If so, it is often an important indicator of their ethics. However, because Big Tobacco has supported many good causes, even if only for their mercenary reasons, I also examine the objective and content of work . For example, did you know that cigarette companies have supported groups calling for progressive taxation policies? It turns out that excise taxes, which hike up the price of cigarettes, have a far bigger impact on the poor than the rich, so the tobacco companies have made common cause with well-meaning groups trying to make the tax system fairer.

Most of the firms I have discussed here have at one time worked for tobacco—Cardno ChemRisk, Exponent, Gradient, Ramboll Environ, TERA, Louis Anthony Cox's firm Cox Associates, Weinberg, and others—in some cases minimizing the risks associated with secondhand smoke in order to defeat regulation proposed by the EPA, FDA, OSHA, and other agencies. Many of their principals have testified for the defense in lawsuits against cigarette manufacturers. I have yet to hear of any of them apologizing for this work. As Michael Dourson explained it, "Jesus hung out with prostitutes and tax collectors. He had dinner with them." He added, "We're an independent group that does the best science for all these things. Why should we exclude anyone that needs help?"[17]

These doubt scientists are analogous to supply-side economists who continually claim that slashing taxes will unleash economic growth that will pay for a tax cut, while raising taxes on the wealthy will crash the economy. Nobel Prize recipient Paul Krugman has called these proponents "Zombies of voodoo economics"—their ideas are dead, yet they keep coming back.[18] The doubt scientists are so often wrong, as eventually the studies (when they can be conducted at all) prove them to be, but by then the doubt champions have moved on to defending a new product, and their previous work has been forgotten.

Regulation *Defends* Capitalism

The catalog of horrors that has necessitated the growth of America's public health regulatory system is long. It includes everything from the conditions in Chicago's slaughterhouses (exposed by novelist Upton Sinclair in *The Jungle*) to cigarettes and asbestos to climate breakdown and the widespread PFAS contamination of drinking water. In each case, corporations making a product caused damage and externalized the costs. Litigation is typically valuable in redressing the public's grievance, but it is not sufficient for changing the root issues, in part because litigation always occurs after the fact. By the time the lawsuit is filed, too many people have been sickened, or maimed, or killed—to say nothing of how the environment has been desecrated.

Our regulatory system is the response to these market failures. The objectives of the new laws and the agencies empowered to enforce them is not only to stop the damage and prevent future harm; it is to maintain and strengthen the free market system. Although many advocates of free market economics refuse to acknowledge this dynamic, law and regulation are the underpinnings of our economic system. They define market structure and property rights while attempting to ensure that property rights don't intrude on personal liberties. Without the regulatory apparatus of the state, our modern economy could not exist. The state fosters a safe space for market growth.[19]

We all value freedom, in particular the freedom to live the lives we choose. But this is not possible unless we are secure from being harmed by others, and in our modern world we individuals cannot bargain with the factory owner or the manufacturer of contaminated food. We generally have little or no knowledge of the effects of a given exposure, or sometimes that such exposures are even occurring. It is our elected representatives and officials who must enact and enforce laws that protect us from individual and collective harm—from violence and from robbery, but also from dangers posed by tainted food, polluted air and water, unsafe drugs, and dangerous workplace exposures.

Science underpins all of these public health and environmental protections. The basic principle of the regulatory system holds that decisions must be made on the basis of the best evidence available at the time. Product defense science doesn't just game our free-market system; it prevents our government from accomplishing one of the reasons for its very existence. It is often unrecognized because it is so ingrained in our understanding that a primary government function is to facilitate some individuals (including the owners of corporations) to benefit by producing or performing something that does not impinge on the freedom and well-being of other individuals. This is the basis of the criminal justice system, as well as our system of public health and environmental protections. We want stronger regulation not because we don't care about freedom, but because we cannot be free without the state's protection from harm. We need to know that our air is safe to breathe, that our food is safe to eat, and that we can return home from work at the end of our shifts no less healthy than when we walked out the door in the morning. That is both the imperative and, alas, the challenge.

DISCLOSURES AND ACKNOWLEDGMENTS

———◆———

Since the failure of scientists to disclose the financial sponsors of their work as well as their conflicts of interest is of importance in this book, it is appropriate that I prominently disclose mine.

While writing this book, I have been a full-time member of the faculty of George Washington University's Milken Institute School of Public Health. My colleagues there, led by School of Public Health Dean Lynn Goldman, welcomed me back from OSHA and eased my return to academia. Part of my salary was supported by grants to the school from the Forsythia Foundation, the Passport Foundation, the Broad Reach Fund of the Maine Community Foundation, and the Bauman Foundation. In addition, I began writing this book during a residency at the Bellagio Center of the Rockefeller Foundation. I am grateful to these foundations for their generous support of my work; none of the foundations had any input into the content of the book.

My research assistants, Alexandra Amman, Brenda Trejo, Sabrina Davis, Delaney MacMath, and Omobolanle Oshinusi, helped with fact checking and reference formatting,

Many scientific journals require the disclosure of any potential conflicts of interest related to the work since the beginning of the period in which the work being published was undertaken. In addition, some publications, like the *Journal of the American Medical Association*, require disclosure for the previous three years of any additional relevant financial activities or relationships.

It is a straightforward exercise to disclose my conflicts of interest for the past ten years, since I was prohibited by law from having any financial conflicts during my tenure at OSHA (2009-2017). Presidentially appointed, senate-confirmed officials are not allowed to earn any money beyond their salary for two reasons: formally, you work 24 hours a day for the federal government, and any of your pronouncements would be considered official statements of the Administration.

Since leaving the government in January 2017, I have been retained to provide expert witness consultation in six legal cases involving individuals who claim to have been made sick by a toxic exposure. In one, I was hired by the plaintiff's attorney for a case involving bladder cancer in a worker exposed to ortho-toluidine. The other five cases all involved mesothelioma following asbestos exposure; in three cases I was retained by attorneys for the defendants and in two by plaintiff's attorneys. I have not actually testified in court or in deposition in any of these six cases.

As I recount in Chapter 9, I was subpoenaed as a fact witness (rather than an expert one) in a trial in which women with ovarian cancer claimed their disease was caused by exposure to talc that was contaminated with asbestiform fibers. I received no financial compensation for that testimony.

Many hands went into editing and shaping this book, and I am grateful for all of them. Chad Zimmerman, my editor at Oxford, waited patiently through my years at OSHA before I could start this book. His thoughtful editing improved the book considerably. Mike Bryan worked with me on the manuscript, helping me make it less dry and hopefully more engaging than most academic efforts. My student research assistants, Alexandra Amman, Sabrina Davis, Delaney MacMath, and Omobolanle Oshinusi, helped with fact checking and reference formatting, and Anita Desikan did invaluable work gathering and summarizing studies. Thanks also to my agent Joe Spieler for helping make it all happen.

I am fortunate to have spent seven plus years in the company of a remarkable group of public servants who were passionate about OSHA's mission. My boundless thanks go to the team that helped me lead the agency: Jordan Barab, who was the longest serving Deputy Assistant Secretary in OSHA's history and was my partner and collaborator in all of our work; Debbie Berkowitz and Dorothy Dougherty, and the agency's two top attorneys during my tenure, Joe Woodward and Ann Rosenthal. Special thanks also to Peg Seminario, the tireless director of the AFL-CIO Safety and Health Department, an unequaled leader in our efforts to improve protections for the nation's workers and someone who never failed to provide me with insightful and sage advice, along with greatly appreciated support; Eric Frumin, Change to Win's Safety and Health Director and Michael Wright, Director of Health, Safety and Environment for the United Steelworkers both of whose wisdom and guidance has been invaluable; and John Howard, Director of NIOSH, a terrific colleague and collaborator.

In trying to ensure OSHA did everything in our (limited) power to protect the safety and health of the nation's workers, we were fortunate to have the enthusiastic support of the leadership of the Obama Administration's Department of Labor:

Secretaries of Labor Tom Perez and Hilda Solis; Deputy Secretaries Chris Lu and Seth Harris; and colleagues who ran other worker protection or support agencies, Sharon Block, Phyllis Borzi, Joe Main, Pat Shui, Patricia Smith, Megan Uzzell, and David Weil.

There is a long list of friends, colleagues, and family members who read chapters, provided me with materials, or otherwise helped me through my writing of this book or advancing the concerns I raise here. My thanks to them and my apologies to those I inadvertently left out. In addition to many of the people named above, they include: Robert Adler, Susan Anenberg, Michael Attfield, Tess Bird, Linda Birnbaum, Kelly Brownell, Gail Dratch, Tony Fletcher, David Goldman, Robert Harrison, Stéphane Horel, Joel Kaufman, Drew Kodjak, Sharon Lerner, Peter Lurie, Steven Markowitz, Joel Michaels, Lila Michaels, Richard Miller, Celeste Monforton, Pete Myers, Naomi Oreskes, Melissa Perry, Mark Petticrew, Lance Price, Josh Sharfstein, Debra Silverman, Dava Sobel, Emily Spieler, Kyle Steenland, Greg Wagner, Wendy Wagner, and Tom Webster.

Despite the best efforts of all of these supportive, dedicated people, there will certainly be mistakes in the book. They are mine.

It may take a village to raise a child, but, as I describe in Chapter 8, it takes an astonishingly large team of experts to produce an OSHA regulation. The standard we promulgated to reduce workplace exposure to respirable silica dust was an almost 20-year effort. This book gives me the opportunity to thank at least some of the federal employees who worked long hours to produce a rule that will save hundreds of lives. At OSHA, they includes (in addition to the people thanked above): Pete Andrews, BJ Albrecht, Paola "Gabby" Arcos, Bill Baughman, Jonathan Bearr, Barbara Bernales, Robert Blicksilver, Davina Brown, Robert Burt, Janet Carter, Joe Coble, Rose Darby, Neil Davis, Tiffany Defoe, Patti Downs, Kathleen Fagan, Casimiro "Cash" Guzman, Mishari Hanible, Michael Hodgson, Annette Iannucci, Dan Johansen, Greg Kuczura, Bryan Lincoln, Tom Mockler, Dalton Moore, David O'Connor, Todd Owen, Lyn Penniman, Bill Perry, Sutton Puglia, Tom Ransdell, Rebecca Reindel, Maureen Ruskin, Kirk Sander, Val Schaeffer, Steve Schayer, Jessica Schifano, Rachel Showalter, Jessica Stone, Robert Stone, Claudia Thurber, Ryan Tremain, David Valiante, and Michelle Walker. With the Solicitor of Labor: Robin Ackerman, Susan Brinkerhoff, Richard Ewell, Anne Godoy, Susan Harthill, Lauren Goodman, Scott Hecker, Chuck James, Allison Kramer, Kristen Lindberg, Juan Lopez, Ian Moar, Kim Robinson, Nate Spiller, Eve Stocker, Radha Vishnuvajjala, and Jordana Wilson. From the policy office: Harvey Fort, Pamela Peters, and Stephanie Swirsky. From the press office: Nancy Cleland, Amanda Kraft, Jesse Lawder, Amanda McClure, Laura McGinnis, and Frank Meilinger. Economists Heidi Shierholz (the chief economist) and Patrick Oakford. And from NIOSH, our sister agency: Andrew Cecala, Chris Coffey, Jay Colinet, Alan Echt, Matt Gillen, Martin Harper, Frank Hearl, Rosa Key-Schwartz, Max Kiefer Robert Park, Faye Rice, Paul Schulte, and David Weissman.

I am grateful to attorneys Gary Dimuzio, Michael Melkersen, and Mark Lanier for providing me with some of the documents cited here and to David Rosner and

Merlin Chowkwanyun of the Mailman School of Public Health of Columbia University and Gerald Markowitz of the City University of New York for facilitating public access to these and other documents by posting them on the Toxic Docs website.

I could not have written this book without the love, encouragement, and enduring support of my wife, Gail Dratch, and my children, Joel and Lila Michaels. I write this book for them and future generations, in the hope they will harness the remarkable powers of science to understand the world in order to make it a safer, more healthy place for all of its inhabitants. For this is what is badly needed, without a doubt.

NOTES

━━━◆◆◆◆━━━

Chapter 1

1. T. W. Wells, B. S. Karp, and L. L. Reisner, *Investigative Report Concerning Footballs Used During the A.F.C. Championship Game on January 18, 2015*, May 6, 2015. https://s3.amazonaws.com/s3.documentcloud.org/documents/2073730/investigative-report-on-a-f-c-championship-game.pdf
2. J. Leonard, "Tom Brady Has Done His Time for Deflategate, but the Science Says He's Not Guilty," *Sports Illustrated*, October 4, 2016. https://www.si.com/nfl/2016/10/04/tom-brady-deflategate-ideal-gas-law
3. J. Leonard, "MIT Professor Debunks Deflategate." https://www.youtube.com/watch?v=wwxXsEltyas
4. S. Jenkins, "NFL Deflated the Truth—and Owes the Court a Correction," *Washington Post*, March 8, 2016.
5. D. J. Paustenbach, A. K. Madl, and J. F. Greene, "Identifying an Appropriate Occupational Exposure Limit (OEL) for Beryllium: Data Gaps and Current Research Initiatives," *Applied Occupational and Environmental Hygiene*, 2001; 16(5): 527–538. doi: 10.1080/10473220121280
6. Brown and Williamson, *Smoking and Health Proposal*, 1969, Brown and Williamson document no. 680561778–1786. http://legacy.library.ucsf.edu/tid/nvs40foo
7. D. J. Paustenbach, "Clever Deception: Judging Science by Funding Source Instead of Intellectual Content," PowerPoint Presentation, March 20, 2009. https://tinyurl.com/ykate9ft
8. D. Michaels, "7 Ways to Improve Operations without Sacrificing Worker Safety," *Harvard Business Review*, March 21, 2018.

9. P. Zoibro, "Hasbro to Make Play-Doh American Again," *Wall Street Journal*, February 25, 2017.

Chapter 2

1. A. Ochsner, "My First Recognition of the Relationship of Smoking and Lung Cancer," *Preventive Medicine*, 1973; 2(4): 611–614. doi: 10.1016/0091-7435(73)90059-5
2. The history of the development of knowledge of carcinogenicity of cigarette smoke, and the role of the tobacco industry in manufacturing uncertainty about the risks associated with smoking, are detailed in A. M. Brandt, *The Cigarette Century*, New York: Basic Books, 2007 and R. N. Proctor, *Golden Holocaust*, Berkeley: University of California Press, 2011.
3. Hill and Knowlton Division of Scientific, Technical and Environmental Affairs circa 1989. https://tinyurl.com/4havmz3b
4. Roper Organization, Inc., *A Study of Public Attitudes Toward Cigarette Smoking and the Tobacco Industry in 1978*, vol. 1. Brown and Williamson document no. 501000285/0340, May 1978. http://legacy.library.ucsf.edu/tid/cns10f00
5. T. Hirayama, "Non-Smoking Wives of Heavy Smokers Have a Higher Risk of Lung Cancer: A Study from Japan," *British Medical Journal*, 1981; 282(6259): 183–85.
6. Tobacco Merchants Association, "Tobacco: Its Economic Performance. Part VIII: Government Impact on Consumption: Executive Summary," October 28, 1983. Lorillard document no. 93137245/7256. http://legacy.library.ucsf.edu/tid/cbc60e00 and "Workplace Smoking Restrictions: Communications and Lobbying Support Program," February 1984. Brown and Williamson document no. https://www.industrydocuments.ucsf.edu/tobacco/docs/#id=hgkv0037
7. P. N. Lee, "'Marriage to a Smoker' May Not Be a Valid Marker of Exposure in Studies Relating Environmental Tobacco Smoke to Risk of Lung Cancer in Japanese Non-Smoking Women," *International Archives of Occupational and Environmental Health*, 1995; 67(5): 287–94.
8. M.K. Hong and L.A. Bero, "How the Tobacco Industry Responded to an Influential Study of the Health Effects of Secondhand Smoke," *British Medical Journal*, 2002; 325 (7377): 1413–16.
9. M.E. Ward, R.J. Reynolds Tobacco Co. to J. Rupp J, Covington and Burling. March 22, 1988. http://legacy.library.ucsf.edu/tid/moq21e00 . Accessed February 26, 2019. G.B.Oldaker III, Center for Indoor Air Research to J.V. Rodricks, ENVIRON Corp. July 14, 1988. http://legacy.library.ucsf.edu/tid/cme04d00. Accessed February 26, 2019. J.R.Viren, R.J. Reynolds to J.A. Goold JA, R.J. Reynolds. "Status report: June to the present". July 18, 1988. http://legacy.library.ucsf.edu/tid/ezj95a00

10. E. T. Fontham, P. Correa, A. Williams et al., "Lung Cancer in Nonsmoking Women: A Multicenter Case-Control Study," *Cancer Epidemiology, Biomarkers & Prevention*, 1991; 1(1): 35–43.

11. A. Baba, D. M. Cook, T. O. McGarity et al. "Legislating 'Sound Science': The Role of the Tobacco Industry," *American Journal of Public Health*, 2005; 95(suppl 1): S20–S27.

12. Meeting transcript: National Toxicology Program Board of Scientific Counselors' Report on Carcinogens subcommittee meeting. December 2–3, 1998. http://legacy.library.ucsf.edu/tid/epw60d00

13. L. P. Dreyer, Wash Tech Conference Call (Handwritten notes of Philip Morris in-house memorializing meeting between Philip Morris in-house counsel and Philip Morris regulatory consultants regarding proposed OSHA rulemaking), April 12, 1994, Philip Morris document no. 2023896207. http://legacy.library.ucsf.edu/tid/cfn12a00

14. J. E. Gulick to R. A. Foos et al. Hill and Knowlton Environmental Public Relations (including attachments), February 23, 1989. https://tinyurl.com/zuw42hwh

15. @Weinberggroup. "Evaluating Product Risk in a Rapidly Changing Environment: bit.ly?QiKfj7 #FDA #productdefense," September 4, 2012. https://twitter.com/weinberggroup/status/243074955464548352

16. H. D. Roth, P. S. Levy, L. Shi, and E. Post, "Alcoholic Beverages and Breast Cancer: Some Observations on Published Case-Control Studies," *Journal of Clinical Epidemiology*, 1994; 47(2): 207–16. doi: 10.1016/0895-4356(94)90026-4

17. North Dakota State Government, LMFS-96–23 *A Survey of Health Effects: Mercury Emissions from North Dakota Lignite-Fired Power Plants*. http://www.nd.gov/ndic/Lrc/Lrcinfo/lmfs-23.pdf

18. Ramboll Foundation, "Our Legacy," 2016. https://rambollfonden.com/-/media/files/ramboll-fonden/l/long-term-priorities-and-aims_2018-1.pdf?la=en

19. P. D. Thacker, "Inside the Academic Journal That Corporations Love," *PacificStandard*, March 28, 2017. https://psmag.com/news/inside-the-academic-journal-that-corporations-love

20. J. J. Zou, "Brokers of Junk Science?" *Center for Public Integrity*, February 18, 2016. https://publicintegrity.org/environment/brokers-of-junk-science/

Chapter 3

1. The story of DuPont's contamination of the drinking water around its facility in Parkersburg, the subsequent health effects activities, and the community's efforts to insist DuPont clean up their waste and compensate their victims has been powerfully recounted by several authors. For more on this subject see M. Blake, "Welcome to Beautiful Parkersburg, West Virginia: Home to One of the Most Brazen, Deadly

Corporate Gambits in U.S. History," *Huffington Post Highline*, August 2015, https://highline.huffingtonpost.com/articles/en/welcome-to-beautiful-parkersburg/; C. Lyons, *Stain-Resistant, Nonstick, Waterproof, and Lethal*, Westport, CT [u.a.]: Praeger; 2007, 1; S. Kelly, "Dupont's Deadly Deceit: the Decades-Long Cover-Up Behind the 'World's Most Slippery Material,'" *Salon*, January 4, 2016. https://www.salon.com/2016/01/04/teflons_toxic_legacy_partner/; and Sharon Lerner's series of articles at the *Intercept*: https://theintercept.com/collections/bad-chemistry/

2. T. Karry and C. Cannon, "Cancer-Linked Chemicals Manufactured by 3M Are Turning Up in Drinking Water," *Bloomberg*, November 2, 2018. https://www.bloomberg.com/graphics/2018-3M-groundwater-pollution-problem/

3. L. Birnbaum, "The Federal Role in the Toxic PFAS Chemical Crisis," September 26, 2018. https://www.govinfo.gov/content/pkg/CHRG-115shrg33955/pdf/CHRG-115shrg33955.pdf

4. Environmental Working Group, "PFCS: Global Contaminants: PFOA Is a Pervasive Pollutant in Human Blood, As Are Other PFCS," April 3, 2003. https://www.ewg.org/research/pfcs-global-contaminants/pfoa-pervasive-pollutant-human-blood-are-other-pfcs

5. Centers for Disease Control and Prevention, *Fourth National Report on Human Exposure to Environmental Chemicals*, 2018.

6. N. Rich, "The Lawyer Who Became DuPont's Worst Nightmare," *New York Times*, January 6, 2016. https://www.nytimes.com/2016/01/10/magazine/the-lawyer-who-became-duponts-worst-nightmare.html

7. D. J. Paustenbach, J. M. Panko, P. K. Scott, and K. M. Unice, "A Methodology for Estimating Human Exposure to Perfluorooctanoic Acid (PFOA): A Retrospective Exposure Assessment of a Community (1951–2003)," *Journal of Toxicology and Environmental Health, Part A*, 2006; 70(1): 28–57. doi: 10.1080/15287390600748815

8. S. Lerner, "Trump's EPA Chemical Safety Nominee Was in the 'Business of Blessing' Pollution," *The Intercept*, July 21, 2017. https://theintercept.com/2017/07/21/trumps-epa-chemical-safety-nominee-was-in-the-business-of-blessing-pollution/

9. P. D. Thacker, "The Weinberg Proposal: a Scientific Consulting Firm Says That It Aids Companies in Trouble, but Critics Say That It Manufactures Uncertainty and Undermines Science," *Environmental Science & Technology*, February 21, 2006. https://www.sourcewatch.org/images/6/67/Weinberg.pdf; A copy of the letter is available at: https://tinyurl.com/29fjwm48

10. S. Lerner, "How DuPont Slipped Past the EPA," *The Intercept*, August 20, 2015. https://theintercept.com/2015/08/20/teflon-toxin-dupont-slipped-past-epa/

11. S. J. Frisbee, A. P. Brooks Jr, A. Maher, et al., "The C8 Health Project: Design, Methods, and Participants." Environmental Health Perspectives 2009; 117(12):1873-82. doi: 10.1289/ehp.0800379

12. C8 Science Panel, "C8 Probable Link Reports." http://www.c8sciencepanel.org/prob_link.html

13. J. Mordock, "DuPont, Chemours to pay $670M over PFOA suits," *Delaware Online*, February 13, 2017. https://www.delawareonline.com/story/news/2017/02/13/dupont-and-chemours-pay-670m-settle-pfoa-litigation/97842870/

14. P. Grandjean, E. W. Andersen, E. Budtz-Jørgensen et al., "Serum Vaccine Antibody Concentrations in Children Exposed to Perfluorinated Compounds," *Journal of the American Medical Association*, 2012; 307(4): 391–397. doi: 10.1001/jama.2011.2034

15. L. R. Zobel, G. W. Olsen, and J. L. Butenhoff, "Perfluorinated Compounds and Immunotoxicity in Children," *Journal of the American Medical Association*, 2012; 307(18): 1910–1911. doi: 10.1001/jama.2012.3599

16. H. Mongilio, "Hidden Studies from Decades Ago Could Have Curbed PFAS Problem: Scientist," *Environmental Health News*, July 31, 2018. https://www.ehn.org/hidden-studies-from-decades-ago-could-have-curbed-pfas-problem-2591289696.html

17. S. Lerner, "Bad Chemistry." https://theintercept.com/collections/bad-chemistry/

18. TP (National Toxicology Program). Monograph on Immunotoxicity Associated with Exposure to Perfluorooctanoic acid (PFOA) and perfluorooctane sulfonate (PFOS). Research Triangle Park, NC: National Toxicology Program. September 2016 https://ntp.niehs.nih.gov/ntp/ohat/pfoa_pfos/pfoa_pfosmonograph_508.pdf

19. American Council of Science and Health, "Regulating Mercury Emissions From Power Plants: Will It Protect Our Health?" September 9, 2005. https://www.acsh.org/news/2005/09/09/regulating-mercury-emissions-from-power-plants-will-it-protect-our-health

20. American Council of Science and Health, "Don't Fear Diesel Fumes," June 13, 2012. https://www.acsh.org/news/2012/06/13/dont-fear-diesel-fumes

21. A. Berezow, "Meet The Scientific Outcasts And Mavericks," June 3, 2016. https://www.acsh.org/news/2016/06/03/meet-the-scientific-outcasts-and-mavericks

22. M. Nestle, "Food Politics," October 15, 2009. https://www.foodpolitics.com/tag/acshamerican-council-on-science-and-health/

23. A. Berezow, "New Alcohol Study Is Mostly Hype: Journal, Authors, Media to Blame," April 13, 2018. https://www.acsh.org/news/2018/04/13/new-alcohol-study-mostly-hype-journal-authors-media-blame-12839

24. American Council on Science and Health, "Teflon and Human Health: Do the Charges Stick?" March 18, 2005. https://www.acsh.org/news/2005/03/18/teflon-and-human-health-do-the-charges-stick

25. American Council of Science and Health, "DuPont Loses Bellwether C8 Teflon Case," July 7, 2016. https://www.acsh.org/news/2016/07/07/dupont-loses-bellwether-c8-teflon-case

26. D. Mondal, R. H. Weldon, B. G. Armstrong, L. J. Gibson, M. J. Lopez-Espinosa, H. M. Shin, and T. Fletcher, "Breastfeeding: A Potential Excretion Route for Mothers and Implications for Infant Exposure to Perfluoroalkyl Acids, *Environmental Health Perspectives*, 2014; 122(2): 187–92.

27. P. Grandjean, C. Heilmann, P. Weihe et al., "Estimated Exposures to Perfluorinated Compounds in Infancy Predict Attenuated Vaccine Antibody Concentrations at Age 5-Years," *Journal of Immunotoxicology*, 2017; 14(1): 188–95.

28. H. K. Knutsen, J. Alexander, L. Barregård et al., "Risk to Human Health Related to the Presence of Perfluorooctane Sulfonic Acid and Perfluorooctanoic Acid in Food," *EFSA Journal*, 2018; 16(12): n/a. doi: 10.2903/j.efsa.2018.5194

29. U.S. Environmental Protection Agency, PFOA & PFOS Drinking Water HealthAdvisories, November 2016. https://www.epa.gov/sites/default/files/2016-06/documents/drinkingwaterhealthadvisories_pfoa_pfos_updated_5.31.16.pdf

30. A. Di Nisio, I. Sabovic, U. Valente et al. "Endocrine Disruption of Androgenic Activity by Perfluoroalkyl Substances: Clinical and Experimental Evidence," *Journal of Clinical Endocrinology & Metabolism*, 2018. doi: 10.1210/jc.2018-01855

31. A. Snider. "White House, EPA Headed Off Chemical Pollution Study," *Politico*, May 14, 2018, https://www.politico.com/story/2018/05/14/emails-white-house-interfered-with-science-study-536950 .

32. Agency for Toxic Substances and Disease Registry, "Per- and Polyfluoroalkyl Substances (PFAS) and Your Health," November 2018. https://www.atsdr.cdc.gov/pfas/mrl_pfas.html

33. S. Lerner, "Lawsuits Charge That 3M Knew About the Dangers of Its Chemicals," *The Intercept*, April 11, 2016. https://theintercept.com/2016/04/11/lawsuits-charge-that-3m-knew-about-the-dangers-of-pfcs

34. State of Minnesota vs. 3M Company. Memorandum in Support of the Plaintiff State of Minnesota's Motion to Amend Complaint. November 17, 2017. https://tinyurl.com/yh2ehcfz

35. *Expert Report of Barbara D. Beck, Ph.D., DABT, ATS, ERT in the Matter of State of Minnesota vs. 3M Company.* November 3, 2017. https://tinyurl.com/mr25sshr

36. National Toxicology Program. Comments Regarding the Systematic Review of Immunotoxicity Associated with Perfluorooctanoic Acid (PFOA) and Perfluorooctane Sulfonate (PFOS): Prepared on behalf of 3M. https://web.archive.org/web/20190718194811/https://ntp.niehs.nih.gov/ntp/about_ntp/monopeerrvw/2016/july/publiccomm/

gradient20160705_508.pdf. July 5, 2016. E .T Chang, H. Adami, P. Boffetta, H. J. Wedner, J.S. Mandel. A critical review of perfluorooctanoate and perfluorooctanesulfonate exposure and immunological health conditions in humans. *Crit Rev Toxicol.* 2016;46(4):279-331. doi: 10.3109/10408444.2015.1122573

37. S. Lerner, Lawsuit reveals how paid expert helped 3m "command the science" on dangerous chemicals. *The Intercept.* https://theintercept.com/2018/02/23/3m-lawsuit-pfcs-pollution/. February 23, 2018. Also see https://www.documentcloud.org/documents/4405489-2004-2005-Project-Priorities.html

38. C. Hogue, "What's GenX Still Doing in the Water Downstream of a Chemours Plant?" *Chemical & Engineering News*, February 12, 2018; 96(7). https://cen.acs.org/articles/96/i7/whats-genx-still-doing-in-the-water-downstream-of-a-chemours-plant.html

39. V. Hagerty, "Deal Would Require Toxicity Studies for 5 Chemicals Released at NC Plant," *Carolina Public Press*, December 11, 2018. https://carolinapublicpress.org/28397/deal-would-require-toxicity-studies-for-5-chemicals-released-at-nc-plant

40. Z. Wang, J. C. DeWitt, C. P. Higgins, and I. T. Cousins. "A Never-Ending Story of Per- and Polyfluoroalkyl Substances (PFASs)?" *Environmental Science & Technology*, 2017; 51(5): 2508–2518. doi: 10.1021/acs.est.6b04806

41. CWAG New Mexico, "Polyfluoroalkyl Substances: Best Practices for Science Policy Decisions," July 24, 2018. https://tinyurl.com/muh7va6w

Chapter 4
1. A. M. Finkel and K. F. Bieniek, "A Quantitative Risk Assessment for Chronic Traumatic Encephalopathy (CTE) in Football: How Public Health Science Evaluates Evidence," *Human and Ecological Risk Assessment: An International Journal*, 2018: 1–26. doi: 10.1080/10807039.2018.1456899

2. J. Mez, D. H. Daneshvar, P. T. Kiernan et al., "Clinicopathological Evaluation of Chronic Traumatic Encephalopathy in Players of American Football," *Journal of the American Medical Association*, 2017; 318(4): 360–370. doi: 10.1001/jama.2017.8334

3. R. O'Brien, "Scorecard," *Sports Illustrated Vault*, December 26, 1994. https://www.si.com/vault/1994/12/26/106787493/scorecard

4. E. J. Pellman, D. C. Viano, A. M. Tucker, I. R. Casson, and J. F. Waeckerle, "Concussion in Professional Football: Reconstruction of Game Impacts and Injuries," *Neurosurgery*, 2003; 53(4): 799–814. doi: 10.1093/neurosurgery/53.3.799

5. E. J. Pellman and D. C. Viano, Concussion in professional football. *Neurosurgical Focus.* 2006;21(4):1-10. doi: 10.3171/foc.2006.21.4.13

6. M. Fainaru-Wada and S. Fainaru, *League of Denial: The NFL, Concussions, and the Battle for Truth*, New York: Random House, 2013.

7. D. C. Viano, I. R. Casson, E. J. Pellman, L. Zhang, A. I. King, and K. H. Yang, "Concussion in Professional Football: Brain Responses by Finite Element Analysis: Part 9," *Neurosurgery*, 2005; 57(5): 891–916.

8. A. Kingsbury, "What Time Is the A.F.C. Championship Game?" *New York Times*, January 18, 2019.

9. D. R. Weir, J. S. Jackson, and A. Sonnega, *Study of Retired NFL Players*, National Football League Player Care Foundation, University of Michigan Institute for Social Research, September 10, 2009. http://ns. umich.edu/Releases/2009/Sep09/FinalReport.pdf

10. A. Schwarz, "Dementia Risk Seen in Players in N.F.L. Study," *New York Times*, September 30, 2009.

11. B. I. Omalu, S. T. DeKosky, R. L. Minster, M. I. Kamboh, R. L. Hamilton, and C. H. Wecht, "Chronic Traumatic Encephalopathy in a National Football League Player," *Neurosurgery*, 2005; 57(1): 128–134.

12. J. D. Silver, "A Life Off-Center: Mike Webster's Battles," *Pittsburgh Post-Gazette*, July 24, 1997.

13. I. R. Casson, E. J. Pellman, and D. C. Viano, "Chronic Traumatic Encephalopathy in a National Football League Player," *Neurosurgery*, 2006; 59(5): E1152. doi: 10.1227/01.NEU.0000249026.95877.F8

14. B. I. Omalu, S. T. DeKosky, R. L. Hamilton et al., "Chronic Traumatic Encephalopathy in a National Football League Player: Part II," *Neurosurgery*, 2006; 59(5): 1086.

15. A. Hamberger, D. C. Viano, A. Saljo, and H. Bolouri, "Concussion in Professional Football: Morphology of Brain Injuries in the NFL Concussion Model, Part 16," *Neurosurgery*, 2009; 64(6): 82; discussion 1182.

16. *In Re National Football Players' Concussion Injury Litigation. Plaintiff's Master Administrative Long-Form Complaint.* June 7, 2012. http://nflconcussionlitigation.com/wp-content/uploads/2012/01/NFL-Master-Complaint1.pdf

17. Tribune News Service, "Supreme Court Leaves $1B NFL Concussion Settlement in Place," *Chicago Tribune*, December 12, 2016.

18. National Football League, "NFL donates $30 million to National Institutes of Health." September 5, 2012. http://www.nfl.com/news/story/0ap1000000058447/article/nfl-donates-30-million-to-national-institutes-of-health

19. US House of Representatives Energy and Commerce Committee, *The National Football League's Attempt to Influence Funding Decisions at the National Institutes of Health*, May 2016, Democratic Staff Report. https://energycommerce.house.gov/sites/democrats.energycommerce.house.gov/files/Democratic%20Staff%20Report%20on%20NFL%20NIH%20Investigation%205.23.2016.pdf

20. L. Wamsley, "NFL, NIH End Partnership for Concussion Research with $16M Unspent," *National Public Radio*, July 29, 2017.

21. K. Belson, "Sony Altered "Concussion" Film to Prevent N.F.L. Protests, Emails Show," *New York Times*, September 1, 2015.

22. J. Macur, "The N.H.L.'s Problem with Science," *New York Times*, February 8, 2017.

23. G. B. Bettman to Senator Richard Blumenthal, July 22, 2016. https:// assets.documentcloud.org/documents/2998884/Commissioner-Bettman-s-C-T-E-Response.pdf

Chapter 5

1. World Health Organization, *Global Status Report on Alcohol and Health— 2018*. http://apps.who.int/iris/bitstream/handle/10665/274603/ 9789241565639-eng.pdf?ua=1

2. Centers for Disease Control and Prevention, "Tobacco Related Mortality," May 17, 2017. https://www.cdc.gov/tobacco/data_statistics/ fact_sheets/health_effects/tobacco_related_mortality/index.htm

3. T. B. Turner and V. L. Bennett. *Forward Together*, Baltimore, MD: Alcoholic Beverage Medical Research Foundation, 1993, 61.

4. T. B. Turner, V. L. Bennett, and H. Hernandez, "The Beneficial Side of Moderate Alcohol Use," *Johns Hopkins Medical Journal*, 1981; 148(2): 53.

5. T. B. Turner, E. Mezey, and A. W. Kimball. "Measurement of Alcohol-Related Effects in Man: Chronic Effects in Relation to Levels of Alcohol Consumption. Part A," *Johns Hopkins Medical Journal*, 1977; 141. doi:10.1097/00006534-197812000-00111

6. P. M. Boffey, "Less Illness Found in Beer Drinkers," *New York Times*, December 18, 1985.

7. A. Richman and R. A. Warren. "Alcohol Consumption and Morbidity in the Canada Health Survey: Inter-Beverage Differences," *Drug & Alcohol Dependence*, 1985; 15(3): 255–282. doi:10.1016/0376-8716(85)90005-5

8. T. F. Babor, "Alcohol Research and the Alcoholic Beverage Industry: Issues, Concerns and Conflicts of Interest," *Addiction* 104, (2009): 34–47. doi:10.1111/j.1360-0443.2008.02433.x.

9. T. F. Babor and K. Robaina, "Public Health, Academic Medicine, and the Alcohol Industry's Corporate Social Responsibility Activities," *American Journal of Public Health*, 2013; 103(2): 206–214. doi: 10.2105/AJPH. 2012.300847

10. R. C. Ellison and M. Martinic, "The Harms and Benefits of Moderate Drinking: Summary of Findings of an International Symposium: Special Issue," *Annals of Epidemiology*, 2007 (17): 1–12.

11. K. M. Fillmore, T. Stockwell, T. Chikritzhs, A. Bostrom, and W. C. Kerr, "Debate: Alcohol and Coronary Heart Disease," *American Journal of Medicine*, 2008; 121(2): e25. doi://doi.org/10.1016/j.amjmed. 2007.09.015

12. International Alliance for Responsible Drinking, "Guide to Creating Integrative Alcohol Policies," January 2016. https://web.archive.org/web/20160323013059/http://www.iard.org/wp-content/uploads/2016/01/TK-Creating-Integrative-Policies.pdf

13. B. MacMahon, S. Yen, D. Trichopoulos, K. Warren, and G. Nardi, "Coffee and Cancer of the Pancreas," *New England Journal of Medicine*, 1981; 304(11): 630–633. doi: 10.1056/NEJM198103123041102

14. M. Shuster, J. Vigna, G. Sinha, and M. Tontonoz, Scientific American Biology for a Changing World. New York: W. H. Freeman and Company, 2012.

15. T. Stockwell, J. Zhao, S. Panwar, A. Roemer, T. Naimi, and T. Chikritzhs, "Do 'Moderate' Drinkers Have Reduced Mortality Risk? A Systematic Review and Meta-Analysis of Alcohol Consumption and All-Cause Mortality," *Journal of Studies on Alcohol and Drugs*, 2016; 77(2): 185–198.

16. F. Prial, "Wine Talk," *New York Times*, December 25, 1991.

17. A. M. Wood, S. Kaptoge, A. S. Butterworth et al., "Risk Thresholds for Alcohol Consumption: Combined Analysis of Individual-Participant Data for 599,912 Current Drinkers in 83 Prospective Studies," *Lancet*, 2018; 391(10129): 1513–1523.

18. M. H. Forouzanfar, L. Alexander, H. R. Anderson et al., "Global, Regional, and National Comparative Risk Assessment of 79 Behavioural, Environmental and Occupational, and Metabolic Risks or Clusters of Risks in 188 Countries, 1990–2013: A Systematic Analysis for the Global Burden of Disease Study 2013," *Lancet*. 2015; 386: 2287–323. and R. Burton and N. Sheron, "No Level of Alcohol Consumption Improves Health," *Lancet*, 2018; 392(10152): 987–988. doi: 10.1016/S0140-6736(18)31571-X

19. R. C. Rabin, "Is Alcohol Good for You? An Industry-Backed Study Seeks Answers," *New York Times*, July 3, 2017.

20. NIH Advisory Committee to the Director, *ACD Working Group for Review of the Moderate Alcohol and Cardiovascular Health Trial*, 2018. https://acd.od.nih.gov/documents/presentations/06152018Tabak-B.pdf

21. ABinBev Foundation, "Our Advisors and Partners." https://abinbevfoundation.org/about/advisors/

22. U.S. National Library of Medicine, *Moderate Alcohol and Cardiovascular Health Trial (MACH15)*, May 30, 2017. https://clinicaltrials.gov/ct2/show/NCT03169530

23. R. C. Rabin, "Federal Agency Courted Alcohol Industry to Fund Study on Benefits of Moderate Drinking," *New York Times*, March 3, 2017.

24. International Agency for Research on Cancer, Monographs on the evaluation of the carcinogenic risks to humans. Alcohol Drinking. Volume 44 [Internet]. Lyon, France: International Agency for Research on Cancer (IARC); 1988. Report No.: Volume 44. Available from: https://

monographs.iarc.fr/ENG/Monographs/vol44/mono44.pdf "Alcohol Drinking." 1988. http://www.inchem.org/documents/iarc/vol44/44.html

25. National Toxicology Program. *Alcoholic Beverage Consumption*, vol. 14, 2016. https://ntp.niehs.nih.gov/ntp/roc/content/profiles/alcoholicbeverageconsumption.pdf

26. International Agency for Research on Cancer, *IARC Monographs on the Evaluation of Carcinogenic Risks to Humans*, vol. 96, 2010. https://monographs.iarc.fr/wp-content/uploads/2018/06/mono96.pdf and B. Secretan, K. Straif, R. Baan et al., "A Review of Human Carcinogens—Part E: Tobacco, Areca Nut, Alcohol, Coal Smoke, and Salted Fish," *The Lancet Oncology*, 2009; 10(11): 1033–1034.

27. V. Bagnardi, M. Rota, E. Botteri et al., "Alcohol Consumption and Site-Specific Cancer Risk: a Comprehensive Dose-Response Meta-Analysis," *British Journal of Cancer*, 2015; 112(3): 580–93. On this subject I want to give a special shout-out to a great piece in *Mother Jones* entitled "Did Drinking Give Me Breast Cancer?" by Stephanie Mencimer. https://www.motherjones.com/politics/2018/04/did-drinking-give-me-breast-cancer

28. American Society for Clinical Oncology, "Alcohol Linked to Cancer According to Major Oncology Organization: ASCO Cites Evidence and Calls for Reduced Alcohol Consumption," November 27, 2017. Survey Finds Most Americans Are Unaware of Key Cancer Risk Factors. Oncology Times: November 25, 2017 - Volume 39 - Issue 22 - p 45–46. doi: 10.1097/01.COT.0000527370.83029.50.

29. P. Buykx, J. Li, L. Gavens et al., "Public Awareness of the Link Between Alcohol and Cancer in England in 2015: A Population-Based Survey," *BMC Public Health*, 2016; 16(1): 1194. doi: 10.1186/s12889-016-3855-6

30. H. D. Roth, P. S. Levy, L. Shi, and E. Post, "Alcoholic Beverages and Breast Cancer: Some Observations on Published Case-Control Studies," *Journal of Clinical Epidemiology*, 1994; 47(2): 207–216. doi: 10.1016/0895-4356(94)90026-4

31. S. Zakhari, "To Say Moderate Alcohol Use Causes Cancer is Wrong," *Dominion Post*, July 22, 2015.

32. J. Connor, "Alcohol Consumption as a Cause of Cancer," *Addiction*, 2016; 112(2): 222–228. doi: 10.1111/add.13477

33. W. Evans, "Alcohol Causes 7 Types of Cancer, New Analysis Confirms," *Deseret News*, July 23, 2016.

34. M. Petticrew, N. Maani Hessari, C. Knai, and E. Weiderpass, "How Alcohol Industry Organisations Mislead the Public About Alcohol and Cancer," *Drug and Alcohol Review*, 2018; 37(3): 293–303. doi: 10.1111/dar.12596

35. National Institute on Alcohol Abuse and Alcoholism, "Women." https://www.niaaa.nih.gov/alcohol-health/special-populations-co-occurring-disorders/women

Chapter 6

1. S. C. Anenberg, J. Miller, D. Henze, and R. Minjares, "A Global Snapshot of the Air Pollution–Related Health Impacts of Transportation Sector Emissions in 2010 and 2015," Washington, DC: International Council on Clean Transportation, February 26, 2019. https://www.theicct.org/publications/health-impacts-transport-emissions-2010-2015

2. National Research Council, *Health Effects of Exposure to Diesel Exhaust: The Report of the Health Effects Panel of the Diesel Impacts Study Committee*, Washington, DC: National Academy Press, 1981.

3. C. Monforton, "Weight of the Evidence or Wait for the Evidence? Protecting Underground Miners from Diesel Particulate Matter," *American Journal of Public Health*, 2006; 96(2): 271–276. http://ajph.aphapublications.org/cgi/content/abstract/96/2/271; doi: 10.2105/AJPH.2005.064410

4. United States Department of Labor, Federal Mine Safety and Health Act. 1977. https://arlweb.msha.gov/REGS/ACT/ACT1.HTM#1

5. B. Furlow, "A New Study Suggests New Mexico's Miners May Be at Risk—but Will Anyone Take Action?" *Santa Fe Reporter*, March 27, 2017. https://www.sfreporter.com/news/2012/03/27/carbon-wars/

6. Mine Safety and Health Administration, "Diesel Particulate Matter Exposure of Underground Metal and Nonmetal Miners," 67 *Federal Register*, 47296 (July 20, 2002).

7. D. T. Silverman, C. Samanic, J. H. Lubin et al., "The Diesel Exhaust in Miners study: A Nested Case-Control Study of Lung Cancer and Diesel Exhaust," *Journal of the National Cancer Institute*, 2012; 104(11): 855–868. doi: 10.1093/jnci/djs034 and M. D. Attfield, P. L. Schleiff, J. H. Lubin et al., "The Diesel Exhaust in Miners study: A Cohort Mortality Study with Emphasis on Lung Cancer," *Journal of the National Cancer Institute*, 2012; 104(11): 869–883. doi: 10.1093/jnci/djs035

8. J. Borak, W. B. Bunn, G. R. Chase et al., "Comments on the Diesel Exhaust in Miners Study," *Annals of Occupational Hygiene*, 2011; 55(3): 339–342. http://dx.doi.org/10.1093/annhyg/mer005

9. B. Furlow, "Industry Group 'Threatens' Journals to Delay Publications," *Lancet Oncology*, 2012; 13(4): 337. https://doi.org/10.1016/S1470-2045(12)70094-3

10. S. Kean, "Journals Warned to Keep a Tight Lid on Diesel Exposure Data," *Science*, February 17, 2012. http://www.sciencemag.org/news/2012/02/journals-warned-keep-tight-lid-diesel-exposure-data

11. W. B. Bunn., T. W. Hesterberg, P. A. Valberg, T. J. Slavin, G. Hart, and C. A. Lapin, "A Reevaluation of the Literature Regarding the Health Assessment of Diesel Engine Exhaust," Inhalation Toxicology. 2004;16(14):889-900. doi: 10.1080/08958370490883783 And T. W. Hesterberg, W. B. Bunn, G. R. Chase et al, "A Critical Assessment of

Studies on the Carcinogenic Potential of Diesel Exhaust," CRC Critical Reviews in Toxicology. 2006;36(9):727-776. doi: 10.1080/10408440600908821

12. E. Garshick, F. Laden, J. E. Hart, M. E. Davis, E. A. Eisen, and T. J. Smith, "Lung Cancer and Elemental Carbon Exposure in Trucking Industry Workers," *Environmental Health Perspectives*, 2012; 120(9): 1301–1306. doi: 10.1289/ehp.1204989

13. L Benbrahim-Tallaa, R. A. Baan, Y. Grosse, et al. Carcinogenicity of diesel-engine and gasoline-engine exhausts and some nitroarenes. Lancet Oncology. 2012;13(7):663-664. doi: 10.1016/S1470-2045(12)70280-2

14. Occupational Safety and Health Administration, "OSHA/MSHA Hazard Alert, Diesel Exhaust/Diesel Particulate Matter." https://www.osha.gov/dts/hazardalerts/diesel_exhaust_hazard_alert.html

15. R. O. McClellan, T. W. Hesterberg, and J. C. Wall, "Evaluation of Carcinogenic Hazard of Diesel Engine Exhaust Needs to Consider Revolutionary Changes in Diesel Technology," *Regulatory Toxicology and Pharmacology*, 2012; 63(2): 225–258. doi: 10.1016/j.yrtph.2012.04.005

16. D. W. Dockery, C. A. Pope, X. Xu et al., "An Association Between Air Pollution and Mortality in Six U.S. Cities," *New England Journal of Medicine*, 1993; 329(24): 1753–1759. doi: 10.1056/NEJM199312093292401

17. A. G. Elaine, "Prevailing Winds," *Harvard Public Health Magazine*, Fall 2012.

18. D. Krewski, R. T. Burnett, M. S. Goldberg et al., "Validation of the Harvard Six Cities Study of Air Pollution and Mortality," *New England Journal of Medicine*, 2004; 350: 198–199. And HEI Diesel Epidemiology Panel, *Diesel Emissions and Lung Cancer: An Evaluation of Recent Epidemiological Evidence for Quantitative Risk Assessment* (Special Report 19), Boston, MA: Health Effects Institute, 2015.s

19. A. Baba, D. M. Cook, T. O. McGarity, and L. A. Bero, "Legislating 'Sound Science': The Role of the Tobacco Industry," *American Journal of Public Health*, 2005; 95(S1): S20. doi: 10.2105/AJPH.2004.050963

20. H. G. Miller and W. H. Baldwin, "A Terse Amendment Produces Broad Change in Data Access," *American Journal of Public Health*, 2001; 91(5): 824–825. doi: 10.2105/AJPH.91.5.824

21. R.O. McClellan. Critique of Health Effects Institute Special Report 19, "Diesel Emissions and Lung Cancer: An Evaluation of Recent Epidemiological Evidence for Quantitative Risk Assessment" (November 2015) https://cdn.ymaws.com/www.ima-na.org/resource/resmgr/Diesel/IMA-NA_ATTACHMENT_10_-_Criti.pdf

22. E. T. Chang, E. C. Lau, C. Van Landingham, K. S. Crump, R. O. McClellan, and S. H. Moolgavkar, "Reanalysis of Diesel Engine Exhaust and Lung Cancer Mortality in the Diesel Exhaust in Miners Study Cohort Using Alternative Exposure Estimates and Radon Adjustment," *American Journal of Epidemiology*, 2018; 187(6): 1210–1219.

doi: 10.1093/aje/kwy038; K. S. Crump, C. Van Landingham,
S. H. Moolgavkar, and R. McClellan, "Reanalysis of the DEMS Nested
Case-Control Study of Lung Cancer and Diesel Exhaust: Suitability for
Quantitative Risk Assessment," *Risk Analysis*, 2015; 35(4):676–700.
doi: 10.1111/risa.12371; S. H. Moolgavkar, E. T. Chang, G. Luebeck et al.,
"Diesel Engine Exhaust and Lung Cancer Mortality: Time-Related
Factors in Exposure and Risk," *Risk Analysis*, 2015; 35(4): 663–675.
doi: 10.1111/risa.12315; and K. S. Crump, C. Van Landingham, and
R. O. McClellan, "Influence of Alternative Exposure Estimates in the
Diesel Exhaust Miners Study: Diesel Exhaust and Lung Cancer," *Risk
Analysis*, 2016; 36(9): 1803–1812. doi: 10.1111/risa.12556

23. K. S. Crump, C. Van Landingham, S. H. Moolgavkar, and R. McClellan,
"Reanalysis of the DEMS Nested Case-Control Study of Lung Cancer
and Diesel Exhaust: Suitability for Quantitative Risk Assessment," *Risk
Analysis*, 2015; 35(4):676–700. doi: 10.1111/risa.12371

24. J. F. Gamble, M. J. Nicolich, and P. Boffetta, "Lung Cancer and Diesel
Exhaust: an Updated Critical Review of the Occupational Epidemiology
Literature," *Critical Reviews in Toxicology*, August 2012; 42(7): 549–98.
doi: 10.3109/10408444.2012.690725

25. J. F. Gamble, "PM2.5 and Mortality in Long-Term Prospective Cohort
Studies: Cause-Effect or Statistical Associations?" *Environmental Health
Perspectives*, 1998; 106(9): 535–549. doi: 10.1289/ehp.98106535

26. P. Taxell and T. Santonen, "149. Diesel Engine Exhaust," The Nordic
Expert Group for Criteria Documentation of Health Risks from
Chemicals and the Dutch Expert Committee on Occupational Safety.
Arbete och Hälsa *(Work and Health)*, June 8, 2016; 49(6). https://gupea.
ub.gu.se/bitstream/2077/44340/1/gupea_2077_44340_1.pdf

27. L. Latifovic, P. J. Villeneuve, M. Parent, K. C. Johnson, L. Kachuri, and
S. A. Harris, "Bladder Cancer and Occupational Exposure to Diesel and
Gasoline Engine Emissions Among Canadian Men," *Cancer Medicine*,
2015; 4(12): 1948–1962. doi: 10.1002/cam4.544

28. Health Effects Institute (HEI) Executive Summary. Advanced
Collaborative Emissions Study (ACES). Boston, MA: Health Effects
Institute; 2015. https://www.healtheffects.org/publication/executive-
summary-advanced-collaborative-emissions-study-aces

29. United States Senate Health, Education and Labor Committee. *Report on
the August 6, 2007 Disaster at Crandall Canyon Mine*, March 6, 2008.
https://eagcg.org/common/pdf/CrandallCanyon.pdf

30. Comment from Edward M. Green, Crowell Moring., Re: RIN 1219-
AB86; Docket No. MSHA-2014-0031, Request for Information on
Exposure of Underground Miners to Diesel Exhaust Comments of
Murray Energy Corporation, the Bituminous Coal Operators'
Association, and Interwest Mining Company. https://www.regulations.
gov/document?D=MSHA-2014-0031-0069

31. United State Environmental Protection Agency. "Repeal of Emission Requirements for Glider Vehicles, Glider Engines, and Glider Kits," *Federal Register* 2017; 82:53442.-53449.

32. T. C. Fitzgerald, D. Petersen, and D. Keener to S. Pruitt, Administrator of Environmental Protection Agency, "Re: Petition for Reconsideration of Application of the Final Rule Entitled 'Greenhouse Gas Emissions and Fuel Efficiency Standards for Medium-and-Heavy-duty Engines and Vehicles - Phase 2 Final Rule' to Gliders," July 10, 2017. https://www.epa.gov/sites/production/files/2017-07/documents/hd-ghg-fr-fitzgerald-recons-petition-2017-07-10.pdf

33. E. Lipton, "University Pulls Back on Pollution Study That Supported Benefactor,". *New York Times*,. February 22, 2018.

34. D. Cutler and F. Dominici, "A Breath of Bad Air: Cost of the Trump Environmental Agenda May Lead to 80,000 Extra Deaths Per Decade," *Journal of the American Medical Association*, 2018; 319(22): 2261–2262. doi: 10.1001/jama.2018.7351

35. E. Lipton, "University Pulls Back on Pollution Study That Supported Benefactor,". *New York Times*,. February 22, 2018.

Chapter 7

1. B. Meier, *Pain Killer*, New York: Random House, 2018.

2. J. Porter and H. Jick, "Addiction Rare in Patients Treated with Narcotics," *New England Journal of Medicine*, 1980; 302(2): 123. doi: 10.1056/NEJM198001103020221

3. P. T. M. Leung, E. M. Macdonald, M. B. Stanbrook, I. A. Dhalla, and D. N. Juurlink, "A 1980 Letter on the Risk of Opioid Addiction," *New England Journal of Medicine*, 2017; 376(22): 2194–2195. doi: 10.1056/NEJMc1700150

4. S. Quinones, *Dreamland*, New York: Bloomsbury Press, 2016.

5. Painful words: How a 1980 letter fueled the opioid epidemic. Stat May 31,2017 https://www.statnews.com/2017/05/31/opioid-epidemic-nejm-letter/

6. *County of Greenville, South Carolina, v. Rite Aid of South Carolina et al.*, C.A. No.: 2018-CP-23-01294, lawsuit, 2018.

7. *State of Ohio vs. Purdue Pharma et al.*, lawsuit, 2017. https://www.ohioattorneygeneral.gov/Files/Briefing-Room/News-Releases/Consumer-Protection/2017-05-31-Final-Complaint-with-Sig-Page.aspx

8. M. S. Greene and R. A. Chambers, "Pseudoaddiction: Fact or Fiction? An Investigation of the Medical Literature," *Current Addiction Reports*, 2015; 2(4): 310–317. doi: 10.1007/s40429-015-0074-7

9. H. Ryan, L. Girion, and S. Glover, "You Want a Description of Hell?" OxyContin's 12-Hour Problem," *Los Angeles Times*, May 5, 2016.

10. C. Conrad, H. M. Bradley, D. Broz et al., "Community Outbreak of HIV Infection Linked to Injection Drug Use of Oxymorphone—Indiana, 2015,"Morbidity and Mortality Weekly Report, 2015; 64:1.

11. A. Schwartz and M. Smith, "Needle Exchange Is Allowed After H.I.V. Outbreak in an Indiana County," *New York Times*, March 26, 2015.

12. United States Food and Drug Administration, "FDA Requests Removal of Opana ER for Risks Related to Abuse," June 8, 2017. Available from: https://www.fda.gov/newsevents/newsroom/pressannouncements/ucm562401.htm

13. T. Caton and E. Perez, "A Pain-Drug Champion Has Second Thoughts," *Wall Street Journal*, December 17, 2012.

14. C. Ornstein and R. G. Jones, "Opioid Makers, Blamed for Overdose Epidemic, Cut Back on Marketing Payments to Doctors," *ProPublica*, June 28, 2018. https://www.propublica.org/article/opioid-makers-blamed-for-overdose-epidemic-cut-back-on-marketing-payments-to-doctors

15. A. Kessler, E. Chen, and K. Grise, "The More Opioids Doctors Prescribe, the More Money They Make," *CNN*, March 12, 2018. https://www.cnn.com/2018/03/11/health/prescription-opioid-payments-eprise

16. G. Chai, J. Xu, J. Osterhout et al., "New Opioid Analgesic Approvals and Outpatient Utilization of Opioid Analgesics in the United States, 1997 Through 2015," *Anesthesiology*, 2018; 128(5): 953–966. doi: 10.1097/ALN.0000000000002187

17. C. Peterson-Withorn, "Fortune of Family behind OxyContin Drops amid Declining Prescriptions," *Forbes*, January 29, 2016.

18. L. Scholl, P. Seth, M. Kariisa, N. Wilson, and G. Baldwin, "Drug and Opioid-Involved Overdose Deaths—United States, 2013–2017," *MMWR. Morbidity and Mortality Weekly Report*, 2018; 67(5152). doi: 10.15585/mmwr.mm675152e1

19. G. M. Franklin, J. Mai, T. Wickizer, J. A. Turner, D. Fulton-Kehoe, and L. Grant, "Opioid Dosing Trends and Mortality in Washington State Workers' Compensation, 1996–2002," *American Journal of Industrial Medicine*, 2005; 48: 91–99.

20. J. Egan, "Children of the Opioid Epidemic," *New York Times*, May 9, 2018.

21. L. Radel, M. Baldwin, G. Crouse, R. Ghertner, and A. Waters, "Substance Use, the Opioid Epidemic, and the Child Welfare System: Key Findings from a Mixed Methods Study, *United States Department of Health and Human Services*, March 7, 2018. https://aspe.hhs.gov/system/files/pdf/258836/SubstanceUseChildWelfareOverview.pdf

22. E. Birnbaum and M. Lora, "Opioid Crisis Sending Thousands of Children into Foster Care," *The Hill*, June 20, 2018.

23. D. Michaels and C. Levine. Estimates of the Number of Motherless Youth Orphaned by AIDS in the United States. JAMA 268:3456-3461, 1992.

24. *Commonwealth of Massachusetts v. Purdue Pharma L.P. et al., First Amended Complaint and Jury Demand.* https://www.documentcloud.org/documents/5715954-Massachusetts-AGO-Amended-Complaint-2019-01-31.html

25. M. K. Delgado, Y. Huang, Z. Meisel et al., "National Variation in Opioid Prescribing and Risk of Prolonged Use for Opioid-Naive Patients Treated in the Emergency Department for Ankle Sprains," *Annals of Emergency Medicine*, 2018. doi://doi.org/10.1016/j.annemergmed.2018.06.003

26. C. M. Jones, P. G. Lurie, and D. C. Throckmorton, "Effect of US Drug Enforcement Administration's Rescheduling of Hydrocodone Combination Analgesic Products on Opioid Analgesic Prescribing," *JAMA Internal Medicine*, 2016; 176(3): 399–402. doi:10.1001/jamainternmed.2015.7799

Chapter 8

1. D. Michaels, "It Takes a Tragedy," *The Pump Handle*, April 20, 2007. https://thepumphandle.wordpress.com/2007/04/20/it-takes-a-tragedy/

2. J. Haughey, "Can Obama's Anti-Gun OSHA Pick Be Stopped?" *Outdoor Life*, September 2009. https://www.outdoorlife.com/blogs/gun-shots/2009/09/can-obamas-anti-gun-osha-pick-be-stopped

3. Occupational Safety and Health Administration, "Permissible Exposure Limits—Annotated Tables." https://www.osha.gov/dsg/annotated-pels/

4. G. Markowitz and D. Rosner, "The Reawakening of National Concerns About Silicosis," *Public Health Reports*, 1998; 113(4): 302–311. https://www.ncbi.nlm.nih.gov/pmc/articles/PMC1308386/

5. IARC Working Group on the Evaluation of Carcinogenic Risks to Humans, "Silica, Some Silicates, Coal Dust and Para-Aramid Fibrils: Lyon, 15–22 October 1996," *IARC Monographs on the Evaluation of Carcinogenic Risks to Humans*, 1997; 68: 1–475.

6. National Toxicology Program, *9th Report on Carcinogens*, Research Triangle Park, NC, 2000.

7. P. Hessel, J. Gamble, J. Gee et al., "Silica, Silicosis, and Lung Cancer: A Response to a Recent Working Group Report," *Journal of Occupational and Environmental Medicine*, 2000; 42(7): 704–720. doi: 10.1097/00043764-200007000-00005

8. P. A. Hessel, J. F. Gamble, and M. Nicolich, "Relationship Between Silicosis and Smoking," *Scandinavian Journal of Work, Environment & Health*, 2003; 29(5): 329–336. doi: 739 [pii]

9. Y. Liu, K. Steenland, Y. Rong et al., "Exposure-Response Analysis and Risk Assessment for Lung Cancer in Relationship to Silica Exposure: A 44-Year Cohort Study of 34,018 Workers," *American Journal of Epidemiology*, 2013; 178(9): 1424–1433. doi: 10.1093/aje/kwt139 [doi]

10. C. Monforton, "Congressman Tells OSHA Chief Not to Use "Buzz" Words Like Cancer," *The Pump Handle*, October 10, 2011. http://www.thepumphandle.org/2011/10/10/congressman-tells-osha-chief-n/#.XBu-5VVKiUl

11. Ibid.

12. K. Steenland and E. Ward, "Silica: A Lung Carcinogen," *CA: A Cancer Journal for Clinicians*, 2014; 64(1): 63–69. doi: 10.3322/caac.21214

13. L. Heinzerling, "Inside EPA: A Former Insider's Reflections on the Relationship Between the Obama EPA and the Obama White House," *Pace Environmental Law (PELR) Review*, 2013; 31(325): 1–35. https://papers.ssrn.com/sol3/papers.cfm?abstract_id=2262337

14. J. Morris, "OSHA Rules on Workplace Toxics Stalled," May 19, 2014. https://publicintegrity.org/workers-rights/osha-rules-on-workplace-toxics-stalled

15. "The Dukes of Workplace Hazard," Wall Street Journal, February 10, 2014.

16. Comments of the American Chemistry Council Crystalline Chemistry Panel February 11, 2014. https://tinyurl.com/4832tzmw

17. J. Plautz, "Trump's Air Pollution Adviser Actually Said That Clean Air Saves No Lives." Mother Jones October 27,2018. https://www.motherjones.com/environment/2018/10/tony-cox-trumps-air-pollution-adviser-clean-air-saves-no-lives/

18. Environmental Protection Agency, "Acting Administrator Wheeler Announces Science Advisors for Key Clean Air Act Committee," EPA Press release, October 10, 2018.

19. S. L. Sessions letter to J. Morrill, "Preliminary Letter Report of Environomics to the American Chemistry Council's Crystalline Silica Panel Regarding the Economic Impact of the Occupational Safety and Health Administration's Proposed Standard for Occupational Exposure to Respirable Crystalline Silica," February 7, 2014. https://tinyurl.com/yc276d5v

20. U.S. Congress, Office of Technology Assessment. Gauging control technology and regulatory impacts in occupational safety and health: An appraisal of OSHA's analytic approach OTA-ENV-635. Washington, DC: U.S. Government Printing Office, 1995.

21. K. A. Mundt, T. Birk, W. Parsons, et al., "Respirable Crystalline Silica Exposure-Response Evaluation of Silicosis Morbidity and Lung Cancer Mortality in the German Porcelain Industry Cohort," *Journal of Occupational and Environmental Medicine*, 2011; 53(3): 282–289. doi: 10.1097/JOM.0b013e31820c2bff [doi]

22. See https://www.documentcloud.org/documents/2816931-Expert-Report-of-Mundt-in-Tobacco-Case.html

23. D. Michaels, C. Monforton, and P. Lurie, "Selected Science: An Industry Campaign to Undermine an OSHA Hexavalent Chromium Standard," *Environmental Health: A Global Access Science Source*, 2006; 5(1): 5.

24. Letter from Construction Safety Coalition to author, March 25, 2015. https://tinyurl.com/rdb86xpp

25. J. F. Werling, "Crystalline Silica Preliminary Economic Analysis: Industry and Macroeconomic Impacts," *Inforum*, November 30, 2011. https://www.osha.gov/silica/Employment_Analysis.pdf

26. 2 North America's Building Trades Unions v. Occupational Safety and Health Admin., et al., No. 16-1105 (D.C. Cir. Dec. 22, 2017), available at https://www.cadc.uscourts.gov/internet/opinions.nsf/03C747A5AB141C9 0852581FE0055A642/$file/16-1105-1710179.pdf
27. H. Berkes, H. Jingnan and R. Benincasa, "An Epidemic Is Killing Thousands of Coal Miners. Regulators Could Have Stopped It," *All Things Considered*, December 18, 2018. https://www.npr. org/2018/12/18/675253856/an-epidemic-is-killing-thousands-of-coal-miners-regulators-could-have-stopped-it

Chapter 9

1. Technology Planning and Management Corporation, *Draft Report on Carcinogens Background Document for Talc Asbestiform and Non-Asbestiform*, December 2000, https://ntp.niehs.nih.gov/ntp/roc/talc_archive/roctalcbg20001213.pdf
2. R. Patric. "Talc Cancer Verdict of $4.6 Billion from St. Louis Jury Sends 'Very Powerful Message.'" *St. Louis Post-Dispatch*, July 13, 2018.
3. G. Lichtenstein. "High Levels of Asbestos Found in 3 Paints and 2 Talcums Here," *New York Times*, June 6, 1972.
4. R. C. Rabin and T. Hsu, "Johnson & Johnson Feared Baby Powder's Possible Asbestos Link for Years," *New York Times*, December 14, 2018.
5. For the investigative reports, see: L. Girion, "Johnson & Johnson Knew for Decades That Asbestos Lurked in Its Baby Powder," *Reuters*, December 14, 2018; R. C. Rabin, T. Hsu, "Johnson & Johnson Feared Baby Powder's Possible Asbestos Link for Years," *New York Times*, December 14, 2018; and S. Berfield, J. Feeley, and M. C. Fisk, "Johnson & Johnson Has a Baby Powder Problem," *Bloomberg Business Week*, March 31, 2016.
6. D. Cramer, W. Welch, R. Scully, and C. Wojciechowski, "Ovarian Cancer and Talc: A Case-Control Study," *Obstetrical & Gynecological Survey*, 1982; 37(11): 686. doi: 10.1097/00006254-198211000-00018
7. International Agency for Research on Cancer IARC monographs on the evaluation of carcinogenic risk of chemicals to humans, Vol. 42, Silica and some silicates. IARC, Lyon 1987.
8. National Toxicology Program, "Toxicology and Carcinogenesis Studies of Talc (CAS No. 14807-96-6)(Non-Asbestiform) in F344/N Rats and B6C3F1 Mice (Inhalation Studies)," TR-421, Research Triangle Park, NC, 1993.
9. S. Jarvis, "Narrative Talc—NTP Regulatory Challenge," undated. https://tinyurl.com/384jz56p
10. E. K. Ong and S. A. Glantz, "Constructing 'Sound Science' and 'Good Epidemiology': Tobacco, Lawyers, and Public Relations Firms," *American Journal of Public Health*, 2001; 91(11): 1749–1757. doi: 10.2105/AJPH.91.11.1749

11. R. Zazenski to R. Bernstein, R. Meli, and E. Turner, "CTFA Conference Call Minutes," October 18, 2000. https://tinyurl.com/cbjyn42p and D. L. Peters to E. D. Holland, *Ingham, et al. v. Johnson & Johnson, et al.*, December 1, 2016 (containing invoice of months October 2000 through January 2001.) https://tinyurl.com/mw2978xj

12. S. D. Gettings to A. P. Wehner, October 18, 1993. https://tinyurl.com/4fn592sz

13. For a sample of Wehner's work for the tobacco industry, see: E. I. Alpen, M. G. Bissell, M. J. Cline et al., "Critiques of EPA External Review Draft 600/6–90/006A. Health Effects of Passive Smoking: Assessment of Lung Cancer in Adults and Respiratory Disorders in Children," Biomedical & Environmental Consultants, Inc., 1991. https://tinyurl.com/fzrzmw2a; and T. Hockaday to H. Bryan, GCI Group London. International Meeting in Europe on Sound Science, May 9, 1994. https://www.industrydocumentslibrary.ucsf.edu/tobacco/docs/#id=yrwb0084. and Biomedical & Engineering Consults, Inc. Proposal to the R.J. Reynolds Tobacco Company, November 11, 1990. https://tinyurl.com/2p98caua

14. A. P. Wehner, "Biological Effects of Cosmetic Talc," *Food and Chemical Toxicology*, 1994; 32(12): 1173–1184.

15. A. P. Wehner to L. J. Loretz. November 2, 2000. https://tinyurl.com/5n8ysd9m

16. R. Zazenski to E. Turner, "RE: Drafting of the EUROTALC submission to NTP," November 13, 2000. https://tinyurl.com/4hrd62u7

17. Daniel M. Cook, Lisa A. Bero, "Identifying Carcinogens: the Tobacco Industry and Regulatory Politics in the United States," *International Journal of Health Services: Planning, Administration, Evaluation*, 2006; 36(4): 747–766.

18. J. J. Tozzi to R. J. Zazenski. November 27, 2000. https://tinyurl.com/3w8xjtpb

19. S. Sharma to M. Greene, "RE: Contractors," October 3, 2011. https://tinyurl.com/3ddk97br

20. P. K. Mills, D. G. Riordan, R. D. Cress, and H. A. Young, "Perineal Talc Exposure and Epithelial Ovarian Cancer Risk in the Central Valley of California," *International Journal of Cancer*, 2004; 112(3): 458–464. doi: 10.1002/ijc.20434; also, see H. Langseth, S. E. Hankinson, J. Siemiatycki, E. Weiderpass, "Perineal Use of Talc and Risk of Ovarian Cancer," *Journal of Epidemiology and Community Health (1979–)*. 2008; 62(4): 358–360. doi: 10.1136/jech.2006.047894

21. W. G. Kelly Jr. to M. S. Wolfe. November 29, 2000. https://tinyurl.com/2p8c7z49

22. National Toxicology Program, *Summary Minutes of the National Toxicology Program Board of Scientific Counselors Report on Carcinogens Subcommittee Meeting*, December 2000. https://ntp.niehs.nih.gov/ntp/roc/twelfth/draftbackgrounddocs/minutes20001213.pdf

23. R. Bernstein to R. Zazenski, "RE: Summary of CRE Meeting—Dec. 15," January 4, 2001. https://tinyurl.com/2p9ch9jp

24. S. Mann to S. Colamarino, C. Linares, and K. O'Shaughnessy, "FW: Talc/NTP-Zazenski," October 7, 2004. https://tinyurl.com/bds7zv4s

25. S. Jarvis, "Narrative Talc—NTP Regulatory Challenge," undated. https://tinyurl.com/384jz56p

26. R. Bernstein R to Zazenski R. "RE: Summary of CRE Meeting—Dec. 15." January 4, 2001. https://tinyurl.com/2p9ch9jp

27. C. Stenneler to E. Turner, R. Zazenski, D. Harris, J. Godla, and J. Roeser. "RE: Confidential—NTP Update and Issues," October 29, 2001. https://tinyurl.com/2u4c2bsx

28. J. J. Tozzi to K. Olden, April 15, 2002. https://tinyurl.com/2p93fyak

29. W. G. Kelly Jr. to K. Weems, U.S. Department of Health and Human Services. March 3, 2004. https://tinyurl.com/5ewcrpnx

30. R. Zazenski to S. Mann, "OMB Letter." January 6, 2005. https://tinyurl.com/2snwxawa

31. A. P. Wehner, "Cosmetic Talc Should Not Be Listed as a Carcinogen: Comments on NTP's Deliberations to List Talc as a Carcinogen," *Regulatory Toxicology and Pharmacology: RTP*, 2002; 36(1): 40–50.

32. R. Zazenski to S. Mann, "More Intelligence," January 12, 2005. https://tinyurl.com/22324enf

33. P. Sterchele to S. Mann, "FW: NTP Withdraws Talc Nomination," October 19, 2005. https://tinyurl.com/bdcmsh3k

34. R. Penninkilampi and G. Eslick, "Perineal Talc Use and Ovarian Cancer: A Systematic Review and Meta-Analysis," *Epidemiology*, 2018; 29(1): 41–49. doi: 10.1097/EDE.0000000000000745

35. R. Bernstein to R. Zazenski, "RE: Summary of CRE Meeting—Dec. 15." January 4, 2001. https://tinyurl.com/2p9ch9jp

36. Statista, "Market Value of Glyphosate Worldwide from 2016 to 2022," Statista, the Statistics Portal, 2018. https://www.statista.com/statistics/791062/global-glyphosate-market-value

37. Monsanto, "Exhibit 42—IARC Carcinogen Rating of Glyphosate Preparedness and Engagement Plan," UCSF Library, Chemical Industry Documents, 2015. https://www.industrydocumentslibrary.ucsf.edu/chemical/docs/#id=xhmn0226

38. K. Z. Guyton, D. Loomis, Y. Grosse, et al. "Carcinogenicity of Tetrachlorvinphos, Parathion, Malathion, Diazinon, and Glyphosate," *Lancet Oncology* 2015; 16(5): 490–491.

39. C. Gillam, *Whitewash. The Story of a Weed Killer, Cancer, and the Corruption of Science*, Island Press, 2017.

40. S. Foucart and S. Horel, "Glyphosate: How Monsanto Conducts Its Media War," *Le Monde*, January 31, 2019.

41. Spinning Science & Silencing Scientists: A Case Study in How the Chemical Industry Attempts to Influence Science. Minority Staff Report, Prepared for Members of the Committee on Science, Space &

Technology U.S. House of Representatives February 2018. https://science.house.gov/imo/media/doc/02.06.18%20-%20Spinning%20Science%20and%20Silencing%20Scientists_0.pdf Many documents detailing Monsanto's efforts to counter IARC's conclusion are posted on the web. For example,
see: https://tobacco.ucsf.edu/ucsf-chemical-industry-documents-adds-monsanto-papers-and-agrichemical-industry-documents

42. C. Hiar, "Under Fire by U.S. Politicians, World Health Organization Defends Its Claim That an Herbicide Causes Cancer," *Science*, February 2018. http://www.sciencemag.org/news/2018/02/who-rebuts-house-committee-criticisms-about-glyphosate-cancer-warning

43. California Office of Environmental Health Hazard Assessment. "Final Statement of Reasons: Glyphosate," https://oehha.ca.gov/media/downloads/crnr/glyphosatensrlfsor041018.pdf

44. E. T. Chang and E. Delzell, "Systematic Review and Meta-Analysis of Glyphosate Exposure and Risk of Lymphohematopoietic Cancers," *Journal of Environmental Science and Health. Part B, Pesticides, Food Contaminants, and Agricultural Wastes.* 2016; 51(6): 402–434.

45. N. Donley, B. Freese, E. Marquez et al. to Editors of *Critical Reviews in Toxicology.* "Dear Editors of *Critical Reviews in Toxicology.*" https://www.biologicaldiversity.org/campaigns/pesticides_reduction/pdfs/Retraction_letter_to_Critical_Reviews_in_Toxicology.pdf

46. J. Rosenblatt, P. Waldman, and L. Mulvany, "Monsanto's Role in Roundup Safety Study Is Corrected by Journal," *Bloomberg.* September 27, 2018.

47. Editor-in-Chief and Publisher "Expression of Concern," *Critical Reviews in Toxicology*, DOI: 10.1080/10408444.2018.1522786

Chapter 10

1. Q. Di, Y. Wang, Y. Wang et al., "Air Pollution and Mortality in the Medicare Population," *New England Journal of Medicine*, 2017; 376(26): 2513–2522. doi: 10.1056/NEJMoa1702747

2. J. Ewing, *Faster, Higher, Farther*, New York; London: W. W. Norton & Company, 2017.

3. G. P. Chossière, R. Malina, A. Ashok, et al., "Public Health Impacts of Excess NOx Emissions from Volkswagen Diesel Passenger Vehicles in Germany," 2017. doi: 10.1088/1748-9326/aa5987

4. S. R. H. Barrett, R. L. Speth, S. D. Eastham et al., "Impact of the Volkswagen Emissions Control Defeat Device on US Public Health," *Environmental Research Letters*, 2015, 10(11): 114005. doi: 10.1088/1748-9326/10/11/114005

5. J. Ewing, "Audi, Admitting to Role in Diesel-Cheating Scheme, Agrees to Pay Major Fine," *New York Times*, October 16, 2018.

6. E. C. Evarts, "VW Bought Back 300,000 Cars After Its Dieselgate Scandal—and Now They're Sitting in 37 Parking Lots Around the US," *Business Insider*, April 18, 2018.

7. C. Rauwald, "VW Agrees to $1.2 Billion Fine as Diesel Crisis Grinds On," *Bloomberg Wire Service*, June 14, 2018.

8. H. Dae-sun, "Audi Volkswagen Korea Criticized After Publically Apologizing for Emissions Scandal," *Hankyoreh*, April 8, 2018.

9. R. Muncrief, "NOx Emissions from Heavy-Duty and Light-Duty Diesel Vehicles in the EU: Comparison of Real-World Performance and Current Type-Approval Requirements," *International Council on Clean Transportation*, 2017. https://www.theicct.org/sites/default/files/publications/Euro-VI-versus-6_ICCT_briefing_06012017.pdf

10. United States Environmental Protection Agency, "News Releases from Headquarters: EPA Notifies Fiat Chrysler of Clean Air Act Violations," January 2017. https://19january2017snapshot.epa.gov/newsreleases/epa-notifies-fiat-chrysler-clean-air-act-violations_.html

11. G. Guillaume and L. Frost, "Renault CEO Ghosn Targeted in French Diesel Probe," *Reuters*, March 15, 2017.

12. A. Sage, "Peugeot Chiefs 'Approved Cheat Devices on 2m Vehicles,'" *Times* (London, England), September 9, 2017.

13. A. White, "VW, BMW, Daimler Face EU Probe Over Clean-Car Collusion," *Bloomberg*, September 18, 2018.

14. European Research Group on Environment and Health in the Transport Sector, "Our Task," EUGT, August 2013. http://web.archive.org/web/20130831020508/http://eugt.org/index.php/start-en.html

15. F. Dohmen, V. Hackenbroch, S, Hage, N. Klawitter, H. Knuth, and G. Traufetter, "A Monkey on Their Back: German Carmakers Have Lost All Moral Standing," *Spiegel Online*, February 2, 2018.

16. M. Spallek to J. McDonald, "AW:," June 11, 2013. https://tinyurl.com/4rjtfrzp

17. P. Morfeld, D. A. Groneberg, and M. F. Spallek, "Effectiveness of Low Emission Zones: Large Scale Analysis of Changes in Environmental NO2, NO and NOx Concentrations in 17 German Cities," *PLoS ONE*, 2014; 9(8): e102999. https://doi.org/10.1371/journal.pone.0102999

18. For information on European Low Emissions Zones, see Urban Access Regulations in Europe website: http://urbanaccessregulations.eu/

19. K. S. Crump, C. Van Landingham, S. H. Moolgavkar et al., "Reanalysis of the DEMS Nested Case-Control Study of Lung Cancer and Diesel Exhaust: Suitability for Quantitative Risk Assessment," *Risk Analysis*, 2015; 35(4): 676–700.

20. P. Morfeld, "Diesel Exhaust in Miners Study: How to Understand the Findings?" *Journal of Occupational Medicine and Toxicology*, 2012; 7(1): 10. doi: 10.1186/1745-6673-7-10 and [20] D. Pallapies, D. Taeger, F. Bochmann, and P. Morfeld, "Comment: Carcinogenicity of Diesel-Engine Exhaust (DE)," *Archives of Toxicology*, 2013; 87(3): 547–549. doi: 10.1007/s00204-012-0955-7

21. B. Stertz to L. Kata and S. Johnson, "FW: Diesel WHO Report Reaction?" June 12, 2012. https://tinyurl.com/4rr4ecm8

22. F. Dohmen, V. Hackenbroch, S, Hage, N. Klawitter, H. Knuth, and G. Traufetter, "A Monkey on Their Back: German Carmakers Have Lost All Moral Standing," *Spiegel Online*, February 2, 2018.

23. Signed agreement between the Europäische Forschungsvereinigung für Umwelt und Gesundheit im Transportsektor (EUGT) and the Lovelace Respiratory Research Institute (LRRI) https://tinyurl.com/3mkyznzp

24. F. Davidoff, C. D. DeAngelis, J. M. Drazen et al. "Sponsorship, Authorship, and Accountability," *New England Journal of Medicine*, 2001; 345(11): 825–827. doi: 10.1056/NEJMed010093

25. J. Ewing, "10 Monkeys and a Beetle: Inside VW's Campaign for 'Clean Diesel,'" *New York Times*, January 25, 2018.

26. J. McDonald to M. Spallek, "RE: Scanned Image from Gilligan," April 10, 2014. https://tinyurl.com/3tbsfuw7

27. H. Irshad to J. McDonald, "FW: Drive Recorder - Signal Booster." November 10, 2014. https://tinyurl.com/2rayedhk

28. Deposition of S. Johnson, August 8, 2017. https://tinyurl.com/y73zbzen

29. Deposition of J.McDonald, August 16, 2017. https://tinyurl.com/bzku8aby

30. F. Dohmen, V. Hackenbroch, S, Hage, N. Klawitter, H. Knuth, and G. Traufetter, "A Monkey on Their Back: German Carmakers Have Lost All Moral Standing," *Spiegel Online*, February 2, 2018.

31. J. Brower to M. Doyle-Eisele, H. Irshad, and J. McDonald, "RE: EUGT abstract," October 7, 2015. https://tinyurl.com/9b2b63hy

32. J. Brower, H. Irshad, M. Doyle-Eisele, Y. Tesfaigzi and J. McDonald, "Exposures to Old Technology Diesel Emissions to Evaluate Biological Response in Non-Human Primates." Society of Toxicology 2016 Annual Meeting Abstract Supplement: Late Breaking Abstract Submissions. https://www.toxicology.org/events/am/AM2016/docs/2016_LB_Supplement.pdf

33. J. Brower to J. McDonald, "EUGT Report" November 25, 2015. https://tinyurl.com/bdzafhvf

34. P. Morfeld and M. Spallek, "Diesel Engine Exhaust and Lung Cancer Risks Evaluation of the Meta-Analysis by Vermeulen et al. 2014," *Journal of Occupational Medicine and Toxicology*, 2015; 10(1): 31. doi: 10.1186/s12995-015-0073-6 and P. Morfeld, U. Keil, and M. Spallek, "The European 'Year of the Air': Fact, Fake or Vision?" *Archives of Toxicology*, 2013; 87(12): 2051–2055. doi: 10.1007/s00204-013-1140-3

35. N. Sawyer to J. Maestas, "EUGT," August 17, 2016. https://tinyurl.com/yckj5byc

36. Deposition of J. McDonald, October 31, 2017. https://tinyurl.com/bzku8aby

37.   J. McDonald to M. J. Campen, "FY14-050_EUGT NHP Diesel Report_23Nov2015," August 29, 2016. https://tinyurl.com/uaese62z

38.   J. McDonald to M. Spallek, "RE: New Proposal Diesel Inhalation Study," February 8, 2017. https://tinyurl.com/t6t7kby5

39.   J. Ewing, "10 Monkeys and a Beetle: Inside VW's Campaign for 'Clean Diesel,'" New York Times, January 25, 2018.

40.   J. McDonald to S. Johnson, June 30, 2017. https://tinyurl.com/3kf9ee33

41.   "VW, BMW and Daimler Denounce Toxic Diesel Fume Tests on Monkeys," *Deutsche Welle*, January 28, 2018.

42.   S. Marks, and J. Posaner, "Monkeygate Doctor Says Car Firms Were Not Kept in Dark," *Politico*. January 31, 2018. And "Automanager Should Have Approved Test." Spiegel Online, January 30, 2018

43.   SEC complaint available from: https://web.archive.org/web/20200422032813/ https://www.sec.gov/files/complaint-2019-03-14_0.pdf

44.   "Volkswagen Engineer Gets Prison in Diesel Cheating Case," *New York Times*, August 25, 2017.

45.   J. Ewing, "Audi, Admitting to Role in Diesel-Cheating Scheme, Agrees to Pay Major Fine," *New York Times*, October 16, 2018.

Chapter 11

1.   S. Begley, "The Truth About Denial," n.d. Begley S. The truth about denial. Newsweek. 2007 Aug 13;150(7):20-7, 29. PMID: 19146210

2.   G. Monbiot, "Climate Breakdown," October 4, 2013. https://www.monbiot.com/2013/10/04/climate-breakdown/

3.   D. Furchtgott-Roth, "Testimony by Diana Furchtgott-Roth on Climate Change," Manhattan Institute for Policy Research, July 18, 2013. https://www.manhattan-institute.org/html/testimony-diana-furchtgott-roth-climate-change-6091.html

4.   D. Furchtgott-Roth, "New Congress Breaks into Action with Smart Bills," Manhattan Institute for Policy Research Economics 21, April 17, 2015. https://economics21.org/html/new-congress-breaks-action-smart-bills-1301.html

5.   National Oceanic and Atmospheric Administration, *Global Climate Report—Annual 2018*. https://www.ncdc.noaa.gov/sotc/global/201813

6.   J. Cook, N. Oreskes, P. T. Doran et al. Consensus on Consensus: A Synthesis of Consensus Estimates on Human-Caused Global Warming. *Environmental Research Letters*. 2016;11(4):48002. doi: 10.1088/1748-9326/11/4/048002.

7.   S. J.Inhofe, *The Greatest Hoax: How the Global Warming Conspiracy Threatens Your Future*, New York: Midpoint Trade Books, 2012.

8.   R. Savransky, "Dem Senator: GOP the Only Major Political Party Dedicated to Making Climate Change Worse," *The Hill* April 8, 2018.

9. C. Borick, B. G. Rabe, N. B. Fitzpatrick, and S. B. Mills. "As Americans Experienced the Warmest May on Record Their Acceptance of Global Warming Reaches a New High," *Issues in Energy and Environmental Policy*, July 2018; 37. https://closup.umich.edu/issues-in-energy-and-environmental-policy/37/as-americans-experienced-the-warmest-may-on-record-their-acceptance-of-global-warming-reaches-a-new-high

10. B. Dawson, "The Beat: The Roots of Conservatives' Environmental View," *Society of Environmental Journalists*, November 15, 2008. https://www.sej.org/publications/sejournal/the-beat-the-roots-conservatives-environmental-view

11. N. Oreskes and E. M. Conway, *Merchants of Doubt*, New York: Bloomsbury Press, 2010, 129.

12. Science & Environmental Policy Project, "Testimony of Dr. S. Fred Singer, Atmospheric Physicist; President, the Science & Environmental Policy Project: To the House Commerce Committee Subcommittee on Oversight and Investigations, August 1, 1995. https://web.archive.org/web/2020*/https://research.greenpeaceusa.org/?a=download&d=3326

13. U.S Department of State, "The Montreal Protocol on Substances That Deplete the Ozone Layer." https://2009-2017.state.gov/e/oes/eqt/chemicalpollution/83007.htm

14. J. Tozzi, "Multinational Business Services Inc., to J. Boland, T. Borelli, and T. Lattanzio," December 29, 1993. https://www.industrydocumentslibrary.ucsf.edu/tobacco/docs/#id=kmxg0117

15. G. Vaidyanathan, "Think Tank That Cast Doubt on Climate Change Science Morphs into Smaller One, *E&E News*, December 10, 2015. https://www.eenews.net/stories/1060029290

16. CO_2 Coalition. http://co2coalition.org/

17. G. Supran and N. Oreskes, "Assessing ExxonMobil's Climate Change Communications (1977–2014)," *Environmental Research Letters*, 2017; 12(8): 84019. doi: 10.1088/1748-9326/aa815f; Climate Investigators Center, "Shell Climate Documents." https://climateinvestigations.org/shell-oil-climate-documents/And B. Franta, "Early Oil Industry Knowledge of CO_2 and Global Warming," *Nature Climate Change*, 2018; 8(12): 1024–1025. doi: 10.1038/s41558-018-0349-9

18. J. Mayer, *Dark Money*, New York: Doubleday, 2016.

19. J. Nesbit, *Poison Tea: How Big Oil and Big Tobacco Invented the Tea Party and Captured the GOP*, New York: St. Martin's Press, 2016.; and A. Fallin, R. Grana, and S. A. Glantz, "'To Quarterback Behind the Scenes, Third-Party Efforts': The Tobacco Industry and the Tea Party," *Tobacco Control*, 2014; 23(4): 322–331. doi: 10.1136/tobaccocontrol-2012-050815

20. Mackinac Center for Public Policy. https://www.mackinac.org/about; Koch funding is documented here: https://www.sourcewatch.org/index.php/Mackinac_Center_for_Public_Policy

21. Good Jobs First, "Subsidy Tracker Parent Company Summary." https://subsidytracker.goodjobsfirst.org/parent/koch-industries
22. E. Scheyder, "Exxon CEO Urges New York Prosecutor to Rethink Climate Change Probe," *Reuters*, May 30, 2018.
23. E. Negin, "Why is ExxonMobil Still Funding Climate Science Denier Groups?" August 31, 2018. https://blog.ucsusa.org/elliott-negin/exxonmobil-still-funding-climate-science-denier-groups
24. R. J. Brulle, "The Climate Lobby: A sectoral Analysis of Lobbying Spending on Climate Change in the USA, 2000 to 2016," *Climatic Change*, 2018; 149(3–4): 289–303. doi: 10.1007/s10584-018-2241-z
25. A. Parker, P. Rucker, and M. Birnbaum, "Inside Trump's Climate Decision: After Fiery Debate, He 'Stayed Where He's Always Been,'" *Washington Post*, June 2, 2017.
26. C. Davenport and E. Lipton, "How G.O.P. Leaders Came to View Climate Change as Fake Science," *New York Times*, June 3, 2017.
27. E. Bolstad, "How Steve Bannon is Shaping Trump's Views on 'Climate Change,'" *E&E News*, November 18, 2016. https://www.eenews.net/stories/1060045998
28. DeSmog "Will Washington Post's Hiring of Former WSJ Opinion Editor Bring Climate Deniers to its Pages?" May 31, 2018. https://www.desmogblog.com/2018/05/31/washington-post-hiring-former-wsj-opinion-editor-mark-lasswell-climate-deniers
29. S. Waldman, "Lawmaker Says Tumbling Rocks Are Causing Seas to Rise," *Science*, May 17, 2018.

Chapter 12

1. A. M. Brandt, *The Cigarette Century*, New York: Basic Books, 2007.
2. R. Hockett, "Application to the TIRC," January 4, 1954. https://www.industrydocumentslibrary.ucsf.edu/tobacco/docs/#id=mgjn0041
3. C. E. Kearns, L. A. Schmidt, and S. A. Glantz, "Sugar Industry and Coronary Heart Disease Research: A Historical Analysis of Internal Industry Documents," *JAMA Internal Medicine*, September 12, 2016. doi:10.1001/jamainternmed.2016.5394
4. H. B. Hass, "What's New in Sugar Research? American Society of Sugar Beet Technologists." https://www.assbt-proceedings.org/ASSBT1954Proceedings/ASSBTVol8p15to22WhatsNewinSugarResearch.pdf
5. R. B. McGandy, D. M. Hegsted, and F. J. Stare, "Dietary Fats, Carbohydrates and Atherosclerotic Vascular Disease," *New England Journal of Medicine*, 1967; 277(4): 186–192, and R. B. McGandy, D. M. Hegsted, and F. J. Stare, "Dietary Fats, Carbohydrates and Atherosclerotic Vascular Disease," *New England Journal of Medicine*, 1967; 277(5): 245–247.

6. M. Nestle, "Food Industry Funding of Nutrition Research: The Relevance of History for Current Debates," *JAMA Internal Medicine*, 2016; 176(11): 1685–1686. doi: 10.1001/jamainternmed

7. D. M. Johns and G. M. Oppenheimer, "Was There Ever a 'Sugar Conspiracy'?" *Science*, 2018; 16(359)6377: 747–750. doi: 10.1126/science. aaq1618

8. P. Barlow, P. Serôdio, G. Ruskin, M. McKee, and D. Stuckler., "Science Organisations and Coca-Cola's 'War' with the Public Health Community: Insights from an Internal Industry Document," *Journal of Epidemiology & Community Health*, 2018; 72(9): 1–3. doi:10.1136/jech-2017-210375

9. R. Applebaum to S. Blair, G. Hand, J. C. Peters et al., "Proposal for establishment of the Global Energy Balance Network," July 9, 2014. https://usrtk.org/wp-content/uploads/2018/03/Establishing-the-GEBN. pdf

10. The Global Energy Balance Network: Getting the Word Out. Share WIK, 2014. https://web.archive.org/web/20150820204330/http://www. sharewik.com/portfolio-items/the-global-energy-balance-getting-the-word-out/

11. A. O'Connor, "Coca-Cola Funds Scientists Who Shift Blame for Obesity Away From Bad Diets," *New York Times*, August 9, 2015.

12. A. O'Connor, "Research Group Funded by Coca-Cola to Disband," *New York Times*, December 1, 2015.

13. A. O'Connor, "Coke Spends Lavishly on Pediatricians and Dietitians," *New York Times*, September 28, 2015.

14. P. Matos Serodio, D. Stuckler, M. Mckee, and D. Cohen, "OP76 Corporate Funding of Scientific Research: A Case Study of Coca-Cola," *Journal of Epidemiology and Community Health*, 2016; 70(Suppl 1): A43. doi: 10.1136/jech-2016-208064.76

15. M.F. Jacobson and W. Willett "Coke's Skewed Message on Obesity: Drink Coke. Exercise More," *New York Times*, August 13, 2015.

16. D. C. Wilks, S. J. Sharp, U. Ekelund, S. G. Thompson, A. P. Mander et al., "Objectively Measured Physical Activity and Fat Mass in Children: A Bias-Adjusted. Meta-Analysis of Prospective Studies," *PLoS ONE*, 2011; 6(2): e17205. doi:10.1371/journal.pone.0017205 And C. Cook and D. Schoeller, "Physical Activity and Weight Control: Conflicting Findings," *Current Opinion in Clinical Nutrition and Metabolic Care*, 2011; 14(5): 419–424. doi: 10.1097/MCO.0b013e328349b9ff

17. S. Caprio, "Calories from Soft Drinks—Do They Matter?" *New England Journal of Medicine*, 2012; 367(15): 1462–1463. doi: 10.1056/ NEJMe1209884

18. "Beverage Industry Addresses Sugar-Sweetened Beverages and Obesity Articles in the *New England Journal of Medicine*." *BevNet*, September 26, 2012. https://www.bevnet.com/news/2012/beverage-industry-addresses-

sugar-sweetened-beverages-and-obesity-articles-in-the-new-england-journal-of-medicine

19. C. Choi, "Nutrition for Sale: How Candy Makers Shape Nutrition Science," *Chicago Tribune*, June 2, 2016.

20. D. Schillinger, J. Tran, C. Mangurian, and C. Kearns. "Do Sugar-Sweetened Beverages Cause Obesity and Diabetes? Industry and the Manufacture of Scientific Controversy," *Annals of Internal Medicine*, 2016; 165(12): 895–7.

21. L. I. Lesser, C. B. Ebbeling, M. Goozner, D. Wypij, and D. S. Ludwig, "Relationship Between Funding Source and Conclusion Among Nutrition-Related Scientific Articles." *PLoS Medicine*, 2007;4(1): e5. doi: 10.1371/journal.pmed.0040005

22. E. A. Litman, S. L. Gortmaker, C. B. Ebbeling, and D. S. Ludwig, "Source of Bias in Sugar-Sweetened Beverage Research: A Systematic Review," *Public Health Nutrition*, 2018; 21(12): 2345–2350. doi: 10.1017/S1368980018000575

23. M. Bes-Rastrollo, M. B. Schulze, M. Ruiz-Canela, and M. A. Martinez-Gonzalez, "Financial Conflicts of Interest and Reporting Bias Regarding the Association Between Sugar-Sweetened Beverages and Weight Gain: A Systematic Review of Systematic Reviews," *PLoS Medicine*, 2013; 10: e1001578 and J. Massougbodji, Y. Le Bodo, R. Fratu, and P. De Wals, "Reviews Examining Sugar-Sweetened Beverages and Body Weight: Correlates of Their Quality and Conclusions," *American Journal of Clinical Nutrition*, 2014; 99: 1096–104. For more on the funding effect in studies on food, see M. Nestle, *Unsavory Truth: How Food Companies Skew the Science of What We Eat*. New York: Basic Books, 2018.

24. S. Lerner, "The Teflon Toxin Part 2," *The Intercept*, August 17, 2015.

25. G. M. Williams, M. Aardema, J. Acquavella et al., "A Review of the Carcinogenic Potential of Glyphosate by Four Independent Expert Panels and Comparison to the IARC Assessment," *Critical Reviews in Toxicology*, 2016; 46(sup1): 3–20, and J. Acquavella, D. Garabrant, G. Marsh, T. Sorahan, and D. L. Weed, "Glyphosate Epidemiology Expert Panel Review: A Weight of Evidence Systematic Review of the Relationship Between Glyphosate Exposure and Non-Hodgkin's Lymphoma or Multiple Myeloma," *Critical Reviews in Toxicology*, 2016; 46(suppl): 28.

26. E. Conneely, American Chemistry Council, to Dr. M. A. Danello, U.S. Consumer Product Safety Commission, September 9, 2014. https://www.cpsc.gov/s3fs-public/2014-09-09_ACC_Letter_to_CPSC_Dr_Danello.pdf

27. D. L. Weed, M. D. Althuis, and P. J. Mink, "Quality of Reviews on Sugar-Sweetened Beverages and Health Outcomes: A Systematic Review," *American Journal of Clinical Nutrition*, 2011; 94: 1340–7.

28. V. S. Malik and F. B. Hu, "Sugar-Sweetened Beverages and Health: Where Does the Evidence Stand?" *American Journal of Clinical Nutrition*, 2011; 94: 1161–62.

29. Sugar Association, "2015 Dietary Guidelines for Americans Recommendation for Added Sugars Intake: Agenda Based, Not Science Based," January 7, 2016. https://web.archive.org/web/20180222140805/ https://www.sugar.org/2015-dietary-guidelines-for-americans-recommendation-for-added-sugars-intake-agenda-based-not-science-based/

30. M. Nestle, "Food Industry Funding of Nutrition Research: The Relevance of History for Current Debates," JAMA Internal Medicine, 2016; 176(11): 1685–1686. doi: 10.1001/jamainternmed. For more of Nestle's important work, see M. Nestle, " Food Company Sponsorship of Nutrition Research and Professional Activities: A Conflict of Interest? *Public Health Nutrition* 2001; 4:1015-1022. doi:10.1079/PHN2001253 and M. Nestle, *Unsavory Truth: How Food Companies Skew the Science of What We Eat.* New York: Basic Books, 2018.

31. J. Belluz, "Dark Chocolate Is Now a Health Food. Here's How That Happened," *Vox*, August 20, 2018.

32. E. Wyatt, "Regulators Call Health Claims in Pom Juice Ads Deceptive," *New York Times*, September 27, 2010.

33. L. Hurley, "U.S. Top Court Rejects POM Wonderful Appeal over Ads," *Reuters*, May 2, 2016.

34. K. D. Brownell and K. E. Warner, "The Perils of Ignoring History: Big Tobacco Played Dirty and Millions Died. How Similar Is Big Food?" *Milbank Quarterly*, 2009; 87(1): 259–294.

35. United States Department of Agriculture, "Research and Promotion." https://www.ams.usda.gov/rules-regulations/research-promotion

36. Centers for Disease Control and Prevention, "Economic Trends in Tobacco," May 4, 2018. https://www.cdc.gov/tobacco/data_statistics/fact_sheets/economics/econ_facts/index.htm

37. K. D. Brownell, T. Farley, W. C. Willett et al., "The Public Health and Economic Benefits of Taxing Sugar-Sweetened Beverages, *New England Journal of Medicine*, 2009; 361: 1599–1605.

38. M. Nestle, *Soda Politics: Taking on Big Soda (and Winning)*, New York: Oxford University Press, 2015.

39. S. A. Roache and L. O. Gostin, "The Untapped Power of Soda Taxes: Incentivizing Consumers, Generating Revenue, and Altering Corporate Behavior," *International Journal of Health Policy and Management*, 2017; 6(9): 489–93. doi:10.15171/ijhpm.2017.69 And C. Sorensen, A. Mullee, and H. Duncan, "Soda Taxes: Old and New," *Tax Advisor*, June 1, 2017. https://www.thetaxadviser.com/issues/2017/jun/soda-taxes.html

40. M. A. Cochero, J. R. Rivera-Dommarco, B. N. Popkin, and S. W. Ng, "In Mexico, Evidence of Sustained Consumer Response Two Years After Implementing a Sugar-Sweetened Beverage Tax," *Health Affairs*, 2017; 36(3): 564–71. doi:10.1377/hlthaff.2016.1231

41. J. Falbe, H. R. Thompson, C. M. Becker, N. Rojas, C. E. McCulloch, and K. A. Madsen. "Impact of the Berkeley Excise Tax on Sugar

Sweetened Beverage Consumption," *American Journal of Public Health*, 2016; 106(10): 1865–1871. doi:10.2105/AJPH.2016.303362

42. Y. Zhong, A. H. Auchincloss, B. K. Lee, and G. P. Kanter, "The Short-Term Impacts of the Philadelphia Beverage Tax on Beverage Consumption," *American Journal of Preventive Medicine*, 2018; 55(1): 26–34. doi: 10.1016/j.amepre.2018.02.017

43. C. Sorensen, A. Mullee, and H. Duncan, "Soda Taxes: Old and New," *Tax Advisor*, June 1, 2017, https://www.thetaxadviser.com/issues/2017/jun/soda-taxes.html

44. Oxford Economics, "The Economic Impact of the Soft Drinks Levy," August 2016. http://www.britishsoftdrinks.com/write/MediaUploads/Publications/The_Economic_Impact_of_the_Soft_Drinks_Levy.pdf

45. B. Richardson and T. van Rens, "Case Against Soft Drink Levy Is Sugar Coated," *The Conversation*, September 27, 2016. https://bsdf-assbt.org/wp-content/uploads/2018/01/ASSBTVol8p15to22WhatsNewinSugarResearch.pdf

Chapter 13

1. A. Waters and E. J. Dionne. "Is Anti-Intellectualism Ever Good for Democracy?" *Dissent*, Winter 2019.

2. Wisconsin Radio Network, "Grothman: More Funding for Anti-Smoking Efforts Is Absurd [transcript]," September 6, 2007. https://www.wrn.com/2007/09/grothman-more-funding-for-anti-smoking-efforts-is-absurd

3. P. Marley, S. Walters, and S. Forster, "Assembly, Senate Pass Indoor Smoking Ban," *Journal Sentinel*, May 13, 2009. http://archive.jsonline.com/news/statepolitics/44913802.html/

4. A. Kaczynski and C. Massie, "Mike Pence Compared Health Risks of Tobacco to Candy in 1997 Op-Ed," *BuzzFeed*, July 18, 2016. https://www.buzzfeednews.com/article/andrewkaczynski/mike-pence-compared-health-risks-of-tobacco-to-candy-in-1997#.veooG38qv

5. A. Kaczynski, "'Smoking Doesn't Kill' and Other Great Old Op-Eds from Mike Pence," *BuzzFeed*, March 31, 2015. https://www.buzzfeednews.com/article/andrewkaczynski/smoking-doesnt-kill-and-other-great-old-op-eds-from-mike-pen#.peNE85VgkG

6. A. S. L. Rodrigues, A. Charpentier, D. Bernal-Casasola et al., "Forgotten Mediterranean Calving Grounds of Grey and North Atlantic Right Whales: Evidence from Roman Archaeological Records," *Proceedings of the Royal Society. Biological Sciences*, 2018; 285(1882): 20180961. doi: 10.1098/rspb.2018.0961

7. Republican Platform 2016. 2016 Republican National Convention. https://prod-cdn-static.gop.com/media/documents/DRAFT_12_FINAL[1]-ben_1468872234.pdf

8. RAND Corporation, "Countering Truth Decay." https://www.rand.org/research/projects/truth-decay.html

9. R. A. Charo, "Alternative Science and Human Reproduction," *New England Journal of Medicine*, 2017; 377(4): 309–311. doi: 10.1056/NEJMp1707107

10. K. Dilanian and M. Memoli, "Top Trump Campaign Aide Clovis Spoke to Mueller Team, Grand Jury," *NBC News*, October 31, 2017.

11. Texas Public Policy Foundation, "Fueling Freedom Project." https://web.archive.org/web/20161113225315/http://fuelingfreedomproject.com/

12. K. Hartnett White, "Energy and Freedom," Texas Public Policy Foundation, June 10, 2014. https://www.texaspolicy.com/energy-and-freedom/

13. D. Michaels, E. Bingham, L. Boden et al., "Advice Without Dissent," *Science*, 2002; 298(5594): 703. doi: 10.1126/science.298.5594.703

14. D. Wray, "TCEQ Scientist Says the Smog Is Fine Because Texans Stay Indoors," *Houston Press*, October 22, 2014. https://web.archive.org/web/20210227133749/https:/www.houstonpress.com/news/tceq-scientist-says-the-smog-is-fine-because-texans-stay-indoors-6719701

15. L. A. Cox Jr., "Do Causal Concentration–Response Functions Exist? A Critical Review of Associational and Causal Relations Between Fine Particulate Matter and Mortality," *Critical Reviews in Toxicology*, 2017; 47(7): 609–637. doi: 10.1080/10408444.2017.1311838 And L. A. Cox Jr., "The EPA's Next Big Economic Chokehold," *Wall Street Journal*, September 1, 2015.

16. T. Cox, MSHA's Draft Quantitative Risk assessment (QRA) of RCMD: Current Flaws and Possible Fixes. February 15, 2011. https://arlweb.msha.gov/regs/comments/2010-25249/AB64-COMM-74-12.pdf

17. P. Collignon, H. C. Wegener, H. P. Braam, and C. Butler, "Reply to Cox," *Clinical Infectious Diseases*, 2006; 42(7): 1053–1054. doi: 10.1086/501134. The Final Decision of the FDA Commissioner can be found at: https://www.regulations.gov/document?D=FDA-2000-N-0109-0137

18. United States Department of Energy, "The Los Alamos National Laboratory Site-Wide Environmental Impact Statement Process." https://www.energy.gov/sites/prod/files/EIS-0238-FEIS-01-1999.pdf

19. United States Department of Energy, "National Environmental Policy Act: Lessons Learned," June 1, 2000. https://www.energy.gov/sites/prod/files/LLQR-2000-Q2_0.pdf

20. C. Horner to T. N. Hyde and R. Tompson, "Federal Agency Science," December 23, 1996. https://www.documentcloud.org/documents/3445520-Horner-to-RJR-Reynolds-1996-Bracewell-Giuliani.html#document/p1

21. D. Michaels and T. Burke, "The Dishonest HONEST Act," *Science*, 2017; 356(6342): 989. doi: 10.1126/science.aan5967

22. Congressional Budget Office Cost Estimate, "HR 1030 Secret Science Reform Act of 2015," December 23, 1996. https://www.cbo.gov/sites/default/files/114th-congress-2015-2016/costestimate/hr1030.pdf

23. Congressional Budget Office Cost Estimate, "HR 1430 Honest and Open New EPA Science Treatment (HONEST) Act of 2017," March 29, 2017. https://www.cbo.gov/system/files?file=115th-congress-2017-2018/costestimate/hr1430.pdf

24. S. Reilly, "Pentagon Fires a Warning Shot Against EPA's "Secret Science" Rule," *Science*, 2018. doi: 10.1126/science.aav2466.

25. D. Cutler and F. Dominici, "A Breath of Bad Air: Cost of the Trump Environmental Agenda May Lead to 80,000 Extra Deaths Per Decade," *Journal of the American Medical Association*, 2018; 319(22): 2261–2262. doi: 10.1001/jama.2018.7351

Chapter 14

1. D. Barnes and L. Bero, "Why Review Articles on the Health Effects of Passive Smoking Reach Different Conclusions," *Journal of the American Medical Association*, 1998; 279: 1566–70, and D. E. Barnes and L. A. Bero, "Scientific Quality of Original Research Articles on Environmental Tobacco Smoke," *Tobacco Control*, 1997; 6: 19–26.

2. R. Smith, "Medical Journals Are an Extension of the Marketing Arm of Pharmaceutical Companies," *PLoS Medicine*, 2005; 2(5): e138. doi: 10.1371/journal.pmed.0020138

3. D. Mukherjee, S. E. Nissen, and E. J. Topol, "Risk of Cardiovascular Events Associated with Selective COX-2 Inhibitors," *Journal of the American Medical Association*, 2001; 286(8): 954–959. doi: 10.1001/jama.286.8.954

4. M. A. Konstam, M. R. Weir, A. Reicin et al., "Cardiovascular Thrombotic Events in Controlled, Clinical Trials of Rofecoxib," *Circulation*, 2001; 104(19): 2280–2288. doi: 10.1161/hc4401.100078

5. M. A. Konstam and L. A. Demopoulos, "Cardiovascular Events and COX-2 Inhibitors," *Journal of the American Medical Association*, 2001; 286: 2809.

6. D. Graham, D. Campen, R. Hui et al., "Risk of Acute Myocardial Infarction and Sudden Cardiac Death in Patients Treated with Cyclo-Oxygenase 2 Selective and Non-Selective Non-Steroidal Anti-Inflammatory Drugs: Nested Case-Control Study," *Lancet*, 2005; 365: 475–481. https://doi.org/10.1016/S0140-6736(05)17864-7

7. H. M. Krumholz, J. S. Ross, A. H. Presler, and D. S. Egilman, "What Have We Learnt from Vioxx?" *British Medical Journal*, 2007; 334(7585): 120–123. doi: 10.1136/bmj.39024.487720.68.

8. G. D. Curfman, S. Morrissey, and J. M. Drazen, "Expression of Concern: Bombardier et al., 'Comparison of Upper Gastrointestinal Toxicity of Rofecoxib and Naproxen in Patients with Rheumatoid Arthritis.'" *New England Journal of Medicine*, 2000; 343: 1520–8, DOI: 10.1056/NEJMe058314. And G. D. Curfman, S. Morrissey, and J. M. Drazen, "Expression of Concern Reaffirmed." *New England Journal of Medicine*, 2006; 354: 1193. DOI: 10.1056/NEJMe068054 .

9. R. Hersher, "Top EPA Science Advisor Has History of Questioning Pollution Research," *All Things Considered*, NPR, February 14, 2018. https://www.npr.org/sections/thetwo-way/2018/02/14/583972957/top-epa-science-adviser-has-history-of-questioning-pollution-research

10. J. J. Zou, "How the Oil Industry Set Out to Undercut Clean Air," *Center for Public Integrity*, December 12, 2017. https://apps.publicintegrity.org/united-states-of-petroleum/fueling-dissent/

11. J. E. Goodman, K. Zu, C. T. Loftus et al., "Short-Term Ozone Exposure and Asthma Severity: Weight-of-Evidence Analysis," *Environmental Research*, 2018; 160: 391–397. doi: 10.1016/j.envres.2017.10.018

12. K. Zu, L. Shi, R. L. Prueitt, X. Liu, and J. E. Goodman, "Critical Review of Long-Term Ozone Exposure and Asthma Development," *Inhalation Toxicology*, 2018; 30(3): 99–113. doi: 10.1080/08958378.2018.1455772

13. J. E. Goodman, S. N. Sax, S. Lange, and L. R. Rhomberg, "Are the Elements of the Proposed Ozone National Ambient Air Quality Standards Informed by the Best Available Science?" *Regulatory Toxicology and Pharmacology*, 2015;7 2(1): 134–140. doi: 10.1016/j.yrtph.2015.04.001

14. N. Satija, "Texas Leading Challenge to New Smog Standards," *Texas Tribune*, June 26, 2015. For Gradient submissions to EPA, see: https://www.api.org/news-and-media/~/media/Files/News/Testimony_Speeches/Gradient_Comments_Ozone_Public_Hearings_Feb2010.ashx and https://www.api.org/~/media/Files/Policy/Ozone-NAAQS/Sax-Testimony-1-29-15.pdf

15. Batteries International, "New Findings on Lead Particles Mean Lower Absorption Rates." http://www.batteriesinternational.com/2017/09/07/new-findings-on-lead-particles-mean-lower-absorption-rates/

16. See: http://www.blackwellsettlement.com/uploads/BRIEF_EXHIBIT_B_-_Findings_of_Fact_and_Conclusions_of_Law_and_Order_Granting_Plaintiffs_Motion_for_C_1_.pdf; and T. Bowers, P. Drivas, and R. Mattuck, "Prediction of Soil Lead Recontamination Trends with Decreasing Atmospheric Deposition," *Soil and Sediment Contamination: An International Journal*, 2014; 23(6): 691–702. doi: 10.1080/15320383.2013.857294

17. White House Office of Management and Budget, *Meeting Record Regarding: Lead NAAQS*, October 2, 2008. https://obamawhitehouse.archives.gov/omb/oira_2060_meetings_792/; and accompanying handout.

18. D. A. Rossignol, S. J. Genuis, and R. E. Frye, "Environmental Toxicants and Autism Spectrum Disorders: A Systematic Review," *Translational Psychiatry*, 2014; 4(2): e360, and M. Arora, A. Reichenberg, C. Willfors et al., "Fetal and Postnatal Metal Dysregulation in Autism," *Nature Communications*, 2017; 8: 15493. https://doi.org/10.1038/ncomms15493

19.   Gradient, "Science and Strategies for Health and the Environment."
      https://gradientcorp.com/alerts/pdf/Lynch%202014%20SOT%20(11x17).
      pdf

20.   M. L. Dourson, B. K. Gadagbui, R. B. Thompson, E. J. Pfau, and
      J. Lowe, "Managing Risks of Noncancer Health Effects at Hazardous
      Waste Sites: A Case Study Using the Reference Concentration (RFC) of
      Trichloroethylene (TCE)," *Regulatory Toxicology and Pharmacology*, 2016;
      80: 125–133. doi: 10.1016/j.yrtph.2016.06.013

21.   Environmental Defense Fund, "Summary of 10 Chemicals Reviewed by
      Dourson and his firm TERA, Paid for by Private Industry, Arguing for
      Less Protective Standards," September 22, 2017. http://blogs.edf.org/
      health/files/2017/09/EDF-10-Dourson-chemicals-summary-and-
      profiles-9-22-17.pdf; Environmental Defense Fund, "EPA Toxics
      Nominee Has Been Paid by Dozens of Companies to Work on Dozens
      of Chemicals," July 24, 2017. http://blogs.edf.org/health/2017/07/24/
      epa-toxics-nominee-has-been-paid-by-dozens-of-companies-to-work-on-
      dozens-of-chemicals/. For more on diacetyl, see: A. Maier, M. Kohrman-
      Vincent, A. Parker, and L. T. Haber, "Evaluation of Concentration-
      Response Options for Diacetyl in Support of Occupational Risk
      Assessment," *Regulatory Toxicology and Pharmacology*, 2010; 58(2):
      285–296. doi: 10.1016/j.yrtph.2010.06.011

22.   D. J. Paustenbach, P. S. Price, W. Ollison et al., "Reevaluation of Benzene
      Exposure for the Pliofilm (Rubberworker) Cohort (1936–1976)," *Journal of
      Toxicology and Environmental Health*, 1992; 36(3): 177–231, and
      M. B. Paxton, V. M. Chinchilli, S. M. Brett, and J. V. Rodricks, "Leukemia
      Risk Associated with Benzene Exposure in the Pliofilm Cohort: I. Mortality
      Update and Exposure Distribution," *Risk Analysis*, 1994; 14(2): 147–154. doi:
      10.1111/j.1539-6924.1994.tb00039.x; and M. B. Paxton, V. M. Chinchilli,
      S. M. Brett, and J. V. Rodricks, "Leukemia Risk Associated with Benzene
      Exposure in the Pliofilm Cohort. II. Risk Estimates," *Risk Analysis*, 1994;
      14(2): 155–161. doi: 10.1111/j.1539-6924.1994.tb00040.x; and K. S. Crump,
      "Risk of Benzene-Induced Leukemia: A Sensitivity Analysis of the Pliofilm
      Cohort with Additional Follow-Up and New Exposure Estimates," *Journal
      of Toxicology and Environmental Health*, 1994; 42(2): 219–242. doi:
      10.1080/15287399409531875; and O. Wong, "Risk of Acute Myeloid
      Leukaemia and Multiple Myeloma in Workers Exposed to Benzene,"
      Occupational and Environmental Medicine, 1995; 52(6): 380–384. doi:
      10.1136/oem.52.6.380; and A. R. Schnatter, M. J. Nicolich, and M. G. Bird,
      "Determination of Leukemogenic Benzene Exposure Concentrations:
      Refined Analyses of the Pliofilm Cohort," *Risk Analysis*, 1996; 16(6): 833–
      840. doi: 10.1111/j.1539-6924.1996.tb00834.x; and K. S. Crump, "Risk of
      Benzene-Induced Leukemia Predicted from the Pliofilm Cohort,"
      Environmental Health Perspectives, 1996; 104 (Suppl 6): 1437–1441; and
      M. B. Paxton, "Leukemia Risk Associated with Benzene Exposure in the

Pliofilm Cohort," *Environmental Health Perspectives*, 1996; 104(suppl 6): 1431–1436. doi: 10.1289/ehp.961041431; and L. Rhomberg, J. Goodman, G. Tao et al., "Evaluation of Acute Nonlymphocytic Leukemia and Its Subtypes With Updated Benzene Exposure and Mortality Estimates: A Lifetable Analysis of the Pliofilm Cohort," *Journal of Occupational and Environmental Medicine*, 2016; 58(4): 414–420. doi: 10.1097/ JOM.0000000000000689

23. R. B. Hayes, S. N. Yin, M. Dosemeci, and G. L. Li, "Benzene and the Dose-Related Incidence of Hematologic Neoplasms in China," *Journal of the National Cancer Institute*, 1997; 89(14): 1065–1071. doi: 10.1093/ jnci/89.14.1065; and Q. Lan, L. Zhang, G. Li et al., "Hematotoxicity in Workers Exposed to Low Levels of Benzene," *Science*, 2004; 306(5702): 1774–1776. doi: 10.1126/science.1102443

24. European Chemicals Agency, "Committee for Risk Assessment Opinion on Scientific Evaluation of Occupational Exposure Limits for Benzene," March 9, 2018 (ECHA/RAC/O-000000-1412-86-187/). https://echa. europa.eu/documents/10162/13641/benzene_opinion_en.pdf/4fec9aac-9ed5-2aae-7b70-5226705358c7

25. F. Mowat, M. Bono, R. J. Lee et al., "Occupational Exposure to Airborne Asbestos from Phenolic Molding Material (Bakelite) During Sanding, Drilling, and Related Activities," *Journal of Occupational and Environmental Hygiene*, 2005; 2: 497–507.

26. D. Egilman, "The Production of Corporate Research to Manufacture Doubt About the Health Hazards of Products: An Overview of the Exponent Bakelite® Simulation Study," *New Solutions: A Journal of Environmental and Occupational Health Policy*, 2018; 28(2): 179–201. doi: 10.1177/1048291118765485

27. D. Paustenbach to D. Nunez Studier, "Re Ford Billing Rates—Proposal from ChemRisk for 2011," December 28, 2010. https://tinyurl. com/3xy43ccu

28. Center for Public Integrity, "Facing Lawsuits over Deadly Asbestos, Paper Giant Launched Secretive Research Program," October 21, 2013. https:// publicintegrity.org/environment/facing-lawsuits-over-deadly-asbestos-paper-giant-launched-secretive-research-program

29. "Corrigenda Y1—2012/01/01," *Inhalation Toxicology*, 2012; 24(1): 80. doi: 10.3109/08958378.2012.655000

30. *Matter of New York City Asbestos Litig., 2013 NY Slip Op 04127* (N.Y. App. Div., 1st Dept., June 6, 2013). http://www.nycourts.gov/reporter/3dser ies/2013/2013_04127.htm

31. P. Boffetta, J. P. Fryzek, and J. S. Mandel, "Occupational Exposure to Beryllium and Cancer Risk: A Review of the Epidemiologic Evidence," *Critical Reviews in Toxicology*, 2012; 42(2): 107–118. doi: 10.3109/10408444.2011.631898

32. J. F. Gamble, M. J. Nicolich, and P. Boffetta, "Lung Cancer and Diesel Exhaust: An Updated Critical Review of the Occupational Epidemiology Literature," *Critical Reviews in Toxicology*, 2012; 42(7): 549–598. doi: 10.3109/10408444.2012.690725

33. H. Checkoway, P. Boffetta, D. J. Mundt, and K. A. Mundt, "Critical Review and Synthesis of the Epidemiologic Evidence on Formaldehyde Exposure and Risk of Leukemia and Other Lymphohematopoietc Malignancies," *Cancer Causes Control*, 2012; 23(11): 1747–1766. doi: 10.1007/s10552-012-0055-2

34. P. Boffetta, H. Adami, P. Cole, D. Trichopoulos, and J. Mandel, "Epidemiologic Studies of Styrene and Cancer: A Review of the Literature," *Journal of Occupational and Environmental Medicine*, 2009; 51(11): 1275–1287. doi: 10.1097/JOM.0b013e3181ad49b2

35. E. T. Chang, H. Adami, P. Boffetta, P. Cole, T. B. Starr, and J. S. Mandel, "A Critical Review of Perfluorooctanoate and Perfluorooctanesulfonate Exposure and Cancer Risk in Humans," *Critical Reviews in Toxicology*, 2014; 44(S1): 1–81. doi: 10.3109/10408444.2014.905767

36. C. La Vecchia and P. Boffetta, "Role of Stopping Exposure and Recent Exposure to Asbestos in the Risk of Mesothelioma," *European Journal of Cancer Prevention*, 2012; 21(3): 227–230.

37. B. Terracini, D. Mirabelli, C. Magnani, D. Ferrante, F. Barone-Adesi, and M. Bertolotti, "A Critique to a Review on the Relationship Between Asbestos Exposure and the Risk of Mesothelioma," *European Journal of Cancer Prevention*, 2014; 23(5): 492–494.

38. C. La Vecchia and P. Boffetta, "Erratum: Role of Stopping Exposure and Recent Exposure to Asbestos in the Risk of Mesothelioma," *European Journal of Cancer Prevention*, 2015; 24(1): 68.

39. Coca-Cola. "Coca-Cola Honors 10 Young Scientists From Around the World," February 4, 2015. https://www.coca-colacompany.com/stories/coca-cola-honors-10-young-scientists-from-around-the-world

40. International Life Sciences Institute, "2015 Member and Supporting Companies." http://ilsi.org/wp-content/uploads/2016/01/Members.pdf

41. See: https://www.usrtk.org/wp-content/uploads/2016/05/ILSI2012donors.pdf

42. J. Erickson, B. Sadeghirad, L. Lytvyn, J. Slavin, and B. C. Johnston, "The Scientific Basis of Guideline Recommendations on Sugar Intake: A Systematic Review," *Annals of Internal Medicine*, 2017; 166(4): 257. doi: 10.7326/M16-2020

43. International Life Sciences Institute, "Nutrition." http://ilsina.org/our-work/nutrition/carbohydrates

44. D. Schillinger and C. Kearns, "Guidelines to Limit Added Sugar Intake: Junk Science or Junk Food?" *Annals of Internal Medicine*, 2017; 166(4): 305.

Chapter 15

1. See: https://www.patagonia.com/blog/2017/02/an-update-on-microfiber-pollution/

2. G. E. Markowitz and D. Rosner, *Deceit and Denial*, New York: University of California Press, 2013.

3. The result was a series of important papers including: B. S. Schwartz, M. P. McGrail, W. Stewart and T. Pluth, "Comparison of Measures of Lead Exposure, Dose, and Chelatable Lead Burden after Provocative Chelation in Organolead Workers." *Occupational and Environmental Medicine*. 1994;51(10):669-673. doi: 10.1136/oem.51.10.669; "K. I. Bolla, B. S. Schwartz, W. Stewart, J. Rignani, J. Agnew and D. P. Ford, "Comparison of neurobehavioral function in workers exposed to a mixture of organic and inorganic lead and in workers exposed to solvents." *American journal of industrial medicine*. 1995;27(2):231-246. doi: 10.1002/ajim.4700270208; M. McGrail, W. Stewart and B. Schwartz, B, "Predictors of Blood Lead Levels in Organolead Manufacturing Workers." *Journal of Occupational and Environmental Medicine*. 1995;37(10): 1224-1229. doi: 10.1097/00043764-199510000-00014

4. R. R. Neutra, A. Cohen, T. Fletcher et al., "Toward Guidelines for the Ethical Reanalysis and Reinterpretation of Another's Research," *Epidemiology*, 2006; 17(3): 335–38.

5. "Full Disclosure: Regulatory Agencies Must Demand Conflict-of-Interest Statements for the Research They Use," *Nature*, 2014; 507(7490). doi: 10.1038/507008a; https://www.nature.com/news/full-disclosure-1.14817

6. D. Salisbury-Jones. "Academic 'hired' by Qataris to undermine US World Cup bid claims Qatar's was 'even stupider'" ITV Report July 30, 2018 https://www.itv.com/news/2018-07-30/academic-hired-by-qataris-to-undermine-us-world-cup-bid-claims-qatars-was-even-stupider/

7. Organisation for Economic Co-operation and Development. "Toward a new comprehensive global database of per- and polyfluoroalkyl substances (PFASs): Summary report on updating the OECD 2007 list of per- and polyfluoroalkyl substances (PFASs)" OECD Series on Risk Management No. 39. May 4, 2018. And Z. Wang, J. C. DeWitt, C. P. Higgins and I. T. Cousins. "A never-ending story of per- and polyfluoroalkyl substances (PFASs)?" *Environmental science & technology*. 2017;51(5):2508-2518. doi: 10.1021/acs.est.6b04806

8. . US Consumer Products Safety Commission. Public Meeting on the Petition Involving Additive Organohalogen Flame Retardants September 14, 2017. https://tinyurl.com/y6z9h44p

9. CPSC Commissioner Robert Adler, personal communication Feb 22, 2019.

10. D. Michaels, C. Monforton, and P. Lurie, "Selected Science: An Industry Campaign to Undermine an OSHA Hexavalent Chromium Standard," *Environmental Health*, 2006; 5: 5.

11. *In Re Elementis Chromium, Inc. TSCA Appeal No. 13–03 FINAL DECISION AND ORDER.* https://yosemite.epa.gov/oa/EAB_Web_Docket.nsf/TSCA-Decisions/C1325F1C5F7B886D85257E07006A88B7/$File/Elementis%20Decision%20Vol%2016.pdf

12. See for example: B. D. Kerger and M. J. Fedoruk, Pathology, toxicology, and latency of irritant gases known to cause bronchiolitis obliterans disease: Does diacetyl fit the pattern? *Toxicology Reports.* 2015;2(C):1463-1472. doi: 10.1016/j.toxrep.2015.10.012. and J. S. Pierce, A. Abelmann, L. J. Spicer, R. E. Adamsand and B. L. Finley. Diacetyl and 2,3-pentanedione exposures associated with cigarette smoking: implications for risk assessment of food and flavoring workers. *Critical Reviews in Toxicology.* 2014;44(5):420-435. doi: 10.3109/10408444.2014.882292

13. M. L. Dourson, B. K. Gadagbui, R. B. Thompson, E. J. Pfau, and J. Lowe, "Managing Risks of Noncancer Health Effects at Hazardous Waste Sites: A Case Study Using the Reference Concentration (RFC) of Trichloroethylene (TCE)," *Regulatory Toxicology and Pharmacology*, 2016; 80: 125–133. doi: 10.1016/j.yrtph.2016.06.013

14. See M. Hawthorne. Officials knew ethylene oxide was linked to cancer for decades. Here's why it's still being emitted in Willowbrook and Waukegan Chicago Tribune. December 20, 2018. And Ramboll. Summary Chicagoland Background Ethylene Oxide Study. December 18, 2018. https://www.sterigenicswillowbrook.com/s/Background-Testing-Methodology_12_18_18.pdf

15. See: https://www.documentcloud.org/documents/5784030-2019-3-29-Sterigenics-Willowbrook-Cancer.html

16. These include K.H. Nguyen, S.A. Glantz, C.N. Palmer and L.A. Schmidt. "Tobacco industry involvement in children's sugary drinks market." *BMJ (Clinical research ed.).* 2019;364:l736 doi:https://doi.org/10.1136/bmj.l736 and Y. van der Eijk and S. A. Glantz, "Tobacco Industry Attempts to Frame Smoking as a 'Disability' Under the 1990 Americans with Disabilities Act," *PLoS One*, 2017; 12(11): e0188188. doi: 10.1371/journal.pone.0188188

17. P. D. Thacker, "Inside the Academic Journal That Corporations Love," *PacificStandard*, June 14, 2017. https://psmag.com/news/inside-the-academic-journal-that-corporations-love

18. P. Krugman, "Zombies of Voodoo Economics," *New York Times*, April 24, 2017. https://www.nytimes.com/2017/04/24/opinion/zombies-of-voodoo-economics.html

19. J. W. Singer, *No Freedom Without Regulation*, New Haven: Yale University Press, 2015.

INDEX

For the benefit of digital users, indexed terms that span two pages (e.g., 52–53) may, on occasion, appear on only one of those pages.

3M (Minnesota Mining and Manufacturing), 27–31, 35–39, 253

AAR (Association of American Railroads), 95
ABA (American Beverage Association), 206–207
ABMRF (Alcoholic Beverage Medical Research Foundation), 58–62, 64, 66–67, 72
ACA (Affordable Care Act), 115, 126–127, 192
ACC (American Chemistry Council), 133–134, 159, 241–242, 263, 267–268
accommodationists, 193
ACEA (European Automobile Manufacturers Association), 94
acid rain, 186–187
Acosta, Alex, 137
ACSH (American Council for Science and Health), 36–37, 261
addiction, 17–18, 104–107, 109–113
Adler, Robert, 263

Administrative Procedures Act, 260
Advancement of Science Coalition, 188–189
advertising, 57–59, 110–111
advisory committees, 224–225, 232
AEM (Association of Equipment Manufacturers), 95
Affordable Care Act (ACA), 115, 126–127, 192
AFL-CIO, 132–133
air pollution
diesel exhaust and, 77–79, 91–93, 96–100
environmental protections and, 220
low-emission zones and, 168–169
lung cancer and, 16–17
NOx compounds and, 162, 166–167
Six Cities Study and, 95
uncertainty campaigns and, 239–240
Volkswagen and, 163–165
see also diesel engines; smog

AIRC (Italian Association for Cancer Research), 247
alcohol, 57–61, 63–75
alcoholic beverage industry, 22, 57–58, 60–75
Alcoholic Beverage Medical Research Foundation (ABMRF), 58–62, 64, 66–67, 72
ALEC (American Legislative Exchange Council), 197–198
Aleve, 235–236
Allergan, 111, 114
Alliance of Automobile Manufacturers (Alliance), 94
Alzheimer's disease, 51–52
American Academy of Pain Medicine, 112
American Beverage Association (ABA), 206–207
American Cancer Society, 125
American Chemistry Council (ACC), 133–134, 159, 241–242, 263, 267–268
American Council for Science and Health (ACSH), 36–37, 261

American Journal of Cardiology,
    63–64
American Journal of Clinical
    Nutrition, 209
American Journal of Medicine,
    63–64
American Journal of Public
    Health, 81
American Legislative Exchange
    Council (ALEC),
    197–198
American Pain Foundation, 110
American Petroleum Institute
    (API), 94, 189–190, 239,
    243–244
American Society of Clinical
    Oncology, 71, 73
American Society of Sugar
    Beet Technologists, 201
American Trucking
    Association (ATA), 94
Anenberg, Susan, 77–78
Anheuser-Busch InBev, 67–68,
    70
animal testing, 96–97, 171–178
Annals of Epidemiology, 63–64
Annals of Occupational
    Hygiene, 88
anti-intellectualism, 217–218,
    232
Anti-Intellectualism in
    American Life
    (Hofstadter), 217
API (American Petroleum
    Institute), 94, 189–190,
    239, 243–244
Appelbaum, Rhona, 203–204
Apuzzo, Michael L. J., 47
asbestiform fibers, 143, 146–147,
    151–153
asbestos
    Johnson's Baby Powder and,
        145–147
    mesothelioma and, 247
    talc and, 143, 151–153
    see also mesothelioma
ASD (autism spectrum
    disorders), 240
aspirin, 234–235
Association of American
    Railroads (AAR), 95
Association of Battery
    Recyclers, 239–240

Association of Equipment
    Manufacturers (AEM), 95
Astroturf groups, 116, 190, 192
ATA (American Trucking
    Association), 94
attorney-client privilege, 150,
    156, 246, 257
Audi, 170, 179–180
autism spectrum disorders
    (ASD), 240
autopsies, 42, 48–49
Azar, Alex, 145

Bakelite, 244–245
Bannon, Steve, 195–196
Barab, Jordan, 122
Battery Council International,
    239–240
Bayer, 160, 224–225, 264–265
Beck, Barbara, 38–39, 240
Begley, Sharon, 181
Belluz, Julia, 210–211
"Beneficial Side of Moderate
    Alcohol Use" (Turner),
    60–61
benzene exposure, 243–244
Bernstein, David, 246
beryllium industry, 7–9, 21
Beth Israel Medical Center,
    109
Bettman, Gary, 55
beverages. *see* alcoholic
    beverage industry; sugar-
    sweetened beverages
Big Tobacco. *see* tobacco
    industry
Bilott, Rob, 30–32
Bingham, Eula, 127
Bituminous Coal Operators'
    Association, 98
Black, Diane, 99–100
Blair, Steven, 204
blood-borne pathogen
    standard, 134
Blumenthal, Richard, 55
BMW, 167–168, 178
Board of Scientific Counselors
    (BSC), 84, 145, 148, 152,
    155–156
Boffetta, Paolo, 246–247
Bosch, 162–163, 168
Boston Collaborative Drug
    Surveillance Program, 106

Boston University, 42, 52–53,
    55, 63
Bradshaw, Terry, 48–49
Brady, Tom, 1–2, 5–6, 47–48
brain injuries, 43–48, 50–52,
    54–55
    see also chronic traumatic
        encephalopathy (CTE);
        head trauma; traumatic
        brain injury (TBI)
Brancheau, Dawn, 221
breast cancer, 68, 70–74
Breitbart News Network,
    195–196
British Soft Drink Association,
    215
Brooks, Mo, 196
Brulle, Robert J., 193–194
Brush Wellman, 21–22
BSC (Board of Scientific
    Counselors), 84, 145, 148,
    152, 155–156
Burke, Tom, 230–231
Burr, Richard, 267–268
Busch, August A., III, 58
Buschon, Larry, 125
Bush, George H. W., 137–138
Bush, George W., 9, 85–87,
    121–122, 184, 224
Butler, William, 19–20

C8 (PFOA), 28, 30–39
Caines, Dwight, 53–54
California, 90
California Air Resources Board
    (CARB), 163, 165–166
Camp Lejeune, North
    Carolina, 267–268
campaign donors, 194–195
cancer
    alcohol and, 64–75
    animal studies and, 96–97
    benzene and, 243–244
    C8 Studies and, 34–35
    causation and, 141–142
    glyphosate and, 157–160
    lung cancer. *see* lung cancer
    product defense industry
        and, 246–247
    see also carcinogens;
        International Agency for
        Research on Cancer
        (IARC)

cap-and-trade, 181–182
capitalism, 251–253, 270–271
    see also free market
CARB (California Air
    Resources Board), 163,
    165–166
carcinogens
    alcohol and, 70–72
    DEP and, 79–80, 89–90,
        161, 168–170
    diesel exhaust and, 95–97
    glyphosate and, 157–160
    identification of, 141–142
    NOx compounds and, 162
    silica and, 123–125, 133
    talc and, 147–156
cardiopulmonary disease, 89, 91
cardiovascular disease, 34–35,
    63–71, 77–78, 89,
    200–202, 210–211, 235–236
Cardno ChemRisk, 23, 270
Carter, Jimmy, 127
Casson, Ira, 49–50
CBO (Congressional Budget
    Office), 230–231
Center for Energy and
    Environment, 194
Center for Indoor Air Research
    (CIAR), 18
Center for Public Integrity, 25
Center for Regulatory
    Effectiveness (CRE),
    149–155
Centers for Disease Control
    and Prevention, 38, 213
Cerro Grande Fire, 227
CFCs (chlorofluorocarbons),
    186–187
Chajet, Henry, 81–82, 87–88
Chamber of Commerce,
    137–138, 197–198, 217–218,
    220–221
Chao, Elaine, 121–122
Charo, R. Alta, 222
Chase, Gerald, 85–86
chemical industry, 119–121,
    133–134, 262–263
chemicals, 28–29, 119–120
Chemours, 34–35, 39
ChemRisk, 32, 34, 135, 245
chlorofluorocarbons (CFCs),
    186–187
chocolate, 210–211

Choi, Candace, 207
Chowkwanyun, Merlin, 269
chronic traumatic
    encephalopathy (CTE),
    41–43, 46–52, 55
    see also concussions; head
        trauma; traumatic brain
        injury (TBI)
CIAR (Center for Indoor Air
    Research), 18
cigarette smoking, 15–20, 81
    see also tobacco industry
cirrhosis, 70–71
Citizens for a Sound Economy
    (CSE), 190, 192
Citizens United decision,
    194–195
City University of New York,
    12–13, 269
civil claims, 33–36
    see also litigation
Clean Air Act, 91
Clean Air Scientific Advisory
    Committee, 133–134,
    224–225
climate change
    accommodationists and, 193
    denial and, 181–183, 194
    doubt and, 12–13
    fossil fuel industry and,
        189–190
    media and, 195–197
    nitrogen and, 77–78
    regulation and, 190–192,
        197–198
climate change denial
    machine, 181–190, 193,
    195–196, 223
clinical studies
    on animals, 97
    back-in-time simulations
        and, 244
    C8 and, 34–35
    DEP exposure and, 79–84
    Diesel Miners Study and,
        81–90
    flaws in, 19
    of lung cancer patients,
        16–17
    observational epidemiology
        and, 65–71
    opioids and, 105
    of PFAS, 29

product defense industry
    and, 3–5, 124
    reanalysis and, 94–95,
        242–243
    risk assessment and, 255
    science and, 233
    uncertainty campaigns and,
        126
    Volkswagen engines and,
        171–178
    see also clinical trials;
        research
clinical trials, 65–67, 234–235
    see also clinical studies;
        research
Clinton, Bill, 6–8, 122,
    137–138, 266
Clovis, Sam, 223
CO2 Coalition, 189
coal industry, 22, 139–140
Coates, Dennis, 261–262
Coca-Cola, 203–206, 208–209,
    248
    see also sugar-sweetened
        beverages (SSBs)
coffee, 64
Cold War, 7–8, 186
Collins, Francis, 69–70
colon polyps, 235–236
colorectal cancer, 70–71
Columbia University, 12–13,
    269
Competitive Enterprise
    Institute, 194
CONCAWE (CONservation
    of Clean Air and Water
    in Europe), 95
Concussion (film), 53–54
concussions, 43–48, 50–52,
    54–55
    see also chronic traumatic
        encephalopathy (CTE);
        head trauma; traumatic
        brain injury (TBI)
Congressional Budget Office
    (CBO), 230–231
congressional committees, 82
Congressional Review
    Act, 136
ConocoPhillips, 117–118
CONservation of Clean Air
    and Water in Europe
    (CONCAWE), 95

construction workers, 118–119,
    122–123, 127–129, 132–133,
    135–136, 139
Consumer Product Safety
    Commission (CPSC),
    141–142, 263
consumers, 142, 220, 251–253
contraception, 222
control banding, 263
Conway, Eric, 186–187
Conway, Kellyanne, 194
Conyers, John, 50–51
Coors, William K., 58
corporations
    AstroTurf groups and, 116
    carcinogens and, 142
    crises and, 2–3
    disclosure and, 261
    disinformation campaigns and,
        228–230
    "independent" research and,
        245–247
    litigation and, 264–266
    litigation support and, 23, 157
    politics and, 193–195
    product defense industry and,
        252–253
    regulation and, 185, 190, 192,
        197–198, 221–222, 267,
        270–271
    Republican Party and, 217–220
    risk assessment and, 255
    SAPROs and, 62–63
    scientific research and, 161
    sustainability movement and,
        254
    uncertainty campaigns and,
        4–5, 92
    workplace safety and, 11
Cosmetic, Toiletry & Fragrance
    Association (CTFA), 145–146,
    148–151, 155
cost-benefit analysis, 129–130,
    134–136, 193, 251–252
Council for Tobacco Research, 16–17
Council on Environmental
    Quality, 223
Covington and Burling, 18
Cox, Louis Anthony (Tony),
    133–134, 224–225, 270
Cox Associates, 270
CPSC (Consumer Product Safety
    Commission), 141–142, 263

CRE (Center for Regulatory
    Effectiveness), 149–155
Critical Reviews in Toxicology, 25,
    38–39, 159
CropLife International, 248
Crowell and Moring, 93, 98
CSE (Citizens for a Sound
    Economy), 190, 192
CTE. see chronic traumatic
    encephalopathy
CTFA (Cosmetic, Toiletry &
    Fragrance Association),
    145–146, 148–151, 155
Cummins Engine, 96

Daimler, 167–168, 178
dark money, 11–12, 261
Dark Money (Mayer), 190
Data Access Act, 19–20, 91–93
data dredging, 94, 258
Data Quality Act, 149–150, 154–155
Deepwater Horizon explosion, 216
defeat devices, 163–174, 178–180
Defense Research Institute, 9–10
Deflategate, 1–2, 5–6
dementia, 51–52
DEP (diesel exhaust particulates),
    78–89, 93–98, 161, 168–170
Department of Agriculture, 216, 223
Department of Defense, 141–142
Department of Energy (DOE),
    6–9, 21, 226–227
Department of Health and Human
    Services, 145–146, 154–155, 222
Department of Justice (DOJ),
    31–32, 113–114, 166, 268–269
Department of Labor, 86, 137–138,
    181–182, 224–225, 266
Department of Transportation,
    181–182, 225–226
Der Spiegel (magazine), 168, 172
deregulation, 129, 228
DeWine, Mike, 110
diabetes, 67–69, 200–201, 206
diesel engines
    Diesel Miners Study and, 81
    emissions and, 77–79
    Europe and, 161–162
    glider kit trucks and, 99–101
    improvements in, 90, 96–98,
        162–163
    Volkswagen and, 163–164,
        170–175, 178–180

diesel equipment industry, 77–79,
    81–83, 88, 90–91, 93–96,
    98–101
diesel exhaust particulates (DEP),
    78–89, 93–98, 161, 168–170
Diesel Miners Study, 81–91, 93–95,
    168–169, 259
Dieselgate, 161, 163–169, 178–180
Dietary Guidelines Advisory
    Committee, 209–210
dioxin, 150
disclosure, 233–234, 246–248,
    259–261
discounting, 129
DISCUS (Distilled Spirits Council
    of the U.S.), 66, 72–73
disease, 7–8, 34–35, 65, 103
Distilled Spirits Council of the
    U.S. (DISCUS), 66, 72–73
distortion, 74
distraction, 74
Division of Metabolism and Health
    Effects (NIAAA), 66
Dodd-Frank Act, 126–127
DOE (Department of Energy),
    6–9, 21, 226–227
DOJ (Department of Justice),
    31–32, 113–114, 166, 268–269
Doll, Richard, 16
doubt
    climate change and, 190–192
    Diesel Miners Study and, 90–91
    PFAS and, 30
    product defense industry and,
        25–26, 168
    public health and, 6–9, 11–12
    Republican Party and, 220
    tobacco industry and, 16–18,
        92–93
    uncertainty campaigns and, 4–5,
        37–38
    see also uncertainty campaigns
Doubt Is Their Product (Michaels),
    9–10, 117
Dourson, Michael, 32, 241–242,
    267–268, 270
Dow AgroSciences, 241–242
Dow Chemical, 27
Drug and Alcohol Review, 73–74
Drug Enforcement Administration,
    115
drug industry. see pharmaceutical
    manufacturers

Duerson, Dave, 41–42
Duffy, Philip, 196
DuPont, 27–39, 157, 241–242,
    255–256, 263–264

Ebell, Myron, 194
Egilman, David, 244–245
EISs (environmental impact
    statements), 225–228
EMA (Truck and Engine
    Manufacturers
    Association), 94
employment. see workers;
    workplace safety
Endo Pharmaceutical, 108,
    110–111, 114
energy balance, 203–206
engine manufacturers, 89–91,
    98–101
Ensminger, Jerry, 267–268
ENVIRON, 18, 23, 246
environmental impact
    statements (EIS), 225–228
Environmental Protection
    Agency (EPA)
    asbestos and, 145–146
    auto industry and, 78
    beryllium industry and,
        21–22
    diesel exhaust and, 90, 96,
        98–100
    disinformation campaigns
        and, 228–231
    DuPont and, 31–34
    Fiat Chrysler and, 167
    HEI and, 91, 256
    NOx compounds and, 163
    NTP and, 141–142
    ozone standards and, 239
    PFAS and, 37–38
    SAB and, 224
    smoking regulation and, 18,
        188–189
    Volkswagen and, 161,
        165–166
environmental protections,
    4–5, 9, 11–13, 220, 267
environmentalists, 186–187,
    197–198
EPA. see Environmental
    Protection Agency (EPA)
epidemiology
    air pollution and, 162

alcoholic beverage industry
    and, 58–60
clinical studies and, 19, 26,
    46–47
defined, 6–7
Diesel Miners Study and,
    85–86
disease causation and, 125
EPA and, 229–230
lung cancer and, 16
observational studies and,
    64–68
PFAS and, 35
science and, 22
silica and, 132–135
talc studies and, 143–144,
    148–149, 153–156
uncertainty campaigns,
    242–243
see also public health
Esiason, Boomer, 44
ethics, 161, 171–175, 178, 212–213,
    242–243, 269–270
ethylene oxide (EtO), 268
EUGT (European Research
    Group on Environment
    and Health in the
    Transport Sector), 94,
    168–179
European Association of
    Internal Combustion
    Engine Manufacturers
    (EUROMOT), 95
European Automobile
    Manufacturers
    Association (ACEA), 94
European Commission, 163
European Food Safety Agency,
    37–38
European Foundation for
    Alcohol Research, 62
European Research Group
    on Environment and
    Health in the Transport
    Sector (EUGT), 94,
    168–179
Ewing, Jack, 165
excise taxes. see taxes
exercise science, 204
Expert Committee on
    Occupational Safety, 95
Exponent, 3, 5–6, 8–9, 38–39,
    93–94, 124, 246

ExxonMobil, 189–190, 193–194,
    197–198

Failure Analysis, 18–20
family planning, 222
Family Smoking Prevention
    and Tobacco Control Act,
    219
Faster, Higher, Farther: The
    Volkswagen Scandal
    (Ewing), 165
fats, 200–203
Fayetteville, North Carolina, 39
FDA (Food and Drug
    Administration), 104–105,
    107–108, 110–111, 115,
    145–146, 224–225, 235
federal agencies, 66–70, 98, 228
Federal Mine Safety and
    Health Act (1977), 82–83
Federal Register, 136
Federal Trade Commission
    (FTC), 211
fentanyl, 103–104, 111–112, 115
fetal alcohol syndrome, 61
Fiat Chrysler, 167
Fitzgerald Glider Kits, 99–100
FOIA (Freedom of
    Information Act), 69,
    91–92, 146–147
Fontham, Elizabeth, 19–20
Food and Drug
    Administration (FDA),
    104–105, 107–108, 110–111,
    115, 145–146, 224–225, 235
football players, 41–52
    see also NFL (National
    Football League)
Ford Motor Company, 245
"forever chemicals." see PFAS
    (per- and polyfluoroalkyl
    substances)
fossil fuel industry
    benzene standard and,
        243–244
    capitalism and, 252
    climate change denial and,
        184, 189–190, 193–194, 198
    Hartnett-White and, 223
    ozone and, 238–239
    regulation and, 190–192
    renewable energy and,
        196–197

foster system, 112–113
Foucart, Stéphane, 158
Foulke, Ed, 121–122
Foundation for Alcohol
    Research, 58
Fox News, 195–196
France, Chet, 99–100
Franklin, Gary, 112, 114–115
free market, 181–182, 185–187,
    190, 192, 214–215,
    252–254, 270–271
    see also capitalism
Freedhoff, Yoni, 204
Freedom of Information Act
    (FOIA), 69, 91–92,
    146–147
French Paradox, 65
Friedman, Milton, 252
front groups, 188, 190–191,
    203–206, 247–248,
    261–262
FTC (Federal Trade
    Commission), 211
funding effect, 207–208, 233,
    248–249, 255–256
    see also motivated reasoning
Furchtgott-Roth, Diana,
    181–182

Gaffney, P. Terrence, 33
Gamble, John F., 95
Garland, Merrick, 137–138, 221
gas industry. see fossil fuel
    industry
GEBN (Global Energy
    Balance Network),
    203–206
General Mills, 211
GenX, 39
George C. Marshall Institute,
    186–188
George Washington
    University, 10–11, 77–78,
    137–138
Georgia-Pacific (GP), 246
Gillam, Carey, 158
Giuliani, Rudy, 113
glider kit trucks, 98–101
Global Energy Balance Network
    (GEBN), 203–206
global warming. see climate
    change
glyphosate, 157–160

Goldstein, Bernard, 229
Goodell, Roger, 2, 5–6, 50–51
Goodling, William, 84–85
Gore, Al, 184–185
Gori, Gio Batta, 24–25
GP (Georgia-Pacific), 246
Gradient, 23, 25, 38–39,
    239–240, 270
Graham, John, 154–155
Grandjean, Philippe, 35, 37
greenhouse gas emissions,
    181–185, 196–198
Grotham, Glenn, 217–218
gun control, 117–118

Haddox, J. David, 109
Halberstam, David, 44
Hand, Gregory, 204
Hartnett-White, Kathleen, 223
Harvard School of Public
    Health, 64, 91, 202–203,
    209
Hasbro, 11
Hass, Henry, 201
head trauma, 12–13, 41–52
    see also chronic traumatic
    encephalopathy (CTE);
    concussions; traumatic
    brain injury (TBI)
Health Effects Institute (HEI),
    91–93, 96–97, 256,
    269–270
healthcare industry, 134
heart disease. see cardiovascular
    disease
HEI (Health Effects Institute),
    91–93, 96–97, 256,
    269–270
Henderson, Karen, 137–138
Hernandez, Aaron, 41–42
heroin, 103, 111–112, 115
n-hexane, 120
Hill, Austin Bradford, 16
Hill, James, 204
Hill, John W., 16–17, 199
Hill & Knowlton, 16–17,
    21–22, 111, 199
Hirayama, Takeshi, 17–19
HIV, 108, 222
HNS (NFL Head, Neck, and
    Spine) Committee, 51–53
Hockett, Robert C., 199–200
Hofstadter, Richard, 217

Holm, Stewart E., 246
Honest and Open New EPA
    Science Treatment Act
    (HONEST Act), 230–231
Honeycutt, Michael, 224, 238
Horel, Stéphane, 158
Horner, Chris, 194, 228–229
House Committee on Science,
    Space, and Technology,
    158
House Education and
    Workforce Committee,
    84–85, 87, 125, 217–218
House Science Committee, 82,
    196, 229
Hu, Frank, 209
hydrocodone, 115
Hyundai-Kia, 166

IARC. see International
    Agency for Research on
    Cancer
ICAP (International Center
    for Alcohol Policy),
    63–64, 74
ICCT (International Council
    on Clean Transportation),
    164–167
Illinois Department of Public
    Health, 268
ILSI (International Life
    Sciences Institute), 152,
    248–249
immune deficiency, 35, 37–39
independent panels, 32–34,
    36–38, 255–256
Industrial Minerals Association -
    North America, 93
infrastructure investment,
    225–227
Inhalation Toxicology, 177
Inhofe, James, 183
Institut de Recherches
    Scientifiques sur Les
    Boissons (Institute for
    Scientific Research on
    Drinks), 62
Institute for Social Research, 48
Institute on Lifestyle and
    Health, 63
International Agency for
    Research on Cancer
    (IARC)

alcohol and, 70–73
cancer causation and,
   141–142
carcinogens and, 157
conflicts of interest and, 259
diesel exhaust and, 80,
   89–90, 95–97, 170
glyphosate and, 157–160
IARC Monographs, 157
silica and, 124–125
smoking and, 24
talc and, 147
International Alliance for
   Responsible Drinking.
   see International Center
   for Alcohol Policy (ICAP)
International Center for
   Alcohol Policy (ICAP),
   63–64, 74
International Council on
   Clean Transportation
   (ICCT), 164–167
International Harvester, 82
International Life Sciences
   Institute (ILSI), 152,
   248–249
International Organization of
   Motor Vehicle
   Manufacturers (OICA), 94
Italian Association for Cancer
   Research (AIRC), 247

J-curve, 59–61, 63–65, 68
JAMA (*Journal of the American
   Medical Association*), 35,
   100, 235
Janey Ensminger Act, 267–268
Janssen Pharmaceuticals, 111
Jarvis, Steve, 148, 152–153
Jastrow, Robert, 186
Jick, Hershel, 106
job safety. *see* workers;
   workplace safety
Johns Hopkins Medical Journal,
   60–61
Johns Hopkins University,
   61–62, 256
Johns Hopkins University
   Medical School, 58
Johnson, Stuart, 173, 177
Johnson & Johnson, 111, 114,
   143–147, 149, 151, 155–156,
   253–254, 264–265

Johnson's Baby Powder, 143,
   145–147
Journal of Inhalation Toxicology,
   246
*Journal of Pain and Symptom
   Management*, 109
*Journal of the American
   Medical Association*
   (JAMA), 35, 100, 235

Karns, Elizabeth, 256
Kavanaugh, Brett, 148, 221–222
Kavanaugh, E. Edward, 148
Kearns, Cristin, 201
Keller and Heckman, 24–25
Koch, Charles, 190
Koch, David, 190
Koch, Fred, 190
Koch Industries, 190–193,
   197–198, 218, 220–221,
   241–242, 261
Koob, George, 66–69
Kraft, Robert, 2
Kristol, Irving, 217
Krugman, Paul, 270

La Vecchia, Carlo, 246–247
labor groups, 137–139, 267
Landesman, Peter, 53–54
Lanier, Mark, 143–145, 156
lead pollution, 239–240, 256
Leonard, John, 6
Lerner, Sharon, 35
Liang, James, 172–173, 178–179
life expectancy, 59–61, 64–72,
   112–113
Lipton, Eric, 99–100
litigation
   3M and, 38–39
   back-in-time simulations
      and, 244
   chemical industry and, 121
   corporations and, 197
   Diesel Miners Study and,
      84–85
   Johnson & Johnson and,
      143–145
   NFL and, 51–52
   NHL and, 55
   pharmaceutical
      manufacturers and,
      113–114, 116
   public health and, 263–266

regulation and, 270–271
silica regulation and,
   137–139
Volkswagen and, 167, 173
see also civil claims
litigation support, 23, 38–39
lobbyists
   climate change denial and,
      193–194, 197–198
   EUGT and, 168–169
   MARG and, 81–84, 86
   Republican Party and,
      220–221
   science and, 12–13, 222–223
   talc industry and, 153–154
Lomborg, Bjørn, 193
London School of Hygiene
   and Tropical Medicine,
   73, 205
Long, Terry, 50
Los Alamos National
   Laboratory, 226–227
Los Angeles Times, 107
Louisiana State University, 19
Lovelace Respiratory Research
   Institute, 96–98, 171–178
Low Emission Zones, 168–169,
   179
lung cancer
   air pollution and, 91
   beryllium and, 21
   DEP and, 78–80, 82–83,
      85–89, 95–97, 170
   secondhand smoke and,
      17–20
   silica and, 119, 123–125,
      132–133
   smoking and, 15–18, 183–188
   talc and, 151–153
   talc miners and, 146–147
   tobacco industry and,
      188–189, 199
Luzenac America, 148–149,
   152–155

MACH (Moderate Alcohol
   and Cardiovascular
   Health) trial, 67–70
MacMahon, Brian, 64, 72
Malaspina, Alex, 248
Malik, Vasanti, 209
Manhattan Institute, 181–182
Manhattan Project, 27–28

Manning, Teresa, 222–223
Marder, Howard, 21
MARG (Mining Awareness
    Research Group Diesel
    Coalition), 81–87
Markowitz, Gerald, 123, 269
Mars Inc., 210–211
Marshall, Ray, 127
Massachusetts Institute of
    Technology (MIT), 6
Materion. see Brush Wellman
Mayer, Jane, 190
McCain, John, 184
McClellan, Roger, 93
McConnell, Mitch, 137–138
McDonald, Jacob, 173–177
McKee, Anne, 42
Medicaid, 20–21, 214, 218–219
medical monitoring, 31–34,
    137–139
Meier, Barry, 113
Melkerson, Michael, 173–174
Merck & Co., 234–237
mesothelioma, 146, 247
    see also asbestos
Methane Awareness Research
    Group Diesel Coalition
    (MARG). see Mining
    Awareness Research
    Group Diesel Coalition
    (MARG)
microplastics, 252–253
Mild Traumatic Brain Injuries
    (MTBI) Committee,
    44–51, 54
Milken Institute School of
    Public Health, 10
Milloy, Steven, 100–101, 194
Mine Safety and Health
    Administration (MSHA),
    80, 82–87, 89–90, 98, 122,
    139–140
Minerals Management Service
    (MMS), 216
miners, 79–87, 90–91, 122,
    139–140, 146–147, 156
Mining Awareness Research
    Group Diesel Coalition
    (MARG), 81–87
mining industry, 81–86, 88, 98
Minnesota, 38–39
Minnesota Mining and
    Manufacturing. see 3M

(Minnesota Mining and
    Manufacturing)
Minnesota Mining and
    Manufacturing (3M),
    27–31, 35–39, 253
MIT (Massachusetts Institute
    of Technology), 6
MMS (Minerals Management
    Service), 216
Moderate Alcohol and
    Cardiovascular Health
    (MACH) trial, 67–70
Monforton, Celeste, 81, 84, 86
Monsanto, 157–160
Montreal Protocol on
    Substances that Deplete
    the Ozone Layer, 187
motivated reasoning, 169,
    207–210, 212, 233–237
    see also funding effect
MSHA (Mine Safety and
    Health Administration),
    80, 82–87, 89–90, 98, 122,
    139–140
Mt. Sinai Medical Center,
    145–146
MTBI (Mild Traumatic Brain
    Injuries) Committee,
    44–51, 54
Mukamal, Kenneth,
    67–68, 70
Muller, Matthias, 178
Multinational Legal Services,
    150
Mundt, Ken, 135
Murdoch, Rupert, 195–196
Murray Energy, 98

n-hexane, 120
NAHB (National Association
    of Home Builders),
    135–138
National Academies of
    Science, Engineering, and
    Medicine, 220
National Asphalt Pavement
    Association, 133
National Association of Home
    Builders (NAHB),
    135–138
National Cancer Center
    Research Institute, 17–19,
    24–25

National Cancer Institute
    (NCI), 80–81, 83–86,
    93–94, 141–142, 208–209
National Environmental Policy
    Act (NEPA),
    226–227
National Football League.
    see NFL
National Hockey League
    (NHL), 55
National Institute for
    Occupational Safety and
    Health (NIOSH), 80–81,
    83–86, 93–94, 120–122,
    132–134, 146, 243–244
National Institute of
    Environmental Health
    Sciences (NIEHS),
    141–142, 154–155
National Institute on Alcohol
    Abuse and Alcoholism
    (NIAAA), 58–59, 66–70,
    72–74
National Institutes of Health
    (NIH), 52–53, 66, 68–70,
    89, 257
National Mining Association,
    224–225
National Rifle Association
    (NRA), 117–118
National Right to Life
    Committee, 222
National Toxicology Program
    (NTP), 19–20, 35, 38–39,
    70–71, 124–125, 141–142,
    145–147
    Executive Committee
    Interagency Working
    Group for the Report on
    Carcinogens, 151–154
Nature, 260–261
Navarro, Peter, 222
Navistar International, 82–83,
    88
NCI (National Cancer
    Institute), 80–81, 83–86,
    93–94, 141–142,
    208–209
NEPA (National
    Environmental Policy
    Act), 226–227
Nesbit, Jeff, 190
Nestle, Marion, 210

neurological disorders, 48, 51–52
Neurosurgery, 45–50
New England Journal of Medicine, 105–106, 115, 202, 206, 236, 243–244
New England Patriots, 1–2, 5–6, 41–42
New York Times, 53–54, 61, 67–69, 99–100, 203
NFL (National Football League), 1–2, 5–6, 12–13, 41–54
  NFL Athletic Trainers Society, 44–45
  NFL Head, Neck, and Spine (HNS) Committee, 51–53
  NFL Players Association, 51–52
  NFL Team Physicians Society, 44–45
NGOs (nongovernmental organizations), 266–267
n-hexane, 120
NHL (National Hockey League), 55
NIAAA (Division of Metabolism and Health Effects), 66
NIAAA (National Institute on Alcohol Abuse and Alcoholism), 58–59, 66–70, 72–74
NIEHS (National Institute of Environmental Health Sciences), 141–142, 154–155
NIEHS Review Committee for the Report on Carcinogens, 151–152
Nierenberg, William, 186–187
NIH (National Institutes of Health), 52–53, 66, 68–70, 89, 257
NIOSH (National Institute for Occupational Safety and Health), 80–81, 83–86, 93–94, 120–122, 132–134, 146, 243–244
Nixon, Richard, 80, 119–120
non-steroid anti-inflammatory drugs (NSAIDs), 234
nondrinkers, 59–60

nongovernmental organizations (NGOs), 266–267
Nordic Expert Group for Criteria Documentation of Health Risks from Chemicals, 95
North American Flame Retardant Alliance, 241–242
North Carolina, 39
NOx emissions, 77–78, 90, 99–100, 161–167, 170–176, 178–179
NOx traps. *see* Selective Catalytic Reduction (SCR)
NRA (National Rifle Association), 117–118
NSAIDs (non-steroid anti-inflammatory drugs), 234
NTP. *see* National Toxicology Program
nuclear waste, 6–8, 226–227
nutritionists, 200, 205–206, 210

Obama, Barack
  Garland and, 137–138
  greenhouse gas emissions and, 193–194
  OSHA and, 10–11, 117
  Secret Science Reform Act and, 230
  silica regulation and, 126–128, 130, 260–261
  Tea Party and, 192
  Trump administration and, 100–101
Obamacare. *see* Affordable Care Act (ACA)
obesity epidemic, 200–201, 203–207, 216
observational epidemiology, 65–71
Occupational Safety and Health Administration (OSHA)
  3M and, 253
  benzene standard and, 243–244
  beryllium and, 8
  diesel exhaust and, 98

Diesel Miners Study and, 89
gun control and, 117–118
NFL and, 54–55
NTP and, 141–142
Obama administration and, 10–11
opioid epidemic and, 112
public hearings and, 130–134
SeaWorld and, 221–222
silica and, 119–120, 126–130, 135–139
smoking regulation and, 18, 20
standards and, 120–123
workplace safety and, 25–26, 262, 265–266
Ochsner, Alton, 15
Office of Information and Regulatory Affairs, 154–155
Office of Management and Budget (OMB), 93, 127, 149–150
Office of Research and Technology, 181–182
Office of Transportation and Air Quality, 99–100
Ogden, Trevor, 88
Ohio, 31–32
OICA (International Organization of Motor Vehicle Manufacturers), 94
oil industry. *see* fossil fuel industry
Olden, Ken, 154–155
Omalu, Bennet, 48–50, 53–54
OMB (Office of Management and Budget), 93, 127, 149–150
Opana ER, 108, 110–111
opioid epidemic, 12–13, 103–107, 110–114
orcas, 221
Oreskes, Naomi, 186–187
organizing, 270–271
OSHA. *see* Occupational Safety and Health Administration
ovarian cancer, 143–144, 146–149, 155–156
Oxford University, 205, 215
oxycodone, 104–105

OxyContin, 104–107, 111, 113–114, 116
ozone, 186–187, 238–239

pain, 103–105, 110, 112, 114–115
Pain (journal), 109
Pain Killer (Meier), 113
painkillers, 103–106
pancreatic cancer, 64
Papadopoulos, George, 223
Paris Climate Accord, 194, 196–197, 219–220
Park, Robert, 133–134
particulates, 78–82
Patagonia, 252–253
Patton Boggs, 81, 87–88
Paustenbach, Dennis, 9–10, 32, 244–245
peer-review, 3, 23–25, 47, 52–54, 106, 155
PELs (permissible exposure limits), 119–122, 126–129
Pellman, Elliot, 45, 47–50, 53
Pence, Mike, 108, 218–219
Pentagon, 231
per- and polyfluoroalkyl substances (PFAS), 27–33, 35–39, 241–242, 253, 262
Perez, Tom, 132, 137
perfluorooctane sulfonate (PFOS), 28, 30–31, 35, 37–39
perfluorooctanoic acid (PFOA), 28, 30–39
permissible exposure limits (PELs), 119–122, 126–129
Pernod Ricard, 68
Perry, Rick, 6–7
Personal Care Products Council. *see* Cosmetic, Toiletry & Fragrance Association (CTFA)
petroleum industry. *see* fossil fuel industry
Petticrew, Mark, 73
PFAS (per- and polyfluoroalkyl substances), 27–33, 35–39, 241–242, 253, 262
PFOA (perfluorooctanoic acid), 28, 30–39
PFOS (perfluorooctane sulfonate), 28, 30–31, 35, 37–39

pharmaceutical manufacturers, 103, 105–107, 109–111, 113–116
Philip Morris, 20, 188–189, 192
physicians, 103, 105–107, 109–110, 115
Pittsburgh Post-Gazette, 49
Poison Tea (Nesbit), 190
politics, 66–70, 81–86, 183–187, 193–195
pollution, 4, 6–8, 23, 28–30, 35–38
polyfluoroalkyl substances (PFAS), 27–33, 35–39, 241–242, 253, 262
POM Wonderful, 211
Portage, Wisconsin, 91
Portenoy, Russell, 109–110, 112
processed foods, 210, 213–214
product defense industry
3M and, 35, 38–39
alcoholic beverage industry and, 58, 60–65, 72–75
back-in-time simulations and, 244
background of, 3–6
beryllium industry and, 21–22
Big Tobacco and, 17–21
carcinogens and, 142
conflicts of interest and, 234–237, 259–261
corporations and, 252–254
diesel equipment industry, 77–79
Diesel Miners Study and, 81–85, 87–88, 90–91, 93–96
documents and, 268–269
DuPont and, 32–34
"equal time" and, 187–188
front groups and, 247–248
glyphosate and, 157–160
gun rights advocates and, 118
IARC and, 157
"independent" research and, 245–247
litigation and, 263–266
manufactured doubt and, 168
MSHA and, 85–86
PFAS and, 36–37

pharmaceutical manufacturers and, 106–110
processed foods and, 210–213
reanalysis and, 242–243
regulation and, 257–258
risk assessment and, 240–242
science and, 23–26, 232–233
scientific literature and, 258
Shelby Amendment and, 91–93
silica and, 119, 133–136, 138
Silica Coalition and, 124
SSBs and, 214–216
talc industry and, 143–145, 148–155
Trump administration and, 12, 223–225
uncertainty campaigns and, 141, 270
Volkswagen and, 174–177
Weed and, 208–209
weight-of-the-evidence analyses and, 237–240
see also uncertainty campaigns
product defense strategies, 74–75
Professional Football Athletic Trainers Society. *see* NFL Athletic Trainers Society
progressive massive fibrosis, 139–140
Prohibition, 58–59
Pruitt, Scott, 99–101, 224, 241–242
pseudoaddiction, 107, 109
public good, 220, 270–271
public health
air pollution and, 91
alcohol consumption and, 57–61, 63–72, 74–75
attacks on, 36–37
Bush administration and, 9
capitalism and, 251–253, 270–271
carcinogens and, 142
climate change and, 184
consumers and, 220
DEP and, 79–80
deregulation and, 228–229

diesel exhaust and, 77–80, 96
doubt and, 4–5, 11–12
epidemiology and, 6–7
gun control and, 117–118
NGOs and, 266–267
obesity and, 203–207
opioid epidemic and, 107
OSHA and, 10–11
PFAS and, 30–32, 37–38
PFOA and, 33
product defense industry
  and, 81–83
public hearings and, 131–132
risk and, 25–26
risk assessment and, 241–242
science and, 22–23
SSBs and, 206–210, 213–215
talc and, 143–144, 155–156
tobacco industry and, 15
uncertainty campaigns and,
  72–73
weight-of-the-evidence
  analyses and, 237–240
see also epidemiology
public hearings, 130–136
public policy, 6–8, 12–13
public relations
  alcoholic beverage industry
    and, 60–62, 74
  beryllium industry and,
    21–22
  climate change and, 183, 194
  Coca-Cola and, 203–206
  doubt and, 4–5
  MACH trial and, 68–69
  misinformation campaigns
    and, 111
  pharmaceutical
    manufacturers and,
    106–110, 113–114, 116
  public health and, 185–187
  SAPROs and, 62–64
  secondhand smoke and,
    188–189
  SSBs and, 204
  sugar industry and, 201–202
  tobacco industry and, 16–18
  Volkswagen and, 170
pulmonary disease, 77–78, 89
  see also air pollution; lung
    cancer
Purdue Pharma, 104–107,
  109–111, 113–116

R. J. Reynolds Tobacco,
  187–188, 228–229
Rabin, Roni Caryn, 68–69
Ramboll Environ, 23, 135, 159,
  268, 270
Rand Corporation, 222
Reagan, Ronald, 149–150
reanalysis, 242–243, 257–258
regulation
  accommodationists and, 193
  ACSH and, 36–37
  Big Tobacco and, 20–21
  Bush administration and,
    121–122
  capitalism and, 270–271
  conflicts of interest and,
    259–262
  corporations and, 197–198,
    254–255, 267
  CRE and, 149–150
  diesel exhaust and, 81–86,
    89–91, 98–101
  disinformation campaigns
    and, 228–231
  at DOE, 8
  doubt and, 2–4
  free market and, 185–187,
    252
  industry and, 126–127,
    129–130
  infrastructure and, 225–227
  Koch brothers and, 190
  litigation and, 263–266
  NOx compounds and,
    163–164
  opioids and, 106
  OSHA and, 120–121
  PFAS and, 35, 38
  processed foods and,
    210–213
  product defense industry,
    134
  product defense industry
    and, 25–26, 257–258
  public health and, 22–23
  public hearings and, 130–131
  public-private work and,
    66–67, 70, 72–73
  safety and, 255
  science and, 12–13
  Shelby Amendment and, 92
  silica and, 119–120, 122–124,
    127–129, 137–138

Supreme Court and,
  220–221
talc and, 155–156
Trump administration and,
  217–220
USDA and, 216
Regulatory Toxicology and
  Pharmacology, 24–25, 155
Renault, 167
renewable energy, 193, 196–197
Report of Carcinogens,
  142–143, 145, 148, 151–152,
  154–157
Republican Party, 183–185,
  194–195, 198, 217–221,
  225–226, 228–232
research
  ABMRF and, 58
  alcoholic beverage industry
    and, 58–62
  conflicts of interest and,
    211–213, 233–237
  front groups and, 247–249
  government funding and,
    257–258
  "independent" research and,
    245–247
  industry and, 92
  NFL head trauma and, 54
  peer-reviewed journals and,
    23–25, 36
  PFAS and, 37
  product defense industry
    and, 23–25, 94–95
  vilification of, 4–5
  see also clinical studies;
    clinical trials
research and promotion
  (R&P) boards, 212–213
respirators, 127–128, 131–132
respiratory disease, 77–78, 89
  see also air pollution; lung
    cancer
responsibility, 57–59, 62–63, 65
Responsible Science Policy
  Coalition, 39
Richardson, Bill, 8
Rinsky, Robert, 243–244
risk, 25–26, 74, 128–129
risk assessment, 65, 123–125,
  240–242, 255, 259
Robert Wood Johnson
  Foundation, 84–85

Rogers, Judith, 221
Romney, Mitt, 190–192
Roper Organization, 17–18
Rosner, David, 123, 269
Roth, H. Daniel, 20, 22, 72
Roundup, 157
R&P (research and
    promotion) boards,
    212–213
Ruckelshaus, William, 240

SAB (Science Advisory Board),
    224
Sackler family, 111, 113–114
Salazar, Ken, 216
Sánchez, Linda, 51
SAPROs (social aspects and
    public relations
    organizations), 62–63,
    73–74
Schatz, Brian, 184
Schmidt, Oliver, 165–166, 173,
    178–179
Schwartz, Alan, 54
science
    alcohol consumption and,
        57–61
    alcoholic beverage industry
        and, 61–62
    animal testing and, 96–97,
        171–174
    anti-intellectualism and,
        217–221
    cancer causation and, 141
    climate change and, 182–185
    climate change denial and,
        195–196
    Coca-Cola and, 203–206
    conflicts of interest and, 212,
        233–237
    corporations and, 161
    CTE and, 42–43
    Diesel Miners Study and,
        85–86
    disinformation campaigns
        and, 228–231
    manufacturing doubt and,
        9, 33, 90–93
    motivated reasoning and,
        169
    NGOs and, 266–267
    opioid epidemic and, 104,
        107–109

policy and, 12–13
product defense industry
    and, 2–5, 22–26, 81–84,
    88, 155
sugar industry and, 202
tobacco industry and, 15,
    20–21, 199
Trump administration and,
    222–225, 232
uncertainty campaigns and,
    36–37
Science Advisory Board (SAB),
    224
Science and Environment
    Policy Project, 188–189
Science (journal), 88
Scientific American, 9
scientific literature
    back-in-time simulations
        and, 244
    climate change and, 182
    Coca-Cola and, 205–206
    conflicts of interest and,
        171–172, 174–177,
        259–260
    disclosure and, 269
    EUGT and, 174–177
    MTBI and, 45–47, 50
    opioids and, 105–106
    peer-reviewed journals and,
        3, 23–25
    product defense industry
        and, 33, 241
    reanalysis and, 243–244
    review of, 141, 258
    silica and, 132–133
    SSBs and, 206–210
    talc and, 149
    weight-of-the-evidence
        analyses and, 237–240
Scotchgard, 28–31, 35
SCR (Selective Catalytic
    Reduction), 163–165
Seau, Junior, 41–42, 44
SeaWorld, 221
SEC (Securities and Exchange
    Commission), 178
secondhand smoke, 17–20,
    24–25, 188–189, 219
Secret Science Reform Act,
    229–231
Securities and Exchange
    Commission (SEC), 178

Seitz, Frederick, 186–189
selection bias, 46–47, 60
Selective Catalytic Reduction
    (SCR), 163–165
Selikoff, Irving, 145–146
Seventh Generation, 252–253
Shelby, Richard, 91–92
Shelby Amendment, 19–20,
    91–93
Shell, 189–190
silica, 118–119, 121–140
Silica Coalition, 123–124
silicosis, 119, 123–125, 131–133
Simons, Joseph H., 27–28
Sinclair, Upton, 169, 258,
    270–271
Singer, Fred, 186–189, 196
Six Cities Study, 91–93, 95, 259
Smith, DeMaurice, 51–52
Smith, Lamar, 196, 229–231
Smith, Will, 53–54
smog, 77–78
    see also air pollution
smoking, 15–20, 81
    see also tobacco industry
Smoking and Health Program,
    24–25
social aspects and public
    relations organizations
    (SAPROs), 62–63, 73–74
Society for the Plastics
    Industry, 24–25
Society of Toxicology, 174–175
Solis, Hilda, 132
Soviet Union, 186
Spallek, Michael, 168–169, 171,
    175–177
Der Spiegel (magazine), 168, 172
SpiritsEUROPE, 68
Sports and Health Research
    Program, 52
Sports Illustrated, 44
SRF (Sugar Research
    Foundation), 199–202
SSBs. see sugar-sweetened
    beverages
Stadler, Rupert, 179–180
State Administration of
    Workplace Safety
    (China), 253
Steenland, Kyle, 124–125
Steg, Thomas, 178
Sterigenics, 268

Stern, Robert, 52–53
Steubenville, Ohio, 91
Stroh, Peter, 58
stroke, 77–78
sugar industry, 199–203,
    208–210, 214, 248–249
Sugar Research Foundation
    (SRF), 199–202
sugar-sweetened beverages
    (SSBs), 206–210, 213–215
    see also Coca-Cola
sulfur, 78
Supreme Court, 194–195,
    220–221
sustainability movement, 254

Tagliabue, Paul, 44–45, 50–51
talc, 143–156
talc industry, 143, 150–156
Tatel, David, 137–138
taxes, 58–59, 161–162, 188–190,
    209, 213–216, 269–270
TBI. see traumatic brain injury
TCE (trichloroethylene),
    267–268
TCEQ (Texas Commission on
    Environmental Quality),
    238–239
Tea Party, 191–194
Teflon, 27–31, 35, 39
    see also PFAS (per- and
    polyfluoroalkyl substances)
Tejeda-Rios, Gabriela, 268
Tennant, Wilbur, 30–32
Tennessee Technological
    University, 99–101
TERA (Toxicology Excellence
    for Risk Assessment), 32,
    34, 37–38, 241–242,
    267–268, 270
Terracini, Benedetto, 247
Teva, 111, 114
Texas Commission on
    Environmental Quality
    (TCEQ), 238–239
Texas Public Policy
    Foundation, 223
Thacker, Paul, 33
Tilikum, 221
Tillis, Thom, 267–268
TIRC (Tobacco Industry
    Research Committee),
    16–17, 199

tobacco industry
    alcoholic beverage industry
        and, 57–58, 72
    climate change denial and,
        185–188
    disclosure and, 261
    disinformation campaigns
        and, 228–229
    documents and, 268–269
    doubt and, 17
    excise taxes and, 213–214,
        269–270
    front groups and, 188
    funding effect and, 233
    litigation and, 264–265
    lung cancer and, 183–185, 199
    Milloy and, 100–101
    public health and, 15, 214
    reanalysis and, 243–244
    regulation and, 192
    Republican Party and,
        217–219
    research and, 24–25
    secondhand smoke studies
        and, 17–20
    Shelby Amendment and,
        92–93
    SSBs and, 206
    uncertainty campaigns,
        149–150, 220–221
    uncertainty campaigns and,
        8–9, 36, 43, 50–51
Tobacco Industry Research
    Committee (TIRC),
    16–17, 199
Toxic Docs, 12–13, 269
toxic products, 22, 26, 28–32,
    119–120, 240–242,
    251–254, 266–267
Toxic Substances Control Act,
    26, 31–32
Toxicology Excellence for Risk
    Assessment (TERA), 32,
    34, 37–38, 241–242,
    267–268, 270
Tozzi, Jim, 149–151, 153–155,
    188–189
traffic accidents, 61
traumatic brain injury (TBI),
    46–48
    see also chronic traumatic
    encephalopathy (CTE);
    concussions; head trauma

trichloroethylene (TCE),
    267–268
Truck and Engine
    Manufacturers
    Association (EMA), 94
trucking industry, 89–90,
    98–101
Trump, Donald
    appointments and, 222–225
    attacks on science and, 12–13
    climate change denial and,
        181–182, 194
    Cox and, 133–134
    deregulation and, 129,
        225–227, 231–232
    Dourson and, 32, 242
    election of, 137
    Fitzgerald family and, 99–100
    greenhouse gas emissions
        and, 196–197
    HONEST Act and, 230–231
    Obama administration and,
        100–101
    PFAS and, 38
    regulation and, 167–168
    Republican Party and, 217
    silica regulation and, 139–140
truth decay, 222
Truth Tobacco Industry
    Documents, 268–269
Turner, Thomas B., 58–61,
    72
Turner, Eric, 154

U-235 (uranium isotope),
    27–28
UCSF (University of
    California - San
    Francisco), 200–202,
    268–269
uncertainty campaigns
    carcinogens and, 141
    climate change and, 183,
        185–186, 189–192
    Diesel Miners Study and,
        83–84, 86
    disclosure and, 260–261
    epidemiology and, 242–243
    front groups and, 247–248
    glyphosate and, 159–160
    Johnson & Johnson and,
        253–254
    litigation and, 266

uncertainty campaigns
(*continued*)
    NFL and, 44–52
    NHL and, 55
    opioids and, 107–109
    product defense industry
        and, 233
    reanalysis and, 257–258
    risk assessment and, 241–242
    silica and, 126, 133–136, 138,
        140
    SSBs and, 209
    sugar and, 199–203
    talc and, 143–144, 152–154,
        156
    tobacco industry and, 36
    Wehner and, 149–150
    weight-of-the-evidence
        analyses and, 237–240
    see also doubt; product
        defense industry
Union Carbide, 244–245
United Mineworkers of
    America, 82–83
United Steelworkers, 87, 132
University of California - San
    Francisco (UCSF),
    200–202, 268–269
University of Colorado, 204
University of Maryland,
    135–136
University of Pittsburgh,
    48–49
uranium isotope U-235, 27–28
US Right to Know, 203

vaccines, 222
Van Houten, Joseph, 253–254
Veneto, Italy, 38
Viano, David, 45, 47–50
Vioxx, 234–236
Virginia Tech massacre, 117
Volkswagen Group, 79, 89,
    99–100, 161–180

Wall Street Journal, 195–196
Warren, Ken, 67
Washington Works, 30–31
water contamination, 28–32,
    34–36, 39
Watson, Andrew, 50
Waxman, Henry, 50–51
Webster, Mike, 48–50, 53–54
Weed, Douglas, 208–209
Wehner, Alfred P., 149–150, 155
Wehrum, William, 138
Weiderpass, Elisabete, 73,
    158–159
weight-of-the-evidence
    analyses, 237–240
Weinberg, Myron, 20
Weinberg Group, 20, 22, 33,
    148–150, 270
West Virginia, 27, 30–35,
    37–39, 112–113
West Virginia University, 165,
    204
Wheeler, Andrew, 101
White, Alan, 131–132
Whitehouse, Sheldon, 194–195
WHO (World Health
    Organization), 70–71, 89,
    124, 141, 170,
    214–215, 259
Will, George, 186
Willowbrook, Illinois, 268
Wine Information Council, 74
Winterkorn, Martin, 178–180
Woods, Darren, 193–194
Woods Hole Research Center,
    196
workers
    beryllium industry and, 21
    compensation and, 266
    employment impact and,
        135–136
    labor groups and, 137
    lead exposure and, 256

opioid epidemic and, 112,
    114–115
    PFOA and, 31
    public hearings and,
        131–133
    radiation exposure and,
        6–8
    respirators and, 127–128
    safety and, 11, 120–122
    silica and, 129–130
    silicosis and, 124–125
    workers' compensation and,
        263–264
workplace safety
    3M and, 253
    DEP exposure and, 79–84,
        89, 95
    football players and, 41,
        54–55
    guns and, 117–118
    opioid epidemic and, 112
    OSHA and, 120
    SeaWorld and, 221–222
    silica and, 118–119, 122–123,
        127–129, 131–136
    see also Occupational Safety
        and Health
        Administration
World Health Organization
    (WHO), 70–71, 89, 124,
    141, 170, 214–215, 259
World War I, 15
World War II, 27–28
Wright, Michael, 87

Yoest, Charmaine, 222–223

Zakhari, Samir, 66,
    72–73
Zatezalo, David, 98, 139–140
Zazenski, Rich, 152–154
Zinke, Ryan, 220
Zymancius, Neringa,
    268